WATER RESCUE
Basic Skills for Emergency Responders

WATER RESCUE
Basic Skills for Emergency Responders

David S. Smith, Ph.D.
Commander, U.S. Coast Guard, (RET)

Sara J. Smith

with 116 *illustrations*

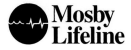

Mosby Lifeline

St. Louis Baltimore Boston Chicago London Madrid Philadelphia Sydney Toronto

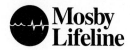

Mosby Lifeline

Dedicated to Publishing Excellence

Publisher: David Culverwell
Executive Editor: Claire Merrick
Developmental Editor: Nancy J. Peterson
Editorial Assistant: Christine H. Ambrose
Project Manager: Carol Sullivan Wiseman
Senior Production Editor: Florence Achenbach
Manuscript Editor: Marilyn K. Wynd
Designer: Betty Schulz
Cover Art and Line Drawings: Donald P. O'Connor

Printed in the United States of America
Composition by Graphic World, Inc.
Printing/binding by R. R. Donnelley & Sons Company, Crawfordsville, IN

Mosby–Year Book, Inc.
11830 Westline Industrial Drive
St. Louis, Missouri 63146

Library of Congress Cataloging in Publication Data

Smith, Davis S. (David Stuart),
    Water rescue : basic skills for emergency responders / David Smith,
Sara J. Smith.
        p.   cm.
    Includes bibliographical references and index.
    ISBN 0-8016-6343-1
    1. Drowning, Restoration from.   2. First aid in illness and injury.
I. Smith, Sara J.   II. Title.
RC88.S549   1994   93-30283
616.02'5 – dc20   CIP
93   94   95   96   97   /   9   8   7   6   5   4   3   2   1

Dedicated to America's modern hero—the wonderful, selfless, and all-too-often unappreciated emergency responder.

D.S.S. and S.J.S.

PREFACE

Water-related accidents are a serious public safety concern. In North America drowning is the second leading cause of accidental death for those under age 44 and is the third leading cause for all ages. Although much has been accomplished in reducing the number of aquatic deaths, a large amount of work remains. A prime requirement is the proper training of emergency service personnel in *modern* water safety and rescue techniques.

Because of the scarcity of accurate information on drowning, many fire, police, and emergency medical service (EMS) providers have not been exposed to adequate knowledge, technique, and equipment to rescue aquatic accident victims while properly protecting themselves. This oversight has been especially telling since emergency service providers respond to most serious water incidents. More importantly, the historical emphasis in aquatic safety has primarily focused on lifesaving and lifeguarding techniques in supervised summer swimming pool and beach environments. The relatively benign, standardized conditions generally assumed in this type of training are met infrequently in actual occurrences.

Hence, even those fire, police, and EMS professionals who have been trained previously in water safety are still placed at potential risk. Additionally, new research has brought about many changes and improved procedures that frequently contradict historical practice.

The text is specifically designed to remedy the foregoing omissions while providing simplified explanations of current research findings. The text defines, on a *basic* level, the aquatic situations most often encountered and fundamental responses required by professional rescuers. References are also provided for *advanced* tactics, training, and equipment.

A central theme repeatedly stressed in this book is that not enough aquatic professionals truly comprehend the causes and behaviors commonly underlying aquatic accidents. Furthermore, the public is even more likely to be misinformed about appropriate water safety approaches. Additionally, despite continuing development of equipment and procedures, the water safety field has been exposed to relatively little research—hence the expectation that there is yet a lot to learn about aquatic accidents. For this reason and to prevent the possibility of apparently minor points growing into major disasters, this text is designed to cover the subject "from the ground (or water) up."

To assist the reader in assessing his or her aquatic IQ, each chapter begins with a pretest. Pretest answers and explanations and important information in the chapter are highlighted. A short list of the correct pretest answers follows each chapter summary.

The student is shown how a relatively small amount of public education can prevent most drownings. Readers will learn how to protect themselves in still water before being exposed to exacting and potentially dangerous procedures such as those used in swift water or ice rescues. In support of this practical approach, readers are encouraged to test the basic safety and survival tips and techniques (initially under safe, well-supervised conditions) presented in the text.

In accord with the foregoing, the information presented is divided into three primary categories: (1) the statistics, causes, common scenarios and settings, and elementary preventive measures normally associated with water accidents; (2) personal safety and self-rescue, including alternatives relating to clothing, protective devices, and environment; and (3) team rescue tactics and organizational considerations covering topics such as equipment requirements; victim extrication, management, and transfer; and legal guidelines.

Appendices list references and resources, equipment and procedural vocabulary, rescue-related medical terminology, drill outlines, and flood rescue planning and preparation pointers. Words that appear in bold type in the text appear in either Appendix II or III.

It is not necessary that an emergency services provider be extremely proficient in the water to use the concepts presented by the text. *But* if you are not the world's greatest swimmer, attempting to improve your aquatic skills will not harm you. In fact, becoming more water oriented can be a distinct help. Similarly, most of the medical information presented herein is rudimentary. However, the more competent you are in emergency medical techniques, the more you will understand the victim's condition, and the more you will be able to assist him or her. You are therefore strongly encouraged to develop both your water and medical capabilities.

The text represents the primary author's extensive experience in developing and presenting a number of the insights now gaining acceptance in aquatics. These insights are based on a lifelong involvement in water safety, including 25 years as a commissioned officer in the U.S. Coast Guard, essentially in the fields of search and rescue and boating safety.

After retirement from the Coast Guard, the Smiths have traveled throughout North America conducting numerous seminars, workshops, and demonstrations for large numbers of emergency service and medical personnel. In addition to writing, lecturing, and appearing on television and radio programs, Dr. Smith (Ph.D., Educational Psychology) frequently is retained as an expert witness in aquatics-related court cases.

As a result of their in-depth exposure to the facts, myths, and misunderstandings surrounding water mishaps, the authors attempt to prepare the potential rescuer for situations he or she may not have previously considered or encountered. This book seeks to provide the most comprehensive yet fundamental aquatic safety information currently available to emergency service personnel.

Reference
Accident facts, 1991, Chicago, 1991, National Safety Council.

Acknowledgements

A number of individuals have been extremely helpful in developing this text. In particular, the authors wish to cite and to thank:

Mr. Jeree Forbes, E.M.I.C.T., coordinator of Emergency Medical Sciences, Hutchinson Community College, Hutchinson, Kansas, for his continuing assistance and encouragement, both as a reality-based reviewer and tireless worker for improvements in all facets of emergency response.

Andrew D. Weinberg, M.D., Assistant Clinical Professor, Yale University School of Medicine, Raynham, Massachusetts, for his timely responses and comprehensive assistance in clarifying medical aspects of this work, especially those dealing with hypothermia.

Mr. Tim Delany, White Water Rescue Consultant/Instructor, Tim Delany Enterprises, Lotus, California, for his instructive comments and characteristic helpfulness in ensuring that all necessary points were properly touched in the chapters dealing with water rescue.

Reviewers whose depth of comment and quality of helpfulness we only hope we can repay in scrutinizing a book they might write: Tom Ferrell, M.S., E.M.T.-P., Education Programs Consultant, Office of EMS, Raleigh, North Carolina; N. Joseph Ketterer, Captain and Public Affairs Officer, Harrisburg River Rescue, Water Safety Division; Battalion Chief Chase N. Sargent, Paramedic in command of Special Operations Section, Public Information Officer, City of Virginia Beach, Virginia; Kenneth C. Henry, Brandon, Florida; Rod Dennison, EMS Program Administrator, Texas Department of Health, Temple, Texas.

Mosby Lifeline editorial staff members participating in development of the text:

Ms. Claire Merrick, Executive Editor, whose natural enthusiasm, professional insight, and contagious good will buoyed the writing process.

Mr. Rick Weimer, Executive Editor, who allowed himself to be talked into the project and greatly aided our early efforts at arranging and focusing information.

Ms. Nancy Peterson, Developmental Editor, whose comments motivated our perserverance.

And finally, our greatest and humblest thanks for her gracious dedication to being and producing only the best: Mosby Editorial Assistant and wonderful person, Ms. Christine Ambrose.

A Note to the Reader

The authors have made every attempt to check this text's rescue procedures and life support protocols for accuracy. The authors and publisher disclaim responsibility for any adverse effect resulting from the use of information contained herein. Readers are strongly advised to seek competent medical advice before undertaking any action that might produce a deleterious or otherwise undesirable result. Attention is directed to repeated admonitions to practice carefully the following procedures in safe, supervised settings before routinely using them. It is also the reader's responsibility to know and to follow local care protocols as provided by his or her medical advisors. Additionally, it is the reader's responsibility to stay informed of emergency care procedure changes.

Contents

Introduction and Overview

Why Water Safety and Rescue for Emergency Service Providers?

A STORY FROM REAL LIFE (AND DEATH)

Even though a similar attempt on the previous afternoon had failed and a rescuer's life was lost, the fire fighters felt confident in their new plan for approaching the "low-head dam." They reasoned that their earlier attempt, which resulted in the rescue boat's being swept uncontrollably into the face of the dam and capsizing, had miscarried because the rescue craft's engine failed.

At sunup on this second day at the rescue site, a passerby had spotted a life jacket bobbing in the **backwash** at the foot of the dam. Since there was a chance of its being attached to the body of the fire fighter drowned on the preceding day, the decision was made to hook the jacket and possibly the missing body.

A camera team from the local television station recorded the scene as the rescue boat, now equipped with a new engine and crewed by the department's rescue chief and two experienced assistants, neared the dam. The boat slowly moved upstream. Conditions apparently were acceptable, and the craft and crew were committed across the **boil line,** or point of no return, before the face of the dam.

Exactly as had occurred the day before, the boat and its occupants suddenly were thrown into the tumbling wall of water. As the craft capsized, its **gunwale** struck and fractured the unprotected skull of the rescue chief. He died in seconds. The fire fighter in the bow was repeatedly swept under the water by the dam's recirculating **hydraulic,** or vertical whirlpool. Because of the unbelievable force of the water, his flotation vest could neither support nor stay on him. He drowned within minutes.

3

The only survivor remained alive because he continuously grasped the lower unit of the overturned boat's outboard engine. Miraculously, he fought the dam for the better part of an hour until another rescue boat crewed by two sheriff's deputies moved across the boil. This boat also was flung into the dam and capsized. Now three men (later rescued) were in danger of dying at the spot where a total of three others had died before.

The television camera crew clearly recorded shoreside cries of disbelief, anguish, and frustration from horrified witnesses. "Don't they have a rescue line tied to shore?" "There goes that boat." "What the hell is going on here?"

Among a host of other things, this tragedy primarily demonstrates that well-intentioned, otherwise competent, reasonable, and experienced rescuers can *easily* kill themselves (and those they are intent on saving) *if they do not understand and properly prepare for the frequently awesome and quite unexpected power of moving water.*[1] (This rescue attempt occurred September 29, 1975, at Binghamton, New York. See "The Drowning Machine" listed in Appendix I.)

These men grew up alongside the river and dam that killed them. They were responsible for river rescue in their community. Yet they clearly demonstrated their lack of appropriate knowledge in dealing with it. The text you are about to use is dedicated to remedying this defect.

You, as a practicing or prospective emergency services provider, are about to discover a number of little known and insufficiently appreciated facts about aquatic accidents. For instance, drowning is a major cause of accidental death. As indicated in Chapter 1, drowning outranks total fatalities caused by fire.

Arguments will be made that:

- Most water rescues are not necessarily accomplished by life-guards but rather by police, fire fighters, and emergency medical service personnel.
- Many, if not most, of these potential water rescuers have relatively little training in aquatic practices.
- A great deal of the information unquestionably accepted by the public as water fact is far closer to myth.

The central aim of this text is to separate aquatic truth from fiction while helping you and your fellow emergency providers to operate safely around the water. We direct a great amount of attention toward explaining and expanding the simpler, basic understandings of what happens to people exposed to aquatic hazards. Similarly, we stress what must be accomplished *before* anyone, rescuer or potential victim, nears the water. In terms of this text, the best, that is, the most desirable, rescue *never happens* or, more importantly, *never has to happen*. The reason? You, your department, and your community can all take the proper, reality-based *preventive* steps to bar or reduce the potential for aquatic accidents.

Foremost among the facts you will encounter in this book is this: drowning and almost all other forms of aquatic mishaps are easily avoidable.

If you and those around you know and practice what is needed to prepare yourself and your community, *drownings do not have to occur!*

REFERENCES
1. Walbridge C: The best of the river safety task force newsletter, 1976-1982, Lorton, Va, 1983, The American Canoe Association, pp 45-46.

P A R T · O N E

Understanding Water Accidents

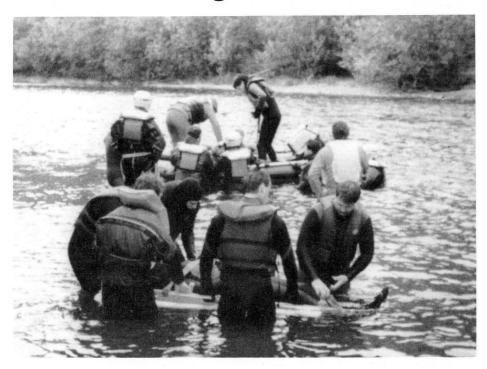

Education, training, and practice are key elements in understanding and responding to water accidents. Rescue personnel properly wearing personal flotation devices (PFDs) is the mark of true professionals.

OVERVIEW

The chapters in Part One provide the foundation for everything that follows. They will increase your understanding of the following:
- Causes of water accidents
- Definitions and types of drowning and other forms of aquatic trauma
- Scenarios and signs of drowning
- Role of alcohol in aquatic mishaps

DISCUSSION

Until the mid-1970s very little detailed research had been applied to water accidents in general and to drowning in particular. One result of this lack of updated information was that many water safety training programs were based on techniques developed and refined in the 1920s. With the passage of the Federal Safe Boating Act of 1973, the U.S. Coast Guard was mandated to reduce boating accident rates and fatalities. The program developed to meet this mandate was labeled the *Three E's: Enforcement, Engineering, and Education.*

The first *E* (enforcement) dealt with writing and carrying out laws that would remove hazardous boat operators from the water while increasing protection for the law-abiding majority. The second *E* (engineering) involved building boats that resisted sinking and equipping them with standardized, tested parts such as lights and horns. This engineering application also focused on developing more wearable, practical personal flotation devices (PFDs). The third *E* (education) pertained to generating and distributing public training programs and informational materials.

Before any of these elements could be put into operation, it was necessary to determine exactly what caused boats to sink or collide and occupants to fall overboard and drown and what made operators unsafe. Then studies were performed to define the best approaches to deal with the causes. Although a number of advances occurred, resulting in the current boating accident rate's falling to less than one third of its 1970 level,[1] the biggest benefit—a much clearer, more precise understanding of what causes *all* water mishaps—is presented in this text.

The following are some of the primary facts learned from the foregoing studies:

- The cause of most boating deaths, which represent a fifth of the overall aquatic total number of deaths, does not differ from that of other drownings.[2] The difference is that someone falls out of a boat rather than off a dock.
- Alcohol may be present, and it plays a major role in most water accidents whether a boat is involved or not.
- Most types of water accidents are highly predictable; therefore they are strongly subject to prevention through education.
- Just as exposure to or immersion in a cold environment can kill, it can also (under certain conditions) allow someone who appears dead to live.

In addition to reenforcing the perception that too little was known about mishaps in the water, these studies also demonstrated the following:

- A great many, if not most, accepted, repeated, and respected rules of water safety and survival were (and in a number of instances still are) *badly* in need of updating.
- Many individuals and institutions continued to believe and to teach concepts and procedures that are as dangerous as they are outdated.
- Most drownings were not inevitable "acts of God" but were based on misunderstanding or lack of appropriate and available information.

To prevent or respond effectively to any accidental occurrence, an emergency services provider *must* understand, as completely as possible, situations actually or potentially involving him or her. Water, because of its dangerous but frequently unappreciated power and changeability, makes this need for understanding even more critical.

The reader must carefully review the information presented in Part One of the text. If you consider yourself an "old hand" at water rescue, it is even *more* imperative that you study these chapters closely. In doing so, you may discover that what has been preached as fact in water safety for so long frequently is fiction.

REFERENCES
1. Boating statistics 1991, COMDTPUB P16754.5, Washington, DC, 1992, US Coast Guard.
2. Accident facts 1991, Chicago, 1991, National Safety Council.

1 Causes of Water Accidents

OVERVIEW

This chapter introduces and analyzes the *where, when, who, why,* and *how* of aquatic mishaps. Interpretations of water accident statistics are emphasized. These interpretations then are used to outline starting points for aquatic accident prevention programs.

OBJECTIVES

After studying this chapter, the reader should understand:
1. The scope of the drowning and water safety problem
2. The locales, seasons, and normal hours of drowning
3. Physical and psychological differences between potential victims
4. Primary factors that interact to cause drowning
5. How to use the foregoing information in developing community-based aquatic accident prevention programs

---

PRETEST

1. Although there are some exceptions, most drownings involve summer-time swimmers who panic in deep water. (True or false?)
2. The majority of fatal aquatic accidents occur (a) at home; (b) at community pools and supervised beaches; or (c) in rural lakes, ponds, waterways, and beaches. (Pick the correct answer.)
3. Which of the following must be removed to keep the wearer afloat: (a) fire fighter turnout gear; (b) chest and hip waders; (c) shoes, shirt, trousers; (d) all of them; or (e) none of them?

---

4. A community's best defense against aquatic accidents is comprehensive safety education. (True or false?)
Pretest answers are at the end of the chapter.

DETERMINING DATA

Water-oriented recreation is the primary outdoor pastime in North America. More than half of the total population of the United States and Canada annually swims, fishes, hunts, or relaxes in some form—on, under, or in the water.[1]

As indicated in Table 1-1, in the United States drowning ranks behind only automobile accidents as a leading cause of accidental death for people under age 44 years. It ranks third for all ages after automobile accidents and falls. The approximately 5000 lives lost annually to water accidents represent a drop in total fatalities of almost 40% since 1973 (Fig. 1-1). This reduction is encouraging, but more effort is needed to diminish this figure further.

The foregoing total is an approximation. Although specific information is garnered through state and federal sources to count exactly every auto, fire, and fall fatality, only 36 states provide drowning statistics to the U.S. Public Health Service's Centers for Disease Control in Atlanta, Georgia.

One segment of the national drowning total that is not approximated is the boating accident input of the U.S. Coast Guard. As part of their boating safety mission, members of the Coast Guard annually tally the numbers displayed in Table 1-1. These boating listings include approximately one fifth of all drownings. An important aspect of the boating

Table 1-1 Accidental Deaths by Age and Type, 1986

Age (yr)	Motor Vehicles	Falls	Drowning	Fire/Burns	Other*
<5	1188	117	754	768	407
5-14	2350	55	649	434	303
15-24	15,227	399	1341	395	1190
25-44	15,884	1035	1665	1003	4019
45-64	6799	1519	716	841	1719
65-74	3096	1554	270	562	1339
>74	3361	6765	305	832	2207

From Accident facts, 1989, Chicago, 1989, National Safety Council.
*Includes ingestion of food or object; firearms; poison; poisonous gas.

computations is that they are divided into smaller subgroups. With minor exceptions, these subgroupings accurately represent the larger overall, non-boat-related drowning population.

Other accurate resources dealing with one aspect of aquatic information are the Consumer Products Safety Council (CPSC) and the National Swimming Pool Safety Committee (NSPSC) (see Appendix I). The CPSC is an agency of the federal government, part of the Commerce Department. The NSPSC is composed of members from the swimming pool plus spa industry and national water safety organizations and representatives from different levels of government. These groups mainly are oriented toward reducing drownings and cerebrospinal (head and neck) diving injuries in swimming pools.

Even though water safety researchers frequently analyze approximate figures, a number of valuable insights have been gained:
- Men drown four times more frequently than women.[12]
- Blacks are twice as likely to die from drowning as whites.[13]
- Thirteen percent of drowning victims are 4 years old or younger.[2]
- Diving-related injuries paralyze an average of 700 people, predomi-

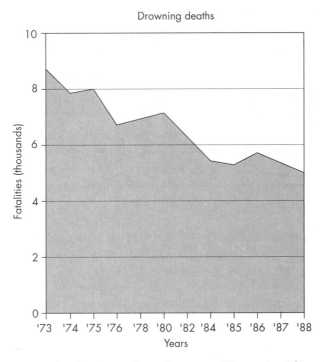

Fig. 1-1 Drowning deaths for selected years. (From Accident facts, 1989, Chicago, 1990, National Safety Council.)

nantly younger males 13 to 23 years of age, annually.[20]

- Estimates of alcohol's involvement in fatalities are as high as two thirds, with possibly 50% legally intoxicated.[10]
- The primary drowning victim is an intoxicated 18- to 24-year-old white male.[26]

> Two out of three drowning victims are *nonswimmers* or poor swimmers, with most fully clothed, usually having *no* intention of entering (deep) water.[6]

- Fifty percent of all water fatalities occur outside the normal June-through-August water recreation season.[13]
- Water accidents peak at 6 PM on summer holidays and summer Saturdays. (This statistic is gleaned from reviewing and interpreting a number of state and municipal reports.)
- Water accidents tend to diminish on the beginning days of the week, tapering to very low overall figures in early winter and slowly resuming in early spring.
- In the average boating accident the craft is 16 feet or less in length and not moving; it has no motor or one with less than 10 horsepower (HP); and the victim usually falls out of or capsizes the boat.[7]
- Eighty-nine percent of those killed in boating accidents would survive if they had *worn* a PFD. According to the 1989 action manual, "How to Conduct a Small Boat Safety Campaign," page 25, published by the National Safe Boating Council in Seattle, 1989, "Of the 1036 people who died in boating accidents in 1987, 89% were not wearing life jackets. Most of the others probably died of traumatic injuries (or underpinnings) from which a life jacket is no protection."
- The primary cause of hunting deaths is drowning or immersion **hypothermia.**
- A person is twice as likely to die from drowning in Canada as in the United States and 10 times as likely to perish from drowning in Alaska as the lower 48 United States.[4]
- Most drownings occur within 10 feet of safety and 50 feet of shore.[14]
- It is estimated that at least 60% of all drownings are witnessed.[19]
- Approximately 70% of all lifeguard rescue attempts resulting in fatalities are post facto (*after* someone tells the guard about the drowning).[15]
- Ten percent of drownings occur at guarded or supervised pools and beaches.

- Thirty percent of drownings happen at home, primarily among small children in pools and elderly people in bathtubs.
- Eighty-five percent of drownings are "wet."
- Ten percent to 15% of drownings are "dry."[17]
- Sixty percent of drownings take place in rural lakes, ponds, streams, and gravel pits.[22,23]
- The toll from secondary drowning may be higher than from primary drowning.[24]
- There may be as many as 10 cases of individuals nearly drowning for every one fatal submersion.[21]
- The longest time for submersion with complete recovery was 66 minutes (June 10, 1986, Salt Lake City, Utah).[8]
- Approximately two thirds to three fourths of all potentially brain-damaged near-drowning survivors *eventually* recover.[18]
- There is no accurate record of the number of near-drowning victims who eventually die.
- Differences of opinion exist in the medical community regarding care of near-drowning victims.[27] (These differences are discussed in Chapter 12.)

INTERPRETING THE DATA

The foregoing insights reveal a number of patterns. For instance, in comparing rural versus urban locations, relatively few fatal accidents occur at guarded pools and beaches. Drownings are much more likely to happen at home or in rural settings. Additional considerations at rural accident sites include the difficulty in gaining access to the scene, searching for and extricating or recovering the victim, and transporting him or her to a clinical facility. All are more difficult than in either the pool or home setting. The rural problem is further complicated if the near-drowning patient is **comatose.** For best results, this patient should be transported as quickly as possible to a trauma center where heart-lung bypass equipment is available.

Children at Home

The majority of younger children (age 4 years and younger) who drown or undergo near-drowning **trauma** are involved in mishaps at home. In those states with large numbers of home pools (Arizona, California, and Florida), drowning is the leading cause of death to 4-year-old and younger children.[5] For this reason, communities having large numbers of home or private pools are encouraged to develop a home water safety program similar to the highly successful "Tot Finder" fire safety approaches. Moreover, individuals with small children at home who read this book should take the initiative, as explained in following chapters, to "waterproof" their home and family.

Alcohol and Drowning or Diving

Particular attention should be given to the major role of alcohol in drownings. Outside of the material presented in this book (see Chapter 4), there is relatively little up-to-date, comprehensive information on alcohol and aquatics available to the general public or safety specialists. However, this situation is improving. (See Appendix I for free brochures and handouts on alcohol and water recreation.)

> Prevention of accidents is far more important than response.

Prevention is based mainly on a person's changing his or her behavior. Behavioral changes generally result from a more complete or altered and expanded perception of facts. For instance, providing detailed information about the interaction of alcohol and water can produce positive results.

Me and the PFD?

The fact that serious water accidents *do not* occur primarily in summer time to swimmers in bathing suits is important. Nonswimmers and poor swimmers who find themselves near the water must be apprised of their risk. They should be coached or coerced into wearing properly fitted and tested (by them in the water) PFDs. There is *no excuse whatsoever* for rescue personnel, especially rescue personnel who swim poorly, not to wear PFDs at a water site. The mark of professional water rescuers is that they are *proud* to wear and to properly use their PFDs

Rescue and Safety

Particular attention must be given to the following facts:

> Most people in serious trouble in the water are *only a few feet* from safety and are poor swimmers or nonswimmers; therefore they tend to trip, slip, stumble, fall or be pushed into an area where they have no intention of going. They do not primarily *swim* into danger.

- A small amount of information indicates that more than half of all drownings, and possibly a much larger portion, are witnessed, but no (or an improper) response is made.
- Lifeguards, presumably trained to recognize drowning persons, frequently fail to notice that anything is wrong until someone brings the situation to their attention.

Can something be done to alert more persons at the scene of an unfolding tragedy that a person in the water needs help? Yes! A community, through public safety programs and providers, can reduce aquatic accidents by using a relatively small amount of educational input. In addition, the more professional rescuers understand and are practiced in knowing and explaining the basic signs of drowning, the greater defense they have against one of their own number becoming an unwanted statistic.

Sportsmen and Weather

There is no statistic accurately indicating the numbers of people involved in outdoor recreation other than water sports (i.e., swimming, diving, wading, waterskiing) who drown. However, U.S. Coast Guard figures indicate that approximately 75% of all boating fatalities occur while the person is going to, returning from, or in the act of fishing. The combination of a nonswimming but drinking fisherman who will not wear a PFD but will go alone to an isolated lake in a small, unstable craft is not hard to imagine.

If half the victims of drowning die outside of the normal summer season, just what are they doing in or on the water? Some of them, especially in the warmer Southern states, are swimming, but the majority are not. They usually are hunters, fishing enthusiasts, and canoeists. They also tend to underestimate the weather, mainly air and water temperatures, and overestimate their own competence. When the rescue professional must deal with them, these potential victims are primarily in hard-to-reach rural locations, which present difficult rescue scenarios.

In the following chapters you are told how to survive in cold, moving water and how best to keep yourself out of the water unless there is no other, better option. Passing this information to local hunters and fishing groups would be of assistance.

Alaskan/Canadian Connection

The differences in drowning rates between people in higher and lower latitudes is easily understood. The farther north, the more cold the air and water become, and in higher latitudes, fewer people are in position to assist a potential victim.

Conversely, the more water activity there is in an area, the more an individual's *probability* of drowning decreases *if* the individual does not increase his or her own risk level through, for example, drinking, not wearing a PFD in hazardous circumstances, or diving into shallow or unknown water. On the other hand, most aquatic accident victims are relatively close to safety. For instance, at a crowded beach when someone steps into a hole, there is a good chance that another person standing nearby can grasp and pull him or her to safety — if the bystander realizes that the person alongside is actually drowning!

RESULTS OF INTERPRETATION AND INTEGRATION

Decreasing Drownings and Boating Fatalities

A multifaceted plan was approved to decrease the number of boating injuries and deaths and was carried out by state and federal agencies. It was comparatively well funded and monitored to ensure it achieved its goals. Its segments were based on carefully applied research programs, the outcomes of which were shared with many state, federal, and private organizations.

Part of the boating safety effort (especially the information on alcohol) has begun to affect the public and the rate of all drownings. The concept that larger numbers of people using the water *aid* safety should be considered. No one knows how many backyard pools there are in North America, but some estimates reach into the millions.[25] Thus more and younger people are exposed to learning how to swim and be relaxed in the water. However, the increased number of pools provides more opportunities for small children to wander unnoticed into unsecured pool areas.

Another primary consideration is that greater numbers of the public are learning and using cardiopulmonary resuscitation **(CPR)**. Although hard facts in this area are extremely difficult to obtain, timely CPR intervention probably is reducing drowning numbers; however, although hard data are not readily available, the number of victims permanently brain-damaged after aquatic incidents, near drowning, and resuscitation has apparently risen.[3]

An additional consideration potentially affecting aquatic accidents may be the aging of America. As the older segment of the population continually increases, the number of comparatively safer, less accident-prone individuals grows; thus this group may moderate the incident and injury rates. Conversely, even though elderly individuals are less exposed to water hazards, they can have some special in-water problems, which are cited in following chapters.

Drowning Profile in Time, Place, Date

Chapter 3 discusses specifics related to drowning and aquatic accident scenarios. However, as you read more of this text, the general patterns involved in understanding drownings should become clearer. The following age-based inferences are broadly valid. Based on Table 1-2:

- Emergency service systems should be prepared to deal with an increase in near drownings of younger children in backyard pools in the summer. Pediatric-oriented CPR training sessions should be scheduled before and during this period. Simultaneously, an informational campaign can be conducted to aid home owners in developing standardized preventive systems to ensure that their own and neighbors' toddlers will not accidentally enter pool areas.[9] Rural providers should review their transport networks with the intention of providing or improving expeditious movement for near-drowning patients to the nearest trauma center.
- Depending on the time of the year, planning should be scheduled to outline response to missing fishermen or hunters. Local outdoor clubs could be contacted for information on areas their membership is most likely to frequent; then a representative of the local fire, police, or emergency medical service (EMS) should visit, as feasible, those areas situated within its geographical zones of responsibility. He or she would note the existing or potential aquatic hazards, making notes on likely equipment access sites, how frequently the area is used, and high water levels and similar considerations.[16] As population increases, accessibility increases. A growing number of water accidents occur at

Table 1-2 Drowning Potential by Age and Locale

Age (yr)	Home			Supervised		Unsupervised		
	Tub	Pool	Pond	Pool	Beach	Beach	Lake	Stream
<1	PRI							
1-4	PRI	PRI	PRI					
5-14		SEC	SEC	SEC	SEC	SEC	PRI	PRI
15-24		SEC	SEC	SEC	SEC	SEC	PRI	PRI
25-64						SEC	PRI	PRI
>64	PRI						PRI	PRI

PRI, Principle drowning locale; *SEC*, secondary drowning locale.

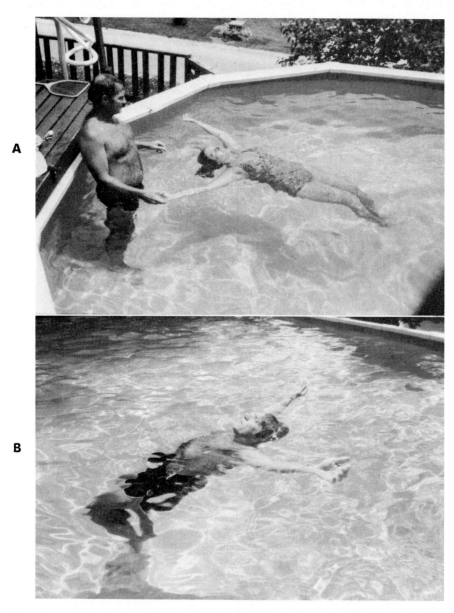

Fig. 1-2 A, Women have little difficulty floating when relaxed. **B,** Most relaxed men will also float, but they assume a different flotation angle than women.

remote, previously unfrequented locations. Many of these sites offer attractive but dangerous aquatic opportunities.

Drowning Differences

The striking disproportion of men to women dying in the water is based on two considerations, one physical and the other psychological.

Physical differences. Weight and relative size have next to no effect on flotation. A person's sinking is far more dependent on his or her body fat content: a person with a higher fat percentage floats better. Women have a thicker layer of **subcutaneous** (beneath the skin) fat than men. Almost all women can float motionlessly flat on their backs (Fig. 1-2). If they relax, it is nearly impossible for them to sink. Males have a slightly higher muscle-to-fat ratio than females. Since approximately three quarters of human body weight is from salt water, the average adult human only weighs 6 to 7 pounds in the water. In addition, with air-filled lungs, the body becomes more buoyant; thus when breath holding, most humans weigh nothing in the water. To confirm this statement, notice how much of a PFD is *out* of the water on a typical wearer (Fig. 1-3). PFDs are usually designed to support a minimum of 15 pounds, and normally half or more of the device is above the water's surface. (Chapter 6 provides

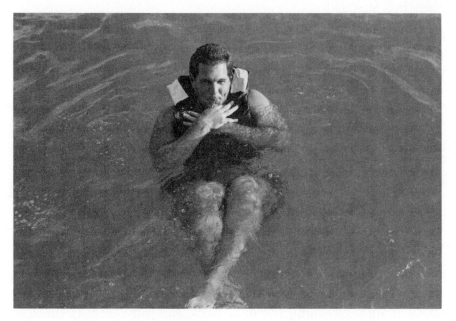

Fig. 1-3 Note how much of this PFD is out of the water. Most of a PFD's buoyancy is actually a reserve for rough or unusual conditions.

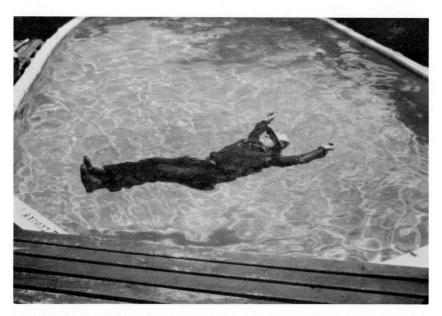

Fig. 1-4 This fully clothed male can float easily as long as he maintains his lung inflation and keeps his mouth shut. However, a PFD would provide a much more secure means of flotation.

details on all the various types and uses of PFDs.) Even without a PFD, most adults can float motionlessly as long as they fully inflate their lungs and keep their mouths closed (Fig. 1-4).

> Almost all types of clothing are neutrally buoyant. They neither sink nor float unless and until something is done to add to or detract from their initial flotation state. Even heavier footwear, including hip and chest waders, tend to follow this rule.

Just as males are slightly heavier in the water than females, men also have more developed, and therefore heavier, leg muscles. For this reason their legs tend to sink. As the legs of the unpracticed, back-floating male sink, he believes that he will continue to travel toward the bottom. This is untrue. Countering this progression requires a small amount of practice, mainly in rolling the head back and fully arching the spine. Younger, thinner, more wiry males are not as buoyant as those with a few more years—and pounds—on them. Conversely, almost every human can float in salt or sea water since it provides more buoyancy than fresh water.

The flotation characteristics of children vary widely. As a general rule, most younger children have sufficient body fat to allow them to float motionlessly. Relaxed back floating, on the other hand, is a *learned* response. Although it is physically simple to master this technique—especially with increases in age and circumference—the psychological barriers, especially for a frightened child, are difficult to overcome without specialized assistance and instruction.[11]

Psychological differences. The primary psychological difference between men and women is that females rarely have to demonstrate being macho. On the other hand, especially when drinking, males "showing off" around the water may perform in a less-than-prudent manner. The potential for drowning of an intoxicated, slender male in cold (i.e., slightly less than body temperature) water is startling.[25] As you become more familiar with this material, you may begin to wonder why so few people actually manage to kill themselves in the water when compared to the huge numbers repeatedly placing themselves at risk!

PRIME DROWNING FACTOR INTEGRATION

Contrary to conventional wisdom, accidents do not in actuality occur suddenly. The final event that we refer to as an *accident* may take very little time to transpire; but the events, behaviors, outlooks, and habits that allow it are fixed into place and *repeatedly* practiced over a far longer period. An *accident* for the purpose of this text is defined as the (usually) undesired result of a highly observable, predictable, and preventable chain of events. This chain of events may also be seen as consisting of certain more-or-less definable factors that interact with or add to each other over time.

The accident-causing factors are divided into two groups: those we can change and those we cannot. Unchangeable factors in aquatic mishaps are environmental and situational elements. For instance, as a person is falling into the water, he or she cannot change it from fresh to salt water to become more buoyant, nor can he or she make it any warmer (although they *can* wear some sort of heat-retentive protective clothing).

The factors that can be modified concern habits and perceptions. This alteration in habits basically is triggered by looking at situations and ourselves differently. When an individual realizes that a six-pack of beer consumed during a 2-hour canoe trip, although traditional, is downright dangerous or that being a fearful nonswimmer on a rescue team is not bright behavior, he or she is taking the first step toward productive behavioral change. The next, bigger step is to form the habit of "parking" the six-pack until the on-water activity *and* the drive home are finished or to take swimming lessons so he or she can be more aquatically dependable.

COMMUNITY ACTION OR WATER DEFENSE PLAN

A leading reason for drowning remaining near the top of public safety concerns is, conversely, not enough public concern. Because of the large number of aquatic myths repeated through conventional wisdom and applied most heavily during the early, most formative years, the public thinks it understands water safety. But does it? As an example, through the years many people have seen the "throw the drunken cowboy into the horse trough" segment in Western movies. Viewers grow up thinking (and probably telling their children) that a cold-water dunking will result in instant sobriety. It does not. What can actually occur is rapid death to an inebriated person in water no deeper than his or her waist.

Similarly, almost everyone growing up in North America has been told the rule about waiting to swim after eating and about the deadly stomach cramps that can occur. This is not really true. Chapter 2 explains more fully.

The foregoing examples illustrate that a large portion of the populace thinks it knows a great deal about water safety. But it does not. Getting someone to learn something entirely new is often difficult. Having them *unlearn* facts embedded into their consciousness and then replace these erroneous concepts with something new and somewhat alien is far more difficult. However, if we want to reduce drownings and other types of water accidents, examination and replacement of faulty ideas provide the best opportunities to do so. This is the rationale behind the repeated injunctions in this text to encourage readers to bring this information to their families and then to the entire community.

Community action and water safety plans have three principle elements:

- Determining which types of hazards exist in the area and analyzing how to best work with them on a preventive, reduction, or removal basis

- Planning to deal with the hazard in an appropriate reactive, rescue-oriented level
- Delivering education and information, usually starting with younger school children, to the community about its water dangers and how to avoid them

Far too many rescuers have risked, and frequently lost, their lives in attempting the rescue of someone who may never have gotten into trouble in the first place—if the danger had been removed, if rescuers were more prepared (e.g., through a preincident visit to the site), or if the victims had heard an explanation of the risks they were creating for themselves and others.

CHAPTER SUMMARY

- Drowning and related aquatic accidents are major public safety concerns.
- The number of water accident deaths and the aquatic accident rates (comparison between those exposed to a hazard and those actually killed or injured) have been decreasing, but more must be done.
- Although the understanding of water accidents needs more research, a number of items can be gathered from present documentation.
- The public believes and follows a number of myths about water, thereby obscuring the true causes of aquatic accidents.
- Unwise alcohol use, the presence of (relatively) cold water, the inability to swim, and not wearing a personal flotation device (PFD) are major interacting factors underlying drowning.
- Community-based, preventive-action plans combining water safety education with inspection and reduction of aquatically hazardous areas or situations are much more valuable and far less dangerous than after-the-fact rescue attempts.

PRETEST ANSWERS

1. False
2. c
3. e
4. True

REFERENCES

1. A.C. Nielson Survey, Swimming pool age and spa merchandiser, October 1982, The Survey.
2. Accident facts, 1989, Chicago, 1990, National Safety Council, p 6.
3. Allman F et al.: Outcome following cardiopulmonary resuscitation and severe pediatric near-drowning, Am J Dis Child 140:6, 1988, pp 571-575.
4. Baker S, O'Neill B, and Karpf R: The injury fact book, Lexington, Mass, 1984, DC Heath, pp 155-165.
5. Barriers for residential swimming pools, spas and hot tubs, Preamble, CPSC Staff Recommendations, Washington, DC, 1990, p 1.
6. Basic rescue and water safety, Washington, DC, 1980, American Red Cross, p 7.
7. Boating statistics 1987, Washington, DC, 1988, US Coast Guard, pp 20-26.
8. Bolte R et al.: The use of extracorporeal rewarming in a child submerged for 66 minutes, JAMA 260:3, 1988, pp 377-379.
9. Children and pools: A safety checklist, Pub No 357, Washington, DC, 1990, US Consumer Safety Commission, pp 3-5.
10. Deluca J: Alcohol and health, Rockville, Md, 1981, National Institute on Alcohol Abuse and Alcoholism, p 83.
11. Freeman M: Teach your child to swim, Gallatin, Tenn, 1981, SEAL Foundation.
12. Gulaid J and Sattin R: Drownings in the United States, 1978-1984, CDC Surveillance Summaries 37(SS-1), Atlanta, 1985, Centers for Disease Control, pp 27-33.
13. Gulaid J and Sattin R: Drownings in the United States, 1978-1984. CDC Surveillance Summaries 37(SS-1), Atlanta, 1985, Centers for Disease Control, p 30.
14. Johnson R: What research has revealed about drowning and diving accidents, 1984, Indiana, Penn, Indiana University of Pennsylvania, p 17.
15. Johnson R: What research has revealed about drowning and diving accidents, 1984, Indiana, Penn, Indiana University of Pennsylvania, pp 8-11.
16. Madison A: Judgement on the water, Chatham, NY, 1987, Alan Madison Productions (videotape).
17. Martin T: Near-drowning and cold-water immersion, Ann Emerg Med 13:263-273, 1984.
18. Nichter M and Everett P: Childhood near-drowning: Is cardiopulmonary resuscitation always indicated? Crit Care Med 17:10, 1989, pp 993-995.
19. North Carolina drownings, 1980-1984, MMWR 35:40, 1986, p 635.
20. Operation water watch sample news release No. 2, Washington, DC, Summer 1990, US Consumer Product Safety Commission, pp 1-2.
21. Perspectives in disease prevention and health promotion aquatic deaths and injuries – United States, MMWR 31:31, 1982, p 417.
22. Pia F: Drowning facts and myths, 1976, Larchmont, NY, Water Safety Films (film).
23. Report: A model state recreational injury control program, Atlanta, 1981, Centers for Disease Control, p A-36.
24. Report: A model state recreational injury control program, Atlanta, 1981, Centers for Disease Control, p BB-9.
25. Smith D: Notes on drowning: The misunderstood preventable tragedy, Physician Sports Med 12:7, 1984, p. 68.
26. Smith D and Smith S: Waterwise, Imperial, Mo, 1984, Smith Aquatic Safety Services, pp 57-71.
27. Spaniol S and Boyd D: Near drowning consensus and controversies in pulmonary and cerebral resuscitation, Heart Lung 18:1, 1989, p 102.

2

Definition of Drowning

OVERVIEW

This chapter defines the primary aquatic and medically related terms encountered in the text. It also describes and explains various types of water injuries. The basic physiological causes of death in drowning are discussed.

OBJECTIVES

After reading this chapter, the reader should understand the fundamental terminology applicable to water injuries and fatalities. This material should also reenforce the underlying premise of Chapter 1 that there is more to comprehend about aquatic accidents than generally suspected. In particular, this chapter aids in discriminating between:
1. Different types of water mishaps
2. Fact and fiction in drowning physiology
3. Precise as opposed to vague reporting and descriptive usage in commenting on or explaining aquatic mishaps
4. Difficulties in determining death in certain water accident victims

PRETEST

1. Eating a large meal immediately before swimming will definitely cause stomach cramps. (True or false?)
2. Persons in the throes of drowning (a) almost always scream for help; (b) cannot verbalize; or (c) are usually mistakenly described as "playing or clowning" in the water. (Which, if any, are correct?)

3. The only infallible way to determine if a drowning victim is dead is to use an **electrocardiograph (ECG)** or brain monitor **(EEG)**. (True or false?)
4. Cold-water near-drowning has next to nothing to do with the time of the year. (More true or more false?)
Pretest answers are at the end of the chapter.

DERIVATION OF A DEFINITION

The term *drowning*, according to *Webster's New World Dictionary*, is derived from the Old Norse word *drukkna*, meaning to die by **suffocation** in water or other liquid. The victim's face, at least the breathing orifices (i.e., nose and mouth), is below the water long enough to allow water to interfere fatally with his or her breathing. In this usage *drowning* is a fairly specific term since it states physical interaction with water was the principle reason for a victim's **mortality.**

Conversely, since many details not yet fully understood or reported and made available for analysis in studies of drowning, other, more comprehensive terms have been coined to describe water-related deaths. One is the word *waterdeath*, which means someone died in the water.

Another somewhat similar word is *hydrocution*, a general, nonspecific term that may also indicate that the exact causes of death in the accident are not fully understood. It is derived from the Greek word for water *(hydro)* and the middle English word *cutten*, meaning either to cut or to kill. *Hydrocution* is a good choice if you wish to avoid saying or writing *drowning* repeatedly. However, it is not as precise as the terminology we are about to examine.

INSPECTING SPECIFIC TERMS

To help reduce future water accidents, individuals responsible for reporting and investigating them must be increasingly precise in defining exactly what has transpired.

A primary reason for this preciseness is the need to provide the best possible information for researchers. Another is to begin peeling away the layers of misconception in the minds of the general public about what actually happens in and how to best protect themselves from water mishaps. The following definitions are intended to sharpen your aquatic perceptions.

People die in the water from four specific types of aquatic injury or trauma (victims may be injured immediately before entering the water, and they may also suffer in-water injuries such as propeller lacerations; however, the following definitions concern *only* what transpires as a result of interacting with water):

- Water covers their breathing passages, enters their throat, and causes an effect called a **laryngospasm,** or blockage of the upper part of the throat by muscular contraction, and they die from suffocation, meaning not being able to get fresh air into or used air out of their lungs. This is called **dry drowning.**
- Laryngospasm is basic to all drownings. However, when the **larynx** immediately relaxes, allowing water to enter the **trachea,** or breathing tube, and the lungs, a person dies from aquatic **asphyxiation.** The lungs are invaded or occluded by water, and he or she cannot obtain air. This is a **wet drowning.**
- Approximately 700 persons suffer permanent, diving-related **cervical** spine injuries or damage to the upper vertebrae and spinal column each year. They are the ones who live, but usually with partial or total loss of use of their limbs and body functions.[8] The victims who die do so because their impact with an underwater obstruction, usually the bottom, is so great that their spinal cord is completely severed. Since most drownings are in rural locations, autopsies, especially for someone assumed to have died from "drowning," are frequently not ordered or requested. This means that the true numbers of deaths due actually to breaking a person's neck are not exactly known.
- The last category of fatal, in-water trauma generally applies to older, fearful, out-of-shape nonswimmers. With sudden and total immersion, usually in very cold water, they suffer from panic-induced and panic-related **cardiac** arrest, which is part of a progression known as immersion syndrome, or immediate disappearance syndrome (IDS). This syndrome involves an overwhelming shock to the **cardiovascular** (heart and circulatory) system, normally resulting from the person's falling overboard, followed by their failing to resurface.

Other physical causes could be added to the above listing; however, cramps, epileptic seizures, and other disease-related factors are assumed to result eventually in one of the four preceding categories. ("Although only 7% of all drowning victims were known to have seizure disorders, persons with seizure disorders accounted for 53% of all drownings resulting from bathing in a bathtub."[10])

Cramping after eating is *not* a major reason for drowning. In actuality, the most common form of eating-related trauma in the water happens after someone *vomits*, then **aspirates** stomach contents, including acid, into the lungs and breathing passages. Eating a large meal before *any* form of vigorous physical activity may produce **regurgitation.** However, although waiting to swim after a large meal is a good idea, eating-induced stomach cramps are *not* greatly related to drowning. In fact, eating *something* before entering the water may be a positive method of maintaining elevated body heat and energy levels (depending on water temperature and length of exposure).

Cramping actually results more from an out-of-shape person's exercising vigorously (and unwisely) in a cold medium. Studies have shown that a very small segment of the population is subject to stomach cramps after eating. This process, medically labeled the *gastrocoronary reflex*, involves increased blood flow to the stomach. In some people the muscle tissue surrounding the stomach is severely deprived of oxygen, and cramps result. With the exception of this relatively rare situation, eating followed by stomach cramping in the water is a general myth.

("Occasionally swimmers suffer abdominal cramps. These, too, are caused by fatigue, cold, or overexertion. They are not caused by swimming too soon after eating, as commonly thought. Severe abdominal cramps are rare."[2])

TYPES OF DROWNING

There is a major difference between primary and secondary drowning.

Primary drowning refers to a person's dying at the accident scene or immediately thereafter as a direct, observable result of the immersion or submersion incident. *Secondary drowning* refers to a death occurring within 72 hours after an aquatic accident.

Secondary drowning usually involves infection or occult, or hidden, damage to the respiratory or cardiovascular systems. Examples of this are adult respiratory distress syndrome **(ARDS)** and/or **pulmonary edema** (Table 2-1). The infection aspect of secondary drowning frequently results from the victim's ingesting water containing fungi or

Table 2-1. Medical Conditions Caused by Near Drowning

Condition	Other Name(s)	Description (Partial)
Acute respiratory distress syndrome (ARDS)	Shock lung Wet lung	Shortness of breath, rapid breathing. Cause: damaged lung tissue; hemorrhage; fluid buildup in lungs.
Acute renal failure	Acute kidney failure	Inability of kidneys to excrete wastes. Cause: hemorrhage; toxic injury. May cause heart failure.
Hemolysis	Hemolytic anemia	Breakdown of red blood cells. Cause: dilution of blood by excessive amounts of hypotonic solutions.
Diffuse intravascular coagulation	Internal clotting	Clotting in blood vessels and organs throughout the body because of breakdown and dilution of blood cells, followed by massive internal bleeding.

Modified from Dive Rescue International: Cold water air drowning—emergency care (slide/tape presentation).

bacteria into the lungs. The victim then gives little or no immediate indication that he or she has been exposed to the threat. After sufficient time has passed to allow the lung contaminants to begin injuring the body, the victim requests help and may even seek aid at a medical facility.

Frequently, since the then **comatose,** or unconscious, victim can no longer explain what has happened to him or her, medical personnel must initiate time-consuming investigatory procedures. Sometimes these tests isolate and identify the cause soon enough to treat it. Too often they do not. Other detrimental progressions such as ARDS involve lung tissue exposed to the highly injurious flushing and diluting action of ingested water. They can also cause lung infections.

The bottom-line notation to rescuers who suspect water has entered a victim's lungs is this: do not delay, but ensure the patient is seen *immediately* at a medical facility.

The term **near drowning** should be mentioned since it is sometimes confused with *secondary drowning.* Near drowning usually means recovery from primary drowning (to review, primary drowning is death from asphyxia, and secondary drowning indicates death from water-induced complications).

It is most important to determine if someone who appears dead from drowning has actually died. The final section of this chapter reviews a number of points specifically dealing with *cold water* near drowning. Do not automatically associate cold water or cold water near drowning *only* with ice and snow, for this term may be grossly misleading. In other words, long-term submersions with resuscitation and complete recovery *do* happen outside the colder months of the year.

TYPES OF SWIMMERS

Just as there is a differentiation among types of drowning, there also are various skill levels in swimming. The terms *nonswimmer* and *drowning nonswimmer* appear frequently in this text. Nonswimmer refers to a person having very poor or nonexistent swimming skills *at the moment of their aquatic accident*. A *drowning* nonswimmer is a person who initiates and sustains classic, recognizable drowning behavior. In addition, nonswimmers' initial skills may be so minimal or ineffective that they cannot maintain themselves on the surface, or something may have interfered with their usual swimming ability.

A person at the outset of the aquatic incident may actually be very

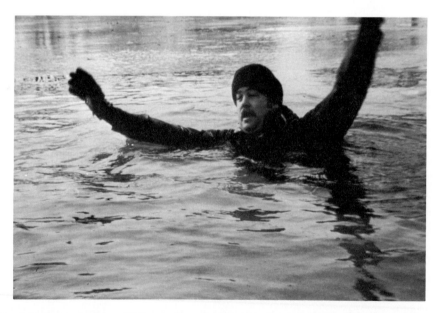

Fig. 2-1 Torso reflex. This person involuntarily inhales while unexpectedly falling into the water. (From Dive Rescue International: Ice rescue [slide/tape presentation].)

proficient in the water *but* has done something to reduce or to obstruct his or her normal skill levels. A non-drug-oriented example is an automatic physiological reaction to suddenly falling into cold(er) water, called a *torso* (or **inhalation**) reflex[6] (Fig. 2-1). Notice that when you step into shower water you thought was warm but it is not, you say something. The initial something you say, or noise you make, is an involuntary gasp, or reflexive sucking in of air, which occurs because your body, through the automatic, bellowlike action of your lungs, is trying to expand oxygen intake rapidly. This increases your **metabolic rate,** building internal warmth in response to the cold's punishing your exterior. You have no control over this except for covering your mouth (Table 2-2).

If someone unexpectedly tumbles into the water, the same reflex may occur, and he or she possibly will inhale a mouthful, or worse, lungful of water. If he or she were swimming strongly and accidently caught a wave in an open, inhaling mouth, the same thing could happen. Even capable, well-practiced swimmers can experience this reflex. When they do, they may panic because they are unable to breathe. If they do panic, they are demoted to nonswimmer status. In this state an individual lapses into unthinking and uncontrollable panic reactions that can kill unless a rescuer, or good fortune, intervenes. These responses are so deeply rooted that a panicked nonswimmer, even when wearing an approved and properly fitted PFD in *shallow* water, can easily lapse into them.

Two other related terms are *passive* and *active drowning*. In the context of this book active drowning infers an observable amount of activity on the part of the person in trouble who requires your professional assistance. Passive drowning means that the victim is in a position of peril but for some reason is not visibly thrashing or reacting

Table 2-2. Torso Reflex or Inhalation Response

The Fire Quadrangle

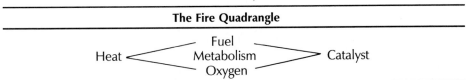

This is an adaptation of the classic fire/rapid oxidation/combustion quadrangle. Humans have an internal oxidation process with similar elements, called *metabolism*. This metabolic process is responsible for maintaining body heat levels. If the brain senses a decrease in body heat, the lungs automatically expand to provide increased oxygen as an aid in developing more internal heat, or "stoking up the fire."

in the water as a sign of distress. The latter condition can occur in cold water in which the victim is so stiffened by exposure to the lower temperature of the water that he or she cannot move. It also can occur in an individual so intoxicated that he or she silently slips under the water surface.

PHYSIOLOGY OF DROWNING

When responding to or investigating an aquatic accident, it is critical for you as a professional emergency services provider to understand as much as possible about what is happening or has happened to the victim(s).

The reasons this knowledge is important are as follows:
- An appropriate, active rescue attempt must be based on exact understanding of the life-threatening situation (including possible problems for the rescuer).
- Medical personnel must be provided as much information as possible, both at the scene and as they make clinical preparations, to care properly for the victim.
- Reporting of the event must be as precise as possible, for this will assist in more specifically defining the causes and defenses involved in water accidents.
- The more that is understood about the actual inner workings of a water accident, the more the public will be correctly advised and educated. As an example: In many outdoorsman drowning cases, emergency responders are quoted as saying, "Heavy clothing pulled the victim underwater." This is not an accurate statement, yet it will be repeated by the media, and the prominent public misconception — that you must remove heavy clothing in the water or die — will be reenforced. This inaccuracy will in turn influence more drownings. Why? Because in most cases, the last thing a person struggling in the water needs to do is to remove his or her clothes. Keeping clothing on is a key to survival.

The following is a general look at the physical stages and events normally encountered in a drowning.

Predrowning Activity
Predrowning events immediately precede the drowning incident. They initiate the victim's life-threatening difficulties in the water and are

scene-setting behaviors. Examples include a person known to suffer from seizures who is swimming alone in deep water and the wader-equipped duck hunter without a PFD who sets out alone in an unstable small craft. This person typically neither tells anyone where he or she is going nor when he or she will return.

Surface Struggle

Conscious, sober humans usually struggle on the surface as a prelude to total submersion. In most cases these struggles are remarkably similar.

Alcohol and drug usage affects the length and intensity of the struggling. The higher the level of impairment or intoxication, the shorter and less vigorous is the surface activity. Persons at 0.2% blood alcohol level and above may not struggle at all. Sudden cardiac arrest or severe trauma before or when entering the water may cancel surface struggling. Once individuals become involved in this surface struggle, they *cannot cry out for help* (Fig. 2-2). This is because they are involuntarily trying to draw in air to breathe, an action that has precedence over crying out. Frequently witnesses are confused by the person's splashing in the water but not yelling for help. Often witnesses state that the victim "looked like he was clowning or playing."

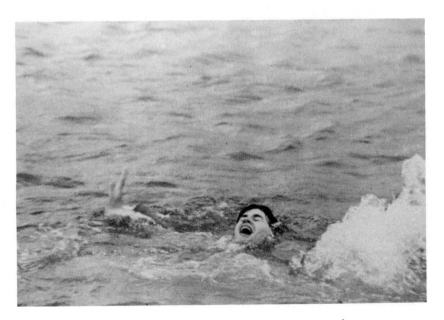

Fig. 2-2 Even though this victim's mouth is wide open, she cannot cry out. (From Flow Graphics: Better think twice [slide/tape presentation].)

Initial Submersion

> The terminal, silent surface struggle normally takes no more than a minute.

During this minute of surface struggling, the victim actually succeeds in expelling enough air from his or her lungs to permit himself or herself to sink. This sinking is also reenforced in most cases by the victim's uncontrollable arm motions. These motions, primarily automatic reactions to draw more air into the lungs, normally result in pushing the victim repeatedly underwater. When the victim sinks below the surface for the final time, he or she attempts to hold his or her breath for as long as possible, but this time is shortened by the exertion. (Also, if the mouth was not closed, increasing water pressure on the chest squeezes out air.) No accurate data are available about humans to indicate how long this breath-holding lasts. Based on reports from resuscitated, near-drowning survivors, 15 seconds probably is the maximum.[7]

Terminal Submersion

When the victim can no longer hold his or her breath, involuntary swallowing begins. Shortly after this point, consciousness is lost because of hypoxia. As previously described, when quantities of water enter the victim's mouth, the muscles at the top of the trachea, including the **pharynx, epiglottis,** and **larynx** (hence the term *laryngospasm*), reactively constrict. One of two actions then occurs. The constriction or spasm relaxes, and water enters the breathing passages and lungs; or the spasm is so severe that it completely prevents water entry.

If the spasm ceases, the body surrenders a large part, but not all, of its total lung-contained air capacity. It then sinks downward. Conversely, if the spasm does not relax, which occurs in approximately 10% to 15% of North American cases, the body remains on the surface. This is an important distinction. If the victim stays on the surface and if rescuers arrive quickly enough, resuscitation opportunities are improved, and lung damage is reduced. However, sinking below the surface might, in some instances, be a greater survival aid than surface floating. As depth increases, temperature and pressure vary. Sudden changes in these variables may trigger the **diving** (or **dive**) **reflex** (see "After Immersion," p. 77), with its potentially protective presence more likely in the submerged victim.[1]

In most instances, dive reflex is coupled with the preservative effect of hypothermia.[12] Acting together, they may actually increase the submerged victim's survival potential as compared to remaining comatose on the surface.

Many factors are involved here: how much the victim struggles (thereby burning or wasting oxygen); water temperature (the deeper the water, the colder its temperature); how long rescuers take in getting to the scene and finding the victim; the rescuers' CPR skill and knowledge level; and equipment. The significant difference to rescuers is that the resuscitation time envelope for underwater victims may be far longer than for those who are not breathing on the surface.

After Submersion Effects

When a person slips below the surface, in most instances the heart is beating very rapidly because of the terrified struggling of the distressed nonswimmer, hypoxia, and the panic-induced release of adrenalin. Although fresh and salt water react somewhat differently with **alveoli,** or lung cells, both types of fluid rapidly proceed through the lungs, into the heart, and into the blood-stream, or **vascular** system.

When a victim goes through this progression, cardiac arrest is caused by a combination of hypoxia and **hemodilution,** or a change in the concentration, components, and acid-base levels of the blood.[11]

It is important to realize what this means in terms of resuscitation and the patient's eventual physical and mental recovery. In the case of dry drowning, next to no fluid enters the victim's body. On the other hand, in a wet drowning when water cooler than body temperature surrounds and also *invades* the body, the victim's internal temperature and concurrent need for oxygen, principally in the brain, are reduced. Therefore the brain and other body organs are better able, in general, to cope with a longer period of hypoxia in a wet, compared to dry, drowning. But as indicated previously, water in the lungs and breathing passages produces additional postresuscitation clinical problems, especially in salt or dirty and contaminated water.

Approximately 10% of all drownings occur in salt water.[9] Distinctions between salt and fresh water are not that important in on-site management and transport of the patient. However, salt water causes absorption of fluid into lung cells, resulting in more severe internal tissue damage, which also complicates clinical resuscitation.

Fouled water such as found in or near many large municipalities is a far greater problem. Agricultural chemicals such as fertilizers and herbicides present similar concerns in rural areas. Another factor is that the water that does enter the body tends to settle in the brain and lungs, thereby causing severe cerebral and pulmonary difficulties.

A sample of the water from the drowning scene should be provided to hospital personnel. It will aid resuscitative procedures and possibly help prevent secondary drowning.

Aquatically Dead or Alive

An essential point is that aquatic accident victims who demonstrate no vital signs whatsoever (including victims receiving cardiac monitoring), may still be resuscitated and live normal lives.[12] Some of the reasons for this were noted in the preceding paragraphs. Nevertheless, not all drowning victims can be resuscitated. At the present state of the art, no one can predict such outcomes with any acceptable degree of confidence. All that can be said is that in most of these instances, *unless* it is overwhelmingly obvious because of accompanying trauma that there is absolutely no chance for survival, you must assume that the victim may be alive if he or she were brought to the surface within 1 hour of the initial underwater disappearance. Some authors go beyond this 1 hour maximum:

DO NOT assume that a person who is **cyanotic** and has no detectable pulse or breathing is dead after cold water exposure, no matter how long it might have been. Seek appropriate medical care to assess and begin the degree of resuscitation indicated based on the individual clinical situation. An absolute time limit beyond which resuscitation is not indicated has not been established. Obvious physical evidence of death would mitigate against beginning resuscitation—gross **evisceration,** decapitation . . .[13]

When trauma, cold, and intoxication are present, determination of vital signs (even with advanced instrumentation) may be difficult. Any one of these factors can cause a reduction of blood flow to the brain, which normally occurs *from the outer layers in*, affecting functioning and—especially when these three conditions are working at the same time—making the victim *appear* dead.

Cerebral death generally is defined as occurring when the brain has completely ceased functioning. This state is usually determined by monitoring only the outer layer of the brain. Since this is the first layer to shut down because of reduced oxygen flow, there is a fair possibility that in the hypothermic patient other inner layers may be functioning but at very low levels. Therefore if cerebral death is indicated, it should be determined that the *whole* brain is no longer functioning. Hence, especially when dealing with colder individuals, halting resuscitative actions on the scene and in a clinical setting may be premature.

In a number of instances well-trained and highly experienced emergency services providers have been misled by this apparent lack of vital signs: " 'City paramedics performed an electrocardiogram on the man showing he was dead,' said Rodney Dreifuss, chief of the Emergency Medical Services."[5] But, the apparently dead man spontaneously revived before transfer to the morgue.

These are very important concepts. For this reason they are discussed from several other viewpoints in later chapters.

CHAPTER SUMMARY

- A number of basic definitions used in describing water accidents were explained.
- A number of the body progressions involved with drowning were described.
- Differences in drowning progressions, particularly as they relate to resuscitation and survival potential, were reviewed.
- A number of elementary factors that may lead experienced rescue and medical providers into mistakenly believing someone is dead were discussed.

PRETEST ANSWERS

1. False
2. b, c
3. False
4. More true

REFERENCES

1. American heat, American Heat Video Productions, St Louis, Jan 1988, (videotape).
2. American Red Cross basic water safety textbook, Washington, DC, 1988, American Red Cross, p 17.
3. American Red Cross lifeguard training, Washington, DC, 1983, American Red Cross, pp 9-1, 9-2.
4. Beach boy spent day drinking, Boston Herald Wire Services, Dec 30, 1983.
5. Bryan B: Heartbeat found in dead man, St Louis Post-Dispatch, Nov 16, 1990.
6. Harnett RM and Bijiani MG: The involvement of cold water in recreational boating accidents, Rep CG-D-31-79, Springfield, Va, 1979, National Technical Information Service, p 1.
7. Lin L: How a medical breakthrough came about—Cold water near-drowning, Ann Arbor, Mich, 1978, Michigan Sea Grant Publications Office, pp. 4-6.
8. Maiman D: Diving-associated spinal cord injuries during drought conditions—Wisconsin 1988, MMWR 37:453-454, 1988.
9. Patetta M: North Carolina drownings, 1980-1984, MMWR 35:635, 1986.
10. Patetta M: North Carolina drownings, 1980-1984, MMWR 35:635-638, 1986.
11. Pearn J: Management of near-drowning, Br Med J 291:1447-1452, 1985.
12. Podolsky ML: Action plan for near drownings, Physician Sports Med 9:46, 1981.
13. Weinberg A and Hamlet M, eds: Cold weather emergencies—Principles of patient management, Branford, Conn, 1990, American Medical Publishing, p 22.

Scenarios and Signs of Drowning

OVERVIEW

This chapter focuses on repeated, predictable chains of events that result in aquatic accidents. Primary topics are:

1. Explanation of four common, time-based scenarios or syndromes for drowning
2. Basics of diving-related accidents and proper responses to them
3. Identification of types of persons most likely to be involved in each scenario and differentiation of the potential for aquatic difficulties
4. Problems in predicting and preventing aquatic accidents
5. Recognition of a human in the act of drowning
6. Introduction to hypothermia

OBJECTIVES

The purpose of this chapter is to provide more information on factors underlying aquatic accidents. This information is divided into categories based on potential intervention time differences and estimated numbers of victims involved. Additional emphasis is placed on identifying what persons do (or apparently are doing) as they place themselves in terminal jeopardy. Another main consideration of this chapter is providing information that may result in water-oriented behavioral change.

PRETEST

1. A fair description of most aquatic accidents is that they are highly unpredictable, following no discernable pattern. (True or false?)

2. In ice water immersion most victims (a) die of cold-induced cardiac arrest; (b) pass out and slip underwater; or (c) drown as a result of cold-impaired swimming skills. (Choose the most *in*correct answer.)
3. A drowning nonswimming child remains on the surface an average of (a) 2 minutes; (b) 20 seconds; or (c) 1 minute. (Choose the correct answer.)
4. Since inner (core) and outer (shell) temperatures fall at the same rate, the concept of "lasting only 30 seconds" in ice water is correct. (True or false?)

Pretest answers are at the end of the chapter.

WATER ACCIDENT PATTERNS

Most water accidents fall into one of four common patterns. Because these patterns deal with repeated, identifiable habits or automatic routines or reactions we all possess, they can be described as **syndromes.** These accident progressions, when compared to each other, are usually quite uniform; therefore the term **scenario,** indicating that the participants act as if they follow a script, can be used. These patterns are as follows:

- Immediate disappearance syndrome (IDS)
- Drowning nonswimmer (DNS)
- Sudden disappearance syndrome (SDS)
- Hypothermia-induced debility (HID)

Table 3-1 describes these classifications.

With IDS, the victim enters the water but does not return to the surface. Companions and/or potential rescuers have little opportunity, once the progression has begun, to intervene on the surface or to offer

Table 3-1. Drowning Versus Time

Type of Drowning	Time for Surface Rescue	Percentage of All Drownings (Estimate)
Immediate	None	20
Drowning nonswimmer	20 seconds (child) 60 seconds (adult)	60
Sudden	5 min	20
Hypothermia-induced	50 × 5	< 1 (outright)

assistance before the victim becomes comatose. Thus the response or intervention time basis for IDS is *0 seconds*. This does not mean that the victim has definitely died because he or she may be subject to underwater search and rescue coupled with resuscitation. However, the emphasis here is on what happens at the beginning of the incident. As previously indicated, data on water accidents are difficult to develop. However, based on the authors' studies of a number of drownings plus comparison with detailed boating accident reports, an estimated 20% of the victims actually were involved in this syndrome. Note that Table 3-1 lists both time and estimated percentages for each of the four accident classifications.

With the DNS pattern, the victim, a struggling nonswimmer or poor swimmer, is observed on the surface for 20 to 60 seconds before sinking under the water. The time basis for most effective rescue or surface intervention averages 40 seconds.

> Most aquatic references agree with the estimate that two out of three drowning victims (approximately 60%) initially are nonswimmers or very poor swimmers.

Undoubtedly there are exceptions to this scenario. For instance, a number of capable swimmers drown because they are injured or incapacitated before entering the water. They may be trapped by sinking debris or undergo some type of *self-*contained *u*nderwater *b*reathing *a*pparatus (scuba) malfunction. Conversely, by reviewing records of witnessed drownings and paying close attention to descriptions of the victims' actions, the 60% estimate appears valid. This percentage is extremely important, for it indicates that with proper educational input (explaining what a drowning person does and how he or she looks), DNS accidents might be greatly reduced. This reduction would occur through increased shore-based or reaching rescues by *trained* passersby or family members. The key element is public understanding of exactly how drowning humans look and act—before they submerge.

In SDS a person who apparently can swim disappears after 5 to 10 minutes' immersion. The name of the syndrome comes from witnesses' repeatedly indicating that the victim was originally seen swimming, usually toward the shore, but when a second look was taken, the victim had "suddenly disappeared." Hard data that might allow a more precise determination of percentages in this classification are not available. On the other hand, a review of detailed boating accident reports (in which someone was in contact with the victim) shows a great number of these instances. Since boating deaths represent an approximation of the larger drowning total and since approximately 20% of boating deaths are in the SDS category, this percentage has been extended to the larger overall total. Because of notification and response time constraints, this syndrome most likely will be occurring as fire, police, and emergency medical service (EMS) personnel arrive on scene. It is the primary rescue scenario you will have to handle as an emergency response team member.

HID begins to affect the average victim seriously after approximately 15 minutes of exposure to relatively cold water. There are two major but widely differing outlooks toward the effects of cold water: (1) hypothermia alone causes water fatalities; and (2) hypothermia has some effect on water fatalities.

In this text hypothermia, acting by itself, is indicated as directly causing less than 1% of all water fatalities. Conversely, the point is continually stressed that coldness of the water has something to do with most aquatic fatalities.

In other words, in the water cold by itself usually does not actually kill the victim. Some other factor normally related to and often initiated by body heat loss provides the terminal event. The latter part of this chapter expands on these points. Additionally, as indicated in Table 3-1, a simple way to remember the time taken by HID to affect the victim fatally is represented by the "50 × 5 rule": an unprotected, untrained *50-year-old individual has 50 minutes in 50° F water before a 50:50 life/death* point is reached.[2] A more detailed description of each classification follows.

IMMEDIATE DISAPPEARANCE SYNDROME

The four main subgroupings in IDS are diving incidents, **hyperventilation, caloric labyrinthitis,** and physiological overload.

Diving Incidents

The primary danger with diving is striking the head or upper torso against the bottom of swimming areas or submerged objects, including other swimmers, with resulting cervical or **cerebroskeletal** trauma. In 1981 the National Safety Council recorded a 29% increase in home pool fatalities.[1] Presumably many of them were due to shallow water diving. Pool chemical levels should always be adjusted for greatest visual clarity, allowing divers to see both the bottom and submerged swimmers.

Similarly, placing highly visible depth markings both on the bottom and on the sides and decks of pools is an effective measure against diving accidents.[7] Pools should be well lighted at night, and all pool users should be informed or warned about the dangers of unwise diving activities.

All pools having diving areas are required to mark the boundary between shallow and deep water with a surface float line. This can be a very important visual clue to both nonswimmers and divers. Be sure that the float line and appropriate, highly visible "No Diving" signs are in place. Additionally, a small but increasing number of diving incidents have been reported from bilingual or multilingual communities. Therefore pool depth markings should be in both feet and meters, with a clear and readily observable distinction made between both systems. Similarly, pool bottom contours and depths can be presented effectively by painting their profile on a wall running alongside the pool deck. International signs using red-crossed circle designs are also effective in warning both non-English-speaking and illiterate pool users.

The predominant age group in diving accidents is composed of 15- to 25-year-old males.[6] A number of these accidents occur in surroundings familiar to the younger victims. In home pool incidents involving adolescents and teenagers, apparently as they grew taller (and heavier), the youngsters failed to realize that the water gets no deeper. Victims in their late teens and early twenties are distributed between home pool and rural settings.

> Prevention should be based on reinforcing the idea of not diving into water of an unknown depth or water shallower than the person is tall.

Research indicates that approximately 50% of all diving accidents involve alcohol.[13] Diving safety depends on precise, split-second interactions between the eyes, balance centers, and muscles. Alcohol, even in amounts well below legal intoxication levels, slows and disrupts these interactions. Statements from paralyzed, alcohol-related diving accident victims are similar. They frequently include something to the effect that the diver, who usually was well practiced, intended to do a flat, shallow dive. However, at the moment of impact, most of these impaired divers were going vertically into the bottom. Alcohol's slowing of reaction time, depending on degree of intoxication, can be so great that a person's head actually is underwater before he or she has adjusted body alignment for the proper or desired angle of entry.[4]

British studies have shown that approximately half of all paraplegics whose condition resulted from an aquatic accident remember *swimming* upward after hitting the bottom.[14] But when the individual reached the surface, a well-intentioned rescuer improperly pulled him or her from the water. Hence methods for dealing with possible spine injuries must always be emphasized. Since, as previously stated, most serious water accidents do not occur near guarded or supervised areas, the first person on the scene with emergency training or responsibility probably will be a non-aquatically prepared policeman or fire fighter. Communities therefore should ensure that both emergency responders and aquatic professionals are proficient in CPR plus in-water management and proper extrication of spinal trauma victims.

Hyperventilation

Hyperventilation most frequently is encountered as a response to stress. It occurs when excited or panicked persons increase their respiratory rate to the point that very little usable air actually enters the lungs. In other words, their rapid inhalation-exhalation cycles actually deprive them of oxygen. This oxygen starvation, or **hypoxia,** is sufficient in some cases to cause unconsciousness.

In the water hyperventilation can involve rapid breathing (e.g., in sudden cold water immersions), or it can involve slowed breathing. Human lungs are designed to absorb a large amount of oxygen and reach saturation levels with each breath. However, many people, especially younger children, have the mental image of their lungs' acting as balloons. They believe their lungs must be pumped up before swimming long distances underwater. This is not true. One good breath is all that is needed. In fact, fully inflating the lungs may make swimming underwater more difficult because of increased buoyancy. If swimmers repeatedly hyperventilate, they may reduce the carbon dioxide content of their bloodstream so much that the normal mechanisms for reminding the lungs to function automatically can be affected. The possible result is sometimes called *shallow water blackout.* In this progression the swimmer repeatedly hyperventilates, swims underwater, passes out, and sinks to the bottom. To prevent this occurrence, a swimmer *should not hyperventilate extensively* before underwater swims. Children especially should be warned of this dangerous practice.

Caloric Labyrinthitis

Caloric means having to do with heat. *Labyrinthitis* refers to an illness of the inner ear or balance center.[9] When combined, they mean that immersion of the head in cold water may interfere with balance, and the individual may not be able to tell up from down when submerged. Small departures from normal body temperature have little affect on sober divers and swimmers. But when a plunging diver penetrates a **thermocline,** or layer of marked temperature difference, he or she may become disoriented, particularly if the water is murky and if he or she is alcohol or drug impaired. Similarly, in colder weather fishermen or hunters who fall deeply into water slightly above freezing may suffer the same inability to orient themselves and in their panicked thrashing might actually swim away from the surface. The fact that the victims are unable to understand which way to swim is only part of the difficulty. They are also rapidly running out of air.

An average adult can hold his or her breath for more than 1 minute when not exercising at room temperature. However, this same person will have only 10 seconds of breath if submerged and exercising in 50°

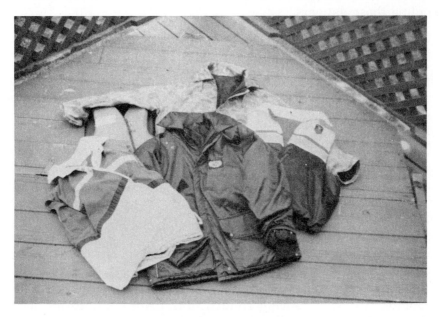

Fig. 3-1 Proper approach to hunting and fishing water safety. Modern, comfortable PFDs are available.

Table 3-2. Physiological Overload Factors

Condition	Process	Result
Cold-augmented	In older person with adverse cardiac history, cardiovascular overload or breakdown	Heart muscle spasms Irregular heartbeat Heart stoppage Immediate disappearance
Undiagnosed enlarged heart	Cold- or panic-induced rapid breathing and hyperventilation	Same as above
Torso reflex (inhalation response)	Gasping as body attempts to increase oxygen uptake to increase internal temperature	Swallows water Ingests water into lungs resulting in blocked breathing passages

F water.[5] As with most other in-water scenarios, a number of factors are at work in the foregoing situations. Conversely, defense is not that hard to imagine. Use of a personal flotation device (PFD) by the outdoorsman is a very big step in the proper direction (Fig. 3-1). Knowledge about the factors involved might also help the unwary in understanding and avoiding these dangers.

Physiological Overload

It is suspected that cold-augmented panic in an older, fearful victim with an adverse cardiac history can result in **fibrillation** (heart muscle spasms), **arrhythmia** (irregular heartbeat), and/or cardiac arrest (heart stoppage) and immediate disappearance (Table 3-2). An undiagnosed enlarged heart (usually affecting teenagers and young adults) suddenly subjected to cold-induced **tachycardia** (rapid beating) and hyperventilation may also be a part of this progression. Seizures of an epileptic or similar nature in victims of any age are also part of this pattern. Wearing a PFD might provide a partial defense in this situation. A complementing option, however, is to ensure that someone who could be injured by these factors is carefully counseled about his or her particular aquatic dangers and then is aided in avoiding them. This might mean boating on colder water only in larger, more stable craft.[11]

Another physiological factor, previously mentioned, is torso reflex, or inhalation response. During sudden, unexpected immersion, even in water that is not much cooler than 90° F, the body automatically attempts to increase its metabolism. Part of this increase hinges on providing more oxygen to the lungs. The outcome is that an unprepared person, responding to an urge to breathe deeply in response to torso reflex, may do so with the mouth underwater. If so, he or she draws water rather

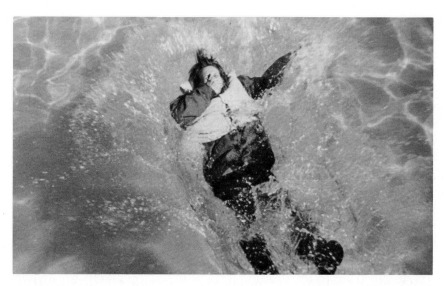

Fig. 3-2 Attempting to cover and/or to keep the mouth away from water in an unexpected plunge is the primary way to defeat torso reflex. (From Dive Rescue International: Waterproof your family [slide/tape presentation].)

than air into the lungs. A workable response to this hazard is training the individual always to cover the nose and mouth as he or she falls into the water. A similar protective measure is attempting to land on the back, thereby reducing facial contact during immersion (Fig. 3-2).

DROWNING NONSWIMMER

> The drowning nonswimmer (DNS) is the most frequently observed type of drowning victim.

The DNS unintentionally steps, trips, falls, slips, or is pushed into deeper water. Depending on age and body size, he or she usually can sustain himself or herself on the surface for no more than 20 to 60 seconds.[8] Children sink more rapidly since they have less reserve lung inflation and buoyancy than adults. This syndrome is evenly distributed among all ages of potential water accident victims.

The first person to analyze, write, and film DNS behavior was Frank Pia. This information was contained in his films "On Drowning," "Drowning Facts and Myths," and "The Reasons People Drown," and in his article "Observations on the Drowning of Nonswimmers." As chief lifeguard at Orchard Beach, Bronx, New York, Pia filmed actual near drownings and rescue sequences during the 1970 bathing season. These films clearly show that in most cases drowning is a relatively rapid occurrence that is often not recognized by nearby swimmers and bathers.

Mr. Pia's research into the behavior of people who are drowning also showed that drowning nonswimmers are unable to control their arm movements. This means that while they are drowning they are unable to reach out for flotation aids or get into a PFD.

To determine if the instinctive arm movements of a drowning victim were subject to voluntary control, Mr. Pia placed himself in several experimental near drowning situations. He cancelled out his swimming skills by placing a 20 pound SCUBA weight belt around his waist. In all the experiments Mr. Pia was unable to stop the drowning episode by reaching down and releasing the emergency buckle on his SCUBA weight belt.

His research led to the modification of throwing assists for drowning victims. Current rescue technique now acknowledges that drowning victims may not be aware that a rescue device has been thrown to them.

In addition to markedly increased respiration and heart rate, the usual outward signs of a distressed nonswimmer's drowning are as follows:

- Head tilted back
- Mouth open (to establish and maintain an airway; seldom any vocalization)
- Arms in unison flailing the water, in and out of the water in a vertical breast stroke, with the younger, smaller person's arms moving very rapidly
- Head bobbing vertically above and below the surface

All of these behaviors stem from drowning persons' immediate, all-compelling drive to breathe. Once they are in this cycle, they cannot hear, think, or usually see. A potential rescuer can neither communicate nor reason with them, and anyone getting within reaching distance will be violently grabbed and frequently pushed underwater by the victims as they attempt to climb upward. Hence this type of behavior often results in multiple drownings.

The following is a detailed analysis of each of the four automatic, uncontrollable victim signs:

- The head is tilted back to establish an airway. Initially the victim's head may be level with the surface, but as he or she loses the battle to maintain air passages above the water, the head tilt increases (Fig. 3-3).
- The mouth is open, again to provide the most effective airway. Understanding the inability to make sounds is paramount. It is

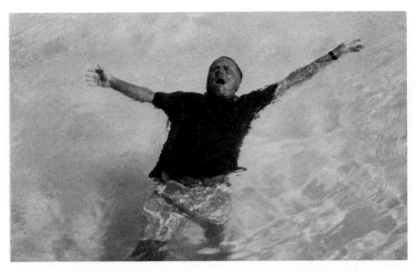

Fig. 3-3 First sign of drowning: head back.

impossible to call for help because of the essential need to draw in air. Try putting your head back, inhaling, and yelling at the same time. It cannot be done (Fig. 3-4).
- The arm motion is another attempt to aid breathing. Raising both arms in unison expands the **thoracic** cavity and increases intake of air. For best results, this should be a slower activity. If performed too rapidly as in a DNS, little usable air enters the lungs. Also, during the part of this cyclic motion while the arms are submerged but moving upward, victims in reality act to drive themselves underwater and to increase their terror further (Fig. 3-5, *A*).
- Bobbing, or a vertical up-and-down motion in which a potential rescuer witnesses the victim's head repeatedly dropping below and then reappearing above the surface, directly relates to the arm motions (Fig. 3-5, *B*). Essentially, the victim is killing himself or herself. A falsehood attached to this part of the drowning progression is the "three sinkings" myth; instead the number of times a victim bobs up and down depends on his or her size, age, and other factors. Children are most active and therefore go under water more quickly than slower moving adults. The normal maximum on-surface time for adults is 60 seconds. Hence, the basic rule is *if you observe someone in this state, you have very little time to react;* therefore your response alternatives must be planned long before you have contact with this type of situation. Chapter 7 and all of Part III aid your developing these alternatives.

It does not appear the DNS is drowning. Such victims look as though

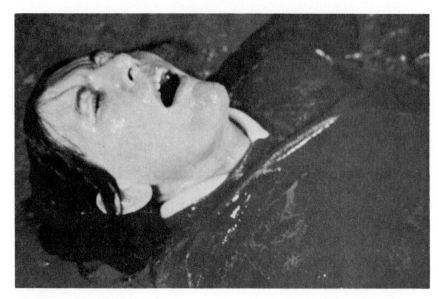

Fig. 3-4 Second sign of drowning: mouth open. (From Dive Rescue International: Waterproof your family [slide/tape presentation].)

they are playing or paddling. Again, they cannot make any sound to indicate their predicament. It is also impossible for them to move horizontally in the water. Particularly in crowded swimming areas, they are usually seen in areas close to shallow water or near drop-offs.

> Alcohol interferes with **psychomotor** performance, balance, and coordination. Depending on a number of variables such as age, drinking experience, prior activity, and water temperature, drinking can markedly reduce swimming ability, thereby causing DNS behavior in an otherwise water-capable person.

Even though this syndrome comprises the majority of water deaths, emergency service providers probably would not be on scene until after it occurred. Possible exceptions include responding to potential accident scenes such as a sinking vessel, winter fishermen on breaking ice, or persons swept downstream by flood waters. Regardless of when you arrive, the primary defense is your knowing and explaining to others exactly what constitutes the four basic signs of drowning as listed previously. As mentioned, most drownings are witnessed; and because the victim rarely swims into danger, he or she normally is close enough

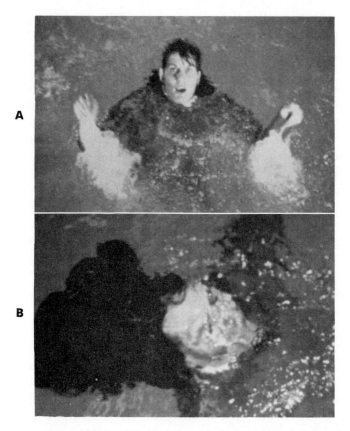

Fig. 3-5 A, Third sign of drowning: both arms raised above the water. **B**, Fourth sign of drowning: head bobbing above, then below the water's surface. (From Dive Rescue International: Waterproof your family [slide/tape presentation].)

to allow a shore- or boat-based rescue. The principle obstacle to rescue is that not enough observers understand what the victim's actions *really* indicate. Study Figs. 3-3 through 3-5 closely. They accurately present the actions and appearance of drowning humans.

If you should arrive at the accident site and find a large number of people in the water but none apparently demonstrating the signs of drowning, are there other clues to consider? Although your first reaction probably would be to assist the potential victims nearest you, there are other signs to notice. Poor swimmers on the verge of lapsing into DNS syndrome demonstrate the following:

- They swim more vertically than horizontally. Their body axis is more perpendicular than horizontal to the water surface.

- They clearly indicate they do not want to put their face in the water.
- Their swimming strokes deteriorate into ineffectual dog paddling.
- They may demonstrate wide-eyed, frightened expressions.

If there are no indications of actual drowning, these people should be the ones most carefully watched and initially aided.

As a final example of productively using DNS information, consider toddler drownings in backyard pools. In many of these cases the child is near the pool with an adult in attendance. A distraction such as a telephone or doorbell ringing takes the adult's attention from the child. The adult responds to the distraction, thinking that the child will call out if he or she gets into trouble. This is completely untrue. Consequently, parents with small children must be told that drowning is as quiet as it is swift.

> Parents must never leave small children unattended around water.[12]

SUDDEN DISAPPEARANCE SYNDROME

Sudden disappearance syndrome (SDS) normally involves the unexpected immersion of poor swimmers or fatigued, cold-debilitated persons who are partially supported by air trapped in their clothing. Either they attempt to swim or to struggle. This motion, combined with the pressure differential of the vertical in-water position, causes air to squeeze rapidly up and out of their clothing. When their reserve of clothing-entrapped air is dissipated, they lapse into DNS behaviors, then rapidly sink below the surface. Since they are frequently in the water with others who are better swimmers or who are wearing PFDs, the victim's "sudden" disappearance is reported by the survivors.

As a responder to an aquatic accident scene, you may notice persons struggling in the water who are kept afloat by air entrapped in clothing or by debris. They should receive priority treatment. As you proceed to assist them, *do not* allow them to be left unobserved. If not closely watched, they may rapidly shift into DNS behavior and disappear, thereby greatly complicating your rescue operation.

> The primary defense to SDS: requiring nonswimmers or poor swimmers to wear PFDs in any situation that might even remotely result in their entering deep water.

Because SDS is frequently boat related, persons using small craft such as canoes, rowboats, or smaller motorboats (especially the **johnboat** variety) should be aware of the flotation characteristics required in their vessel. Any watercraft less than 20 feet long and manufactured or sold in the United States is required by the federal government to float upright and level when completely filled with water. It must support as many people when swamped as it is rated to carry when dry. This requirement allows those who have been thrown into the water when their boat capsizes or swamps to crawl back into it and sit on the bottom *inside* the upright craft. This is a far better option than trying to hold onto the small keel of an overturned boat. Unfortunately, in many boating accidents the occupants are unaware of this option, and their first, unwise, decision is to swim for shore.

If you or your rescue squad own a small craft other than an inflatable one, test it in safe, shallow conditions to ensure it will float and support the required number of occupants when swamped. The U.S. Coast Guard capacity plate, usually fastened to the **transom,** or flat inside surface at the **stern** (rear), gives occupant numbers, total weight, and horsepower limits for the craft. Horsepower has an important relationship to level flotation. When a craft is overpowered, it is usually overweight, and the calculations for flotation material needed to keep the craft level and above the surface are invalidated.

SDS most frequently affects adults who fall out of boats or from above-water locations; therefore informing local hunting and fishing clubs of this danger could result in preventive action and lives saved.

HYPOTHERMIA-INDUCED DEBILITY

Hypothermia-induced debility (HID) encompasses a number of cold-related physiological phenomena. Suddenly falling into cold water produces three primary effects. The first is a sudden involuntary gasp. This torso reflex is deadly if it occurs when the head is immersed. Second, cardiac arrest or ventricular complications often occur in fearful, older, out-of-shape persons in this situation. Third, muscle performance and stamina are quickly reduced by cold water. Different levels of hypothermia are described in Table 3-3.

In this text unless otherwise stipulated, *cold* means a temperature less than normal body level, which is approximately 98.6° F. This temperature does not seem terribly dangerous, and for sober, healthy, well-rested, well-nourished individuals, water 10° or 15° below body temperature is not overly menacing. But by factoring in a few other elements, the situation can rapidly change. Heat is lost to still water 25

Table 3-3. Levels of Hypothermia: Average Responses for Otherwise Healthy, Sober Persons

State	F°	C°	Physical Impact
Mild (awake with shivers)	99.6	37.6	"Normal" rectal temperature
	96.8	36	Increased metabolic rate
	95.0	35	Maximum shivering
	93.2	34	Patients usually responsive; maximum BP*
	91.4	33	Increasing severity of hypothermia
Moderate (awake without shivers)	89.6	32	Consciousness clouded; shivering stops
	87.8	31	Blood pressure difficult to obtain
	86.0	30	Approaching unconsciousness/rigidity
	85.2	29	Slow pulse/respiration; cardiac irregularity (arrhythmia) may develop
Major (unconscious; may look dead)	82.4	28	Ventricular fibrillation may occur
	80.6	27	Voluntary motion lost; appears dead
	78.8	26	Victims seldom conscious
	77.0	25	Spontaneous ventricular fibrillation
	75.2	24	Pulmonary edema develops
	71.6	22	Maximum risk of fibrillation
	69.8	20	Heart standstill

From Resuscitation from hypothermia: A literature review, Rep CG-D-26-79, Springfield, Va, 1979, National Technical Information Service, p 3.
NOTE: See Appendix III for explanation of medical terms.
*BP, Blood pressure.

times as fast as to still air of the same temperature. When the water moves, heat loss rate jumps markedly. For instance, at a current flow of approximately 5 mph, human bodies may lose 250 times as much heat to the water as to still air of a similar temperature. If someone is injured or impaired (intoxicated) or both, this heat loss rate skyrockets. This phenomenon is similar to windchill. But in the water, a much heavier, denser medium is carrying off calories.

In aquatics two types of immersion, or in-water, hypothermia are studied. The first is *shell*, or skin and muscle, temperature levels. The second is *core*, or internal body, temperature.

Shell Hypothermia

Most observers are familiar with shell hypothermia. Place a hand in or under cold, flowing water, and a number of changes occur. Your skin turns a paler color; you have difficulty manipulating objects with your fingers. Depending on how long your hand is immersed, you may have intense pain, followed by a loss of feeling. Each of these observations represents the body's working to protect itself from cold. Because the exposed limb loses heat faster than it can be replaced, the exterior blood vessels shut down, or constrict, which causes the skin coloring change. Next blood flow to muscles and connective tissues is diminished, and with cooling-induced thickening of the blood, you cannot work your extremities properly. Last, as the **vasoconstriction** becomes **acute,** you experience severe pain caused by oxygen deprivation and then numbness.

Core Hypothermia

Core hypothermia follows somewhat the same progression but at a slower pace.

Shell hypothermia immediately begins to affect exposed portions of the body. However, our inner body (core) temperatures, because of outer fat and muscle insulation, are maintained at an elevated level longer.

Even when immersed in ice water, healthy adults do not begin to exhibit an internal temperature drop until they have been in the water for 15 to 20 minutes.[10] A number of factors influence both types of hypothermia. The larger, more insulated a person, the slower he or she loses heat. Women, who generally have a deeper layer of subcutaneous fat, cool more slowly than men of the same size. Children cool much more rapidly than adults.

Just as there are two different types of hypothermia, there are also two different ways that hypothermia causes death in the water. Fatalities resulting from core, or inner body, cooling result from heart stoppage or cardiac arrest, which generally happens when the inner body temperature drops to approximately 70° F. Even in extremely cold water, this first fatal process takes some time to transpire.

Conversely, the second fatal progression involving cold occurs more rapidly. In this far more frequent scenario, shell, or outer body, hypothermia renders the muscles ineffective, and a person can no longer swim, grasp a flotation aid, or in some way maintain himself or herself on the surface.

Even if wearing certain types of PFD, a victim may not be able to float with his or her nose and mouth above the surface. This could be because of breaking waves or due to the action of some flotation devices in tipping the wearer's face forward. This latter example can be corrected by proper training and by trying different devices as explained later in the text. However, once a person becomes too cold to move, he or she is totally dependent on the PFD to hold the face out of the water. The two types of hypothermia can combine, with the victim passing out as a result of pain and oxygen deprivation caused by reduction of inner body blood circulation to the brain. If not wearing a PFD, the victim will then drown. As these examples demonstrate, the victim will probably become unconscious and drown before suffering cold-induced cardiac arrest.

> The best protection from immersion hypothermia is to remove the body's primary heat loss areas from the water and cover or insulate them.

The primary heat loss areas are the head, neck, and face; armpits; and groin. The victim should try to conserve energy and body heat by not moving. Of major importance is learning about the *heat escape lessening position* (HELP), which involves floating with the head out of the water and the body in a fetal tuck. If others are in the water, victims should *huddle* or float facing each other with arms wrapped around each others' waists, with at least half the group wearing PFDs (see Chapter 7).

Hypothermia affects different people in a number of highly variable ways, and peripheral, or shell, hypothermia rapidly immobilizes and saps the strength of even strong swimmers who are not experienced in and adapted to cold water. A good swimmer can proceed for only approximately 12 minutes in 50° F water before becoming exhausted.[3]

CHAPTER SUMMARY

The preceding observations focused on understanding causes of drowning from a behavioral viewpoint. The primary focus has been on understanding initiating factors before formulating defenses. A working knowledge was presented of the primary elements involved in immediate disappearance syndrome (IDS), the drowning nonswimmer (DNS), sudden disappearance syndrome (SDS), and hypothermia-induced debility (HID). The general types of persons involved in each of the foregoing were indicated. In addition, preventive suggestions were given to use on a family, departmental, or community basis.

PRETEST ANSWERS

1. False
2. a
3. b
4. False

REFERENCES

1. About life jackets and EMP, St Cloud, Minn, 1981, Stearns Manufacturing Co, p 1.
2. Accident facts, 1980. Chicago, 1981, National Safety Council, p 81.
3. Collis M: Survival behavior in cold water immersion, Toronto, 1976, The Royal Life Saving Society Canada, p 25.
4. Egstrom G et al.: Alcohol and diving performance, Los Angeles, 1988, University of California Los Angeles, Department of Kinesiology, pp 4-7.
5. Hayward J: Hypothermia update, Washington, DC, 1985, National Safe Boating Council, p 156.
6. Head and spinal cord injury prevention, Atlanta, July 1988, National Coordinating Council on Spinal Cord Injury, p 54.
7. NSPI-1 Standard for public swimming pools, Alexandria, Va, 1989, National Spa and Pool Institute, pp 24-25.
8. Pia F: Drowning facts and myths, Larchmont, NY, 1986, Water Safety Films (film).
9. Pipkin G: Caloric labyrinthitis: A cause of drowning, Am J Sports Med 7:4, 1979, pp 260-261.
10. Pozos R and Born D: Hypothermia—Causes, effects, prevention, Piscataway, NJ, 1982, New Century Publishers, p 70.
11. Praleck B: Boating for the handicapped, Washington, DC, 1985, National Safe Boating Council, p 144.
12. Present P: Child drowning study, Washington, DC, September 1987, US Consumer Product Safety Commission, p 7.
13. Safe diving means checking water depth first . . . , Operation water watch sample news release No 2, Washington, DC, Summer 1990, US Consumer Product Safety Commission, p 2.
14. Smith D and Smith S: Waterwise, Imperial, Mo, 1984, Smith Aquatic Safety Services, p 30.

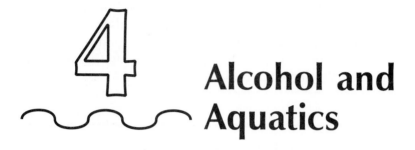

Alcohol and Aquatics

OVERVIEW

This chapter focuses on general effects of alcohol as it affects balance, vision, sensory integration, and judgment. Statistics dealing with the presence of alcohol in water-related fatalities are examined. Scenarios are presented indicating how intoxication or impairment can produce aquatic accidents.

OBJECTIVES

This material should aid your understanding of:
1. The basics of ethanol impairment or intoxication as influenced by immersion
2. Additive effects of environmental stressors, cold, and trauma
3. Specific progressions (and indications) of intoxication in swimming, diving, and boating accidents
4. Alcohol's impact before, during, and after (sudden) immersion or submersion
5. Intoxication and resuscitation
6. Influence of other recreational drugs in aquatic situations

---

PRETEST

1. An intoxicated person may not be able to distinguish the colors of lights and signs at night. (True or false?)
2. At legal intoxication levels, reaction time is (a) unchanged; (b) increased slightly; or (c) doubled. (Pick the correct answer[s].)

3. Cooling intoxicated persons through immersion (a) wakes them; (b) substantially increases their metabolism; (c) speeds sobriety; (d) all of the above; or (e) none of the above.
4. In a small boat or canoe, balancing ability can be dangerously degraded by drinking one or two cans of beer. (True or false?) *Pretest answers are at the end of the chapter.*

ALCOHOL AND AQUATICS: HISTORICAL OVERVIEW

Drugs used in social, religious, or nonmedicinal roles have been part of the human experience since the beginning of societies. Ethanol, or grain alcohol, in its fermented forms as beer or wine has been traced back as far as the Neolithic age, approximately 8000 BC. In more aquatically specific usage, the word *grog*, from which we derive the term *groggy*, denoted a ration of rum prescribed for sailors in most of the world's navies a few hundred years ago.

The nautical toddy remains as an ever present part of water-oriented recreation. Most recreational boats equipped with more than basic amenities have some type of built-in cup holders. Surveys of what the average fisherman takes on a day's outing frequently list a cooler and one or more six-packs of beer.[16] A large amount of major breweries' advertising is allotted to water-oriented displays of their products. With fishermen, hunters, or frolicking surfers in the foreground, some view of still or moving water provides the backdrop. The purpose of the aquatic inclusion is twofold: (1) to increase the viewer's thirst and (2) to condition potential users to associate relaxing and enjoyable water pastimes with alcohol-based beverages (Fig. 4-1).

For the most part, there is nothing wrong with enjoying an occasional libation near the water. But when the imbibing becomes too relaxing and the imbiber approaches too close to water deep enough to cause trouble, unnecessary tragedy if not embarrassment often follows. The exact scope of this trouble is still not exactly known. As the statistics in the following paragraphs indicate, researchers do not agree completely about the role of intoxication in accidents, particularly water accidents. However, almost everyone with experience in studying aquatic mishaps agrees that alcohol plays some part in at least half of all water deaths.[21]

The reason for this relationship between alcohol and water deaths is also historical. For years the presence of intoxication in drowning statistics was completely missed. Until relatively recently, warnings

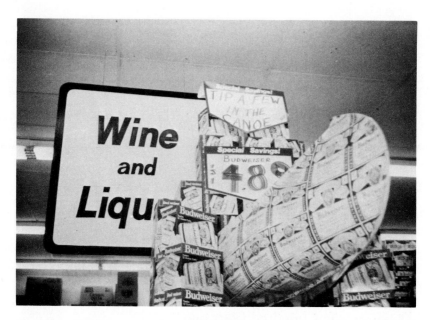

Fig. 4-1 This display was photographed in a large supermarket. Are we conditioning people to kill themselves in the water?

about drinking and water sports were nonexistent. In fact, the opposite interpretation reigned. People tended to laugh at the drunk's struggling in the water or nodded in agreement with the notion that a cold plunge induced instant sobriety. Neither of these impressions is true. The struggling intoxicant may be dying, and that cold plunge only generates a startled and far more incapacitated drinker.[25]

STATISTICAL REVIEW

As previously stated, gathering specific information about water mishaps is difficult. In addition to there not being enough conformity or effort placed into data gathering, several other factors intervene. For instance, when comparing aquatic to land-based accidents, terrestrial victims (not to mention their vehicles and related evidence) do not disappear through the surface of their surroundings.[22] When attempting to determine intoxication levels, surface decomposition does not itself produce ethanol, but underwater decomposition generally does.

The U.S. Coast Guard has comparatively tight control over boating accident information. However, as demonstrated in Tables 4-1 and 4-2, between one fifth and one fourth of all the data collected falls into the

Table 4-1 USCG Boating Accident Statistics: Causes of Accident

Category	Total Boats	Deaths
Loading of passengers or equipment	295	171
Free water in boat	135	6
Equipment failure or malfunction	635	22
Operation of vessel	3268	268
Environment (wave, visibility, current)	1394	250
Other vessel at fault	1813	28
Ignition	94	1
Other	1142	69
UNKNOWN	244	221
TOTAL	9020	1036

From Boating Statistics, 1987, Washington, DC, 1988, U.S. Coast Guard, p 21.

Table 4-2 USCG Boating Accident Statistics: Vessel Information

Category	Total Boats	Deaths
Type of boat		
Known	8114	924
Unknown	906	112
Hull Material		
Known	8051	887
Unknown	969	149
Propulsion		
Known	7985	882
Unknown	1035	154
Horsepower		
Known	7113	882
Unknown	1907	154
Year Built		
Known	6912	482
Unknown	2108	554
Length		
Known	7784	862
Unknown	1236	174
TOTAL	9026	1036

From Boating Statistics, 1987, Washington, DC, 1988, U.S. Coast Guard, p 23.

"unknown" category. This has been particularly true of estimates of alcohol involvement. In 1982 researchers found only 7% of all fatal boating accidents were alcohol related.[21] Two years later, however, after comprehensive revision of reporting procedures, this estimate grew to 38%, with another 20% suspected as involving alcohol but unconfirmed.

In a further study, covering the years 1986 to 1991, the National Transportation Safety Board reported alcohol involvement in approximately one half of all boating deaths.[16a] The National Safety Council also indicated in 1982 that alcohol was a serious problem in aquatic mishaps, but it could not pin its figures to anything more precise than 34% to 78%. However, when state and city officials have given sufficient attention to the situation, the figures have been compelling. Table 4-3 contains results gathered from such efforts.

An encouraging aspect of accident prevention in North America is that *all* forms of accidental deaths, with the exception of automobile accidents, have decreased approximately 25% since 1980.[1] Even with driving mishaps, although the totals of killed and injured have remained roughly the same, the actual rates (comparison of numbers affected to

Table 4-3 Drowning and Alcohol Statistics From Selected Areas

Study	Drownings (% Tested)	Using (%)	Intoxicated (%)
North Carolina, 1980-1984	1052 (80)	48	34
Georgia, 1981-1983	573	50 (estimated)	Unknown
Oklahoma, 11/1/87-10/31/88	95	40 (estimated)	Unknown
South Carolina, 5/75-4/76	21 (100)	52	48
New York City, 1980-1981	298	56	Unknown
Baltimore, Md, 1/72-12/72	45 (100)	47	38

Table 4-4 Alcohol Involvement

Accident/Incident	Percentage
Automobile fatalities	50
Fire deaths	80+
Drownings	**65**
Home accidents	22
Pedestrian accidents	36
Criminal arrests	55
Murder	65
Suicide	30
Domestic fights or assaults	55
Child abuse	60
Airplane accidents	44

Modified from Safety tips. In USAA aide, San Antonio, Spring 1982, U.S. Automobile Association, p 24.

numbers exposed) have decreased measurably. As shown in Table 4-4, alcohol plays a major role in all accidents; yet serious accidents have decreased. Are we becoming more educated about alcohol? The answer, especially when considering the growing amount of drug awareness information now available, must be "yes." But is there more to learn? Again, the answer is in the affirmative, particularly where water is concerned.

GENERAL ALCOHOL EFFECTS

Grain alcohol, or ethanol, can be found in two beverage forms: (1) fermented as in beer and wine or (2) distilled as in liquors, whiskey, and spirits. The amount of alcohol in fermented drinks is usually given by percentage and in distilled drinks by proof. To find the ethanol content of the latter group, divide the proof by two; for example, 50 proof beverages contain 25% alcohol by content.

> A reigning myth is that "hard" liquors, or distilled spirits, induce intoxication quicker than wine or beer. This is not true. One 12-ounce can of beer, one 5-ounce glass of wine, and one highball with 1½ ounces of 86 proof liquor are equally intoxicating.

Table 4-5 shows the effects of alcohol consumption. Differences in type of drinks consumed have little effect.

Another prevalent myth, especially with younger users, is that "kiddie beer" (3.2% or less alcohol content) affects the user less than higher

Table 4-5 Effects of Alcohol Per Drink

Alcohol		Normal Measure	Alcohol Content (oz)	Body Weight in Lb			
Beverages	Content (%)			100	140	180	220
				Blood alcohol level or content			
Beer	4	12 oz bottle	0.48	0.04	0.03	0.02	0.02
Wine	12	5 oz glass	0.36	0.03	0.03	0.02	0.02
Liqueur	40	1 oz glass	0.40	0.03	0.03	0.02	0.02
Distilled spirits	45	1 oz glass	0.45	0.04	0.03	0.02	0.02
Mixed drinks	30	3½ oz glass	1.05	0.08	0.06	0.04	0.04

Driver Magazine, Washington, DC, June 1977, U.S. Air Force.

percentage beverages. There might be some slight, overall differences in effect; but when a younger, smaller, less drug tolerant, less experienced person is drinking, 3.2% brew is sufficient to induce impairment and intoxication. Another disturbing aspect of the lower alcohol content beverages is that in some locales they are labeled as "nonintoxicating."

The belief that eating while consuming alcohol slows its effects is partially correct. Alcohol is unique in that it requires no digestion and can be absorbed rapidly from the stomach into the bloodstream. It is taken even more rapidly into the bloodstream from the small intestine. Food in the stomach slows absorption. However, over time the results on blood level accumulation are the same.

> Since alcohol is so easily absorbed into the bloodstream and the body's tissues, it rapidly permeates and affects all of our nerve systems.

Clinically, ethanol is described as a central nervous system **(CNS) depressant.** The basic outcome of this effect is that messages to and from the brain to other parts of the body are slowed, with the slowing proportionate to the amount of alcohol consumed. The blood alcohol level (BAL) is reported as the number of grams of alcohol in each 100 ml of blood and are expressed as a percentage. Table 4-6 lists a way of viewing the behavioral effects of an increasing BAL. Alcohol levels in the blood may also be expressed as blood alcohol content (BAC). The terms *BAC* and *BAL* are equal and interchangeable. Most states have 0.1% BAC as a legal intoxication level, whereas others have opted for 0.08% BAC.

Besides acting as a CNS depressant, ethanol is a muscle and vascular (blood distribution system) relaxant. One result of the vascular effect is that human brains, especially in their higher, outer levels, receive less oxygenated blood when alcohol is consumed. Another effect is that the body's normal ability to shrink circumferentially, or vasoconstrict its outer blood vessels to retain internal heat, is compromised by ethanol. Thus individuals become cold and clumsy more quickly when drinking. Understanding the double effect of ethanol (i.e., nervous system slow down and reduced oxygen supply to the brain cells) is important in appreciating the inner workings of accidents. Adding the effects of chilling further completes the picture.

Table 4-6 Behavioral Effects of Alcohol

Blood Alcohol Level	Behavioral Effects
0.05	Lowered alertness, usually good feeling, release of inhibitions, impaired judgment
0.10	Slowed reaction times and impaired motor function; less caution
0.15	Large, consistent increases in reaction time
0.20	Marked depression in sensory and motor capability; decidedly intoxicated
0.25	Severe motor disturbance, staggering; sensory perceptions greatly impaired; smashed!
0.30	Stuporous but conscious; no comprehension of the world around them
0.35	Surgical anesthesia; near lethal dose (LD) 1 (i.e., LD in 1% of population); minimum level causing death
0.40	Near LD 50 (i.e., LD in 50% of population)

Modified from Oakley R: Drugs, society and human behavior, St Louis, 1983, CV Mosby Co, pp 166-167.

SPECIFIC AQUATIC EFFECTS

Studies concerning the effects of alcohol on boaters were the first efforts to define clearly alcohol's aquatic aspects. Using extensive automobile driver research as a basis, these programs examined a number of water-related issues. Initial and follow-up boat and water-related findings have dealt with balance, vision, sensory integration, and judgment.

Before reviewing each of these factors, the difference between *impairment* and *intoxication* is defined. Although both physiology and behavior are involved with it, impairment in this text is treated primarily as a behavioral term. Conversely, intoxication is defined in its physiological or legal meaning: an illegal or unlawful level of blood alcohol. Understanding and properly using this difference is important. Despite increasing awareness of the problems alcohol's unwise use creates, its accident-causing aspects still are not sufficiently familiar. Enough research has been done to predict what happens to a person at different BALs. The behavior of a person over the legal limit is familiar. However, most of ethanol's dangerous effects (particularly around the water) begin to develop well below legal intoxication levels. The person may not be observably affected, yet he or she can definitely be impaired.[5]

Another, even finer, distinction is that the behavioral aspects of alcohol begin to manifest themselves and to interfere measurably with the performance of the average drinker at a BAL of 0.035%.[26] Conversely, the presence of alcohol can be detected at a BAL of as low as 0.02%. Thus as an individual drinks, there is, in general, no sudden arrival of higher levels of intoxication. If attention is paid to drinking and to the potential for aquatic trouble inherent even in the lower levels, possible dangers should be avoidable. With these two concepts in mind—(1) impairment or interference with mental and physical actions occurs at relatively low BALs and (2) a person can learn to appreciate where his or her behavior may be headed—the four factors listed above are investigated.

Balance

Watching toddlers as they slowly learn to stand and to move in an upright posture awakens an appreciation of standing and walking as two of the most difficult, yet commonplace physical manipulations humans perform. Supporting an unbalanced, dynamic, elevated center of gravity in both stationary and moving modes is an impressive trick and uses a large number of muscle groups, several balancing systems, and a very sensitive, finely tuned program of automatic responses. Is it any wonder that when alcohol begins to slow the transmissions and feedback within the nervous systems, an individual has trouble standing? It is not surprising that most deaths in boating accidents result from falls from or capsizings of smaller craft 16 or fewer feet long.[20] Tests have shown that a person attempting to stand or move around in a small craft or canoe is readily affected by alcohol, even at levels well below legal intoxication (Fig. 4-2).

Balancing systems have been cited previously in discussions of caloric labyrinthitis, or underwater disorientation, and of the inability of an impaired diver to carry out an intended plan of action. To complete this picture, the inebriated person in shallow water not much deeper than his or her waist should be studied. For the following scenario to occur, the drinker's BAL should be elevated, probably 0.15 or above. The coldness of the water also may play a role, with colder water increasing muscle stiffness, thereby reducing physical flexibility and performance. For this example, the scene is a normal summer afternoon in the middle United States. The specific balance and orientation requirements of the human are carried out, in order of decreasing importance, by the eyes; inner ear balancing centers; and gravity sensors located in various parts of the body. Eyes are most important because they provide orientation cues from seeing nearby horizontal and vertical surfaces. To confirm this fact, note what happens to a person in an amusement park's fun house

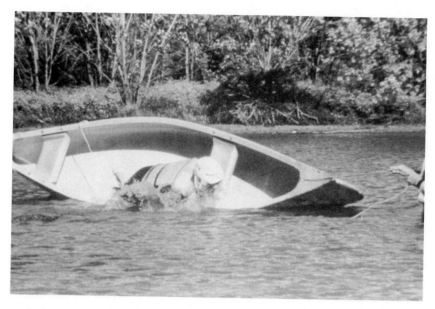

Fig. 4-2 Testing balance after alcoholic beverages have been drunk reveals dangerous impairment at levels well below the legal intoxication point. (From Better think twice . . . A look at alcohol use while boating, Delaware, Ohio, 1985, FlowGraphics Photography.)

that has slanted floors, doors, and windows: the individual normally cannot stand erect *until* his or her eyes are shut. Another test is to shut your eyes and attempt to walk perfectly upright, or try to stand perfectly still with your eyes shut. Have someone observe your balancing movements.

Inebriated persons in shallow water have two vision-related problems affecting balance. First, they cannot see clearly, especially if looking toward the light or sun if out of doors, and what they *can* see is a moving surface. Labyrinthic, or semicircular, canals are located in the inner ears, and gravity detection sensors are spread throughout the body. With sighted people, these are backup systems. If these backup systems are affected by alcohol as much as vision, it is easy to grasp how someone could fall in shallow water and drown.[17] Completing this example is the balancing disturbance caused by suddenly placing the ears under (relatively) cold water.

Vision

A number of psychologists believe that in a sighted person 80% to 90% of all information comes through the eyes. If something interferes with or degrades vision, especially something not normally noticed, a number of difficulties can result.

> Alcohol not only slows the transmission of information from the eyes to the brain, but just as importantly it directly affects the eye itself and its surrounding muscles.

Depending on how impaired the viewer may be, he or she cannot accurately discern what it is he or she is looking at or how to respond to it. At higher levels of intoxication (e.g., >0.2% BAL), the average person has difficulty seeing the colors red and green at night.[2] He or she may know that a light source is ahead but is not sure what its colors are. This can produce tragic consequences when power boats, which have red and green running lights, are closing on each other.

Ethanol interaction produces a number of results on the eye itself. The iris is an adjustable shutter located directly behind the eye's lens. This shutter expands or contracts to allow varying amounts of light to enter the eye and to interact with the optic nerve. (In addition to the iris, the cornea and lens are also subject to alcoholic interference.) Because of ethanol's relaxing effects, the iris **dilates,** allowing excessive light to overpower the optic nerve. This may be one reason most drinking establishments have subdued lighting. It is also a prime reason for impaired drivers having accidents at night; they are blinded by oncoming vehicles.

Boating studies have indicated other serious aspects of the vision problem. As muscles relax and reaction times slow, it is extremely difficult for a viewer in a bobbing, vibrating craft to concentrate on a distant object. The eyes tend to bounce down when the boat comes up and vice versa. Similarly, peripheral vision, especially at night, may be completely degraded at 0.1% BAC. The actual field of view is 210 degrees. To test this, extend your arms horizontally out from your shoulders. Look straight ahead; then wiggle your thumbs. Note when you can no longer detect your thumbs' movement. The thumbs should be on a line *behind* your eyes. This means that humans can detect motion in objects slightly behind them; that is, if they are sober. The total effect of all these muscle and focusing difficulties is to reduce the legally intoxicated person's visual field to approximately 25% of normal.[14]

That is only part of the problem. Although humans tend to think that they see everything around them simultaneously, they do not. A sober person makes five to ten eye fixations per second. In other words, the eyes are in constant motion, taking snapshots of the surroundings. Then these separate pictures are arranged and combined by the brain to provide a panorama. At legal intoxication levels, eye fixations may be reduced by 50%. A drunken person then can see only half of what was seen when sober. If you doubt this, study the face of someone who is visibly intoxicated. Note how much his or her eyes *do not* move. One way of appreciating this is to realize that objects may be perceived as moving twice as fast toward an intoxicated person.

As another example, distances are judged through two main visual processes. The first has to do with parallax and the second with comparisons to known objects. In this first process, the minute, slightly different angles from which the eyes view the same target are calculated by the vision centers of the brain, and a distance to the object is computed. In turn, this computation is subject to the second process in which the target is compared to similar objects in the memory and to the sizes of familiar objects near the target. This information is analyzed, and an idea is developed of how far away the target is. This input is next passed, for instance, to the arm muscles if the individual is going to reach for or to throw at the target that is seen. The minuscule angular differences involved in determining distances through parallax are extremely precise and easily disrupted by the effects of alcohol. Memory of sizes and outlines of objects also is important; but ease and accuracy of their recall are progressively reduced as impairment heightens. Pondering this, remember that this discussion has been about computing distances to *stationary* objects. Consider what alcohol does to parallax computations of a *moving* target such as an approaching car or boat; and, the problem of automatically computing distances to a moving target has another, separate aspect that is readily degraded by ethanol.

A primary facet of our ocular abilities is immediate awareness of and attraction to any movement in our visual surroundings. Here again, ethanol greatly degrades this most important capability. As part of one's total visual degradation, a drinker may suffer a severe loss in perception of objects suddenly moving into his or her field of vision. The impaired viewer will eventually become aware of the objects; however, this might occur too late to avoid a collision.

In addition to causing the foregoing interruptions in the normal viewing processes, alcohol further disturbs the visual centers of the brain. In these centers the fragmented, slowly arriving optic information must undergo one further step in which the brain attempts to make sense of what the eyes are seeing. Depending on BAC, this final process may eventually bog down in total confusion or disregard. Diving accidents are especially likely as a direct result of this whole progression. Diving is highly dependent on visual cues and split-second timing. Warning signs, if visible, are disregarded or ignored. Normal appreciations of water depth and bottom contour are jumbled, if perceived. In such situations the all too frequent final outcome is highly predictable.[9]

Sensory Integration

Psychologists state that in spite of the tremendous computational abilities of the human brain, most of the time humans do not think, meaning that most human behavior is depressive. This is not the same as being depressed. It is a clinical term indicating that approximately 60% of the time, the average person does not actively participate in what is happening in his or her brain. To substantiate this, remember that a large portion of what the body does is automatically controlled. In the foregoing section, the simple acts of standing and walking were discussed. However, how much do you *consciously* tell your muscles to do as you go about these activities? Another way of viewing this concept is that humans tend to use preprogrammed mental tapes in a stimulus-response mode. In this mode new behavior that requires extensive introspection or external analysis is rarely initiated. What we primarily tend toward is perpetuating habits and ingrained routine. For this reason, especially when we are impaired, if something, new, different, or unexpected suddenly intrudes, we may not be able to respond as quickly as needed.

The unending flow of information being gathered by the physical sensing apparatus underlies what may or may not be happening in the higher thought-processing centers of the mind. Although the majority of perceptions are gathered by sight, a myriad of other sensing systems act to confirm visual impressions and to add their own special inputs. Normally, we believe that these details are provided by five senses: sight, sound, smell, touch, and taste. If so, where do the gravity detectors, used in telling up from down, fit? They do not. They are part of what may actually number more than 35 sensing mechanisms now recognized as operating within the body.[13] If the human body is being bombarded by so many continuous information channels that the sober person neatly integrates and uses, what happens when ethanol begins to affect an individual?

One way of appreciating normal cerebral operations is to think of a telephone exchange in which all the incoming and outgoing calls are simultaneously processed and cross fed. Suppose something were to interrupt or impede this exchange. To carry out its mission, the system would have to slow down; prioritize certain transmissions; and let lower priority information wait until sufficient lines were clear. In other words, the operation would deteriorate from simultaneous to sequential. Essentially, this is what happens when intoxication levels increase. This also means that instead of taking in and working with all the available input at the same time, the brain may only be capable of dealing with *one input at a time!* Remember, too, that there are 35 sensing mechanisms, not five.

Studies indicate that one of the basic outcomes of the shift to sequential mental operations is that the inebriate may become totally locked in on one process. For instance, at 0.1% BAC an experienced driver may make his or her way from one location to another without major problems *if* (1) he or she is familiar with the route and has driven it a number of times and (2) nothing distracting happens such as an unexpected vehicle approaching from the side or an obstacle appearing in the road. On the other hand, if something does unexpectedly appear and he or she must swerve to avoid a collision and then return to the proper lane, he or she has, at best, a 50/50 chance of safely carrying out the two-step maneuver.[18] Why? Sequential thinking locks him or her into (slowly) responding to one item at a time.

Another way to consider this scenario is through reaction time. Although several standards may be applied to its definition, *reaction time* in this context is the delay between the instant a decision begins to be made to act or react and the time when the physical force is applied to carry out the ordered response. To return to the automobile analogy, if a sober, rested driver perceives an object in the road, he or she must proceed through a number of cerebral steps to evaluate it properly and then respond. This process may seem instantaneous, but it can take upward of three fourths of a second. Part of this time is devoted to ordering the muscles in the arms and legs to steer and brake the car, a subprocess taking approximately two tenths of a second. If the driver is at 0.1% BAC, his or her reaction may be delayed to *twice* its normal time. This means that the physical part is now extended to four tenths of a second.

If BAC is increased, reaction time increases proportionately until a point is reached at which the drinker can no longer react because he or she is unconscious. In other words, ethanol is not only an effective depressant and relaxant, it is also an anesthetic.

Time and motion studies using high speed photographic methods have put this occurrence in an aquatic context. They show that a person

6 feet tall diving from a platform or deck (level with the water) immerses his or her head approximately three tenths of a second after initiating the dive; thus as noted in the preceding paragraph, the time required for an intoxicated person to carry out physical commands is longer than it takes to hit the water. In diving, the body follows where the head leads. But even before the head enters the water, hands and arms should be out in front. They act as aquaplanes or flat surfaces, steering the diver up and away from the bottom. Yet based on reaction time considerations, it is evident that an inebriated person does not have sufficient time to aim the head (and body) accurately or to place the hands and arms properly. The predictable result is the individual's slamming straight into the bottom.

In another aquatic context, if a passenger should fall off the bow of a 16-foot power boat cruising at 25 mph, an intoxicated operator would be unable to react in time to avoid running over the victim. This is assuming the operator is at a BAC of 0.1%. In the case of an operator at 0.2% BAC, the chance is good, especially at night, that the operator will not know that the victim fell overboard or even that the boat struck him or her.

In a final context, consider all the various, coordinated actions that allow a person to swim. To remain on the surface, the average human has to maintain some degree of lung-inflation buoyancy. This is only part of this process because the swimmer, to proceed through the water, must properly time breathing and swimming strokes. He or she must also orient himself or herself to the destination (which most of the time cannot be seen clearly) and with the surface of the water. If not swimming at the best angle, he or she will become fatigued. In the worst case, the individual will go nowhere. The basic integration of leg and arm motions in swimming must also fit into these actions, with timing of the highest importance. But at increasingly elevated levels of impairment, the probability of accurate integration drops off until some point is reached at which swimming, even with a simple dog paddle, is impossible.

Judgment

A side effect of the sensory integration impact of ethanol is its ability to modify judgment and risk-taking behavior. As pointed out previously, men drown four times as frequently as women, partly because some individuals need to display their macho, or manly, behavior. How and where persons choose to demonstrate such facets of their makeup depend usually on situation and personality. Since society does not tend to condone continuous displays of this nature, the individual has to train or program himself regarding when such actions and activities are proper and accepted. This is fine until something such as ethanol intervenes to reduce inhibitions and social sanctions.[19] This is a double action since alcohol also acts to impair judgment. Although both reduced inhibitions and judgmental impropriety appear similar, they spring from somewhat different alcohol-related factors. Judgment has to do with sensory integration. Inhibitions have to do with specific habits of memory and practice.

Judgment in the sense of decision making depends on the ability to compare and analyze situations and possible outcomes. Judgment can also relate to psychomotor skills such as hand-eye coordination and interactions or physical movements. In both these areas judgment is dependent on the quality and quantity of information presented to and processed by an individual.

An impaired person's ability to acquire information is increasingly degraded by ethanol, and the time taken to make determinations increases.[15] These increases may induce pressure to act without complete review of all the increasingly degraded available data.

The effect of alcohol on judgment in terms of disregarding prohibitions, or outside rules, and inhibitions, or inner guidelines, also has to do with memory interruptions and the inability to make fine interpretations of what is remembered. One of the most telling aspects of impairment is that the imbibing individuals lapse into an increasingly fixed and limited style of behavior. Since they can handle fewer and fewer concepts or sensory inputs, they tend to fix on a single idea and little else. They may have been warned about attempting certain acts or may have reasoned by themselves why and how to avoid such hazards while sober. But these memories increasingly fail to intervene or to interrupt the chosen singular alcohol-influenced path. Anyone who has attempted to reason with impaired individuals quickly realizes that he or she may be conducting a losing battle. Little can be done at this stage outside of physical intervention and/or restraint and allowing the alcohol in the persons' bloodstream to oxidize. (This metabolic dissipation process usually removes 0.015% to 0.017% BAC per hour, and very little can be done to speed the conversion.[10])

With this consideration of judgment, it would appear that a circle has been closed. As this text began, the point was repeatedly emphasized that prevention is far better than intervention. Little can be done on scene to deter or to enhance the thinking mechanisms of an inebriated person. What can be done *before* this point is reached is to attempt to provide sober individuals as much detailed information about potential outcomes as possible. Experience, especially in dealing with the truths and myths involved in drowning, has clearly shown that the more the potential accident victims (even those who unwisely use alcohol) are exposed to factual information, the better they respond and the fewer accidents they precipitate.[8]

DO NOT LET ALCOHOL TAKE YOU DOWN

What happens to an impaired person before, during, or after immersion? This detailed review condenses and combines the points thus far covered.

Before Immersion

Alcohol affects balance, vision, information processing and integration, and risk-taking behavior. In many instances a younger person, because of drinking inexperience, lower alcohol tolerance, smaller physical size, and, higher levels of metabolism and activity, may decide to go boating, canoeing, or rafting in what otherwise would represent less-than-safe conditions. Then since most boating fatalities occur in small craft (older folks in dinghies are not immune to this situation either), balance becomes critical, and environmental clues and warnings that are simultaneously integrated and acted on when the individual is sober become slowed and unclear. Thus the normally prohibitive sound of and increased inertial flow near a waterfall may be perceived and processed too late to prevent a fatal plunge.

In an impaired individual, the number of eye fixations, or snapshots, taken of what is happening around him or her can be markedly reduced. Hence results the potentially truthful term—*blind drunk*.

During Immersion

Vasodilation (expansion of blood vessels) caused by the relaxing aspects of alcohol may result in a greater-than-average amount of warm blood circulating near the skin's surface, causing increasingly rapid loss of body heat. (This peripheral flow makes the skin's heat sensors believe that the body is warmer than it actually is.) Also, a similar dilation of the blood vessels in the brain results in decreased oxygen loading of brain cells. This mental oxygen deficiency explains why an individual becomes tipsy and undergoes behavioral and psychomotor changes. Therefore the following may happen:

- Caloric labyrinthitis
- Torso reflex, or inhalation response

- Cold water shock, interrupting the autonomic nervous system's signals to the heart and lungs and leading to rapid unconsciousness or cardiac arrest
- Thermal interactions, including peripheral or shell hypothermia, rapidly reducing even a champion swimmer's in-water capabilities
- Greatly decreased breath-holding times resulting from the effect of cold water magnified by alcohol
- Coordination or psychomotor (physical) skills and controls immediately compromised by drinking

After Immersion

Should one or more of the above occur, the individual may sink below the surface and apparently drown. However, amazing advances have been made in reviving and resuscitating the apparently dead drowning victim. But if the victim has been drinking, the probability of recovery apparently is reduced. For example, reports have indicated that intoxicated individuals underwater for periods as short as 1 to 2 minutes have been extremely difficult to revive.[3]

Since medical researchers are still investigating and debating protocols for restoration of long-term submersion patients, the overall impact of alcohol is indistinctly perceived. However, it appears that intoxication interferes with the diving reflex. This reflex triggers protective metabolic slowdown and redistribution of oxygen-rich blood to the brain, heart, and lungs of a nonbreathing, submersed individual. Additional research indicates that alcohol and similar depressive drugs may act to drive the victim, in both aquatic and terrestrial situations, into an even more profound, quickly developing state of suspended animation.[12a] (REMEMBER: Alcohol is a general anesthetic.) This near-death, yet survivable, level is extremely hard to diagnose and treat without special training and equipment. Unfortunately, these procedures and understandings are not yet widespread. The result is that the inebriate may have squandered his or her last reprieve from death.

OTHER RECREATIONAL DRUGS AND AQUATICS

Although a number of aspects about alcohol's aquatic effects are known, presumed present, or can be inferred (mainly from auto accident studies), researchers still have much more work to do. In addition, the difficulty of determining exactly what happens in the common water fatality is heightened by a number of factors, including location, finding the body, and decomposition.

If these factors cloud the perception of ethanol's presence, other recreational, as opposed to prescription, drugs' involvement is even less clear. Although a great deal has been written about the total drug picture in this society, estimates are often in disagreement. For instance, the number of full-time, hard-core alcohol abusers is, in some drug studies, indicated as 10 times the figure representing the users of other recreational drugs.[11] Other similar studies state that 25% of alcohol overusers or abusers also use additional recreational drugs.[6] Since actually determining the number of water accidents involving alcohol is so difficult, tracking the in-water presence of other drugs is almost impossible. However, the effects of other drugs are well known. Hypothetically, translating them into aquatics is not out of the question.

For instance, marijuana is the third most popular psychoactive drug in North America, ranking behind only tobacco and alcohol in overall use. Reports indicate that close to 60% of all Americans have tried marijuana, with approximately 20 million considered regular users.[7]

> Short-term marijuana effects that could directly affect a user's water accident potential are dulling of time, depth, distance, and speed perception; a tendency toward thinking lags; and impairment of mental tasks requiring concentration and attention.

These traits of marijuana are also included in the effect of almost all other recreational drugs, thus altering perception of time and space and seriously interfering with an individual's perceptive and reactive abilities.

The following statement from Hafen and Frandsen[12] can be transferred to the aquatic environment:

Most of the depressants — alcohol, barbiturates, and some of the inhalants — result in severe loss of motor coordination, which affects an individual's ability to drive a car safely, operate machinery, or even control simple motor reflex actions. A person who regularly uses drugs can quickly lose the ability to control even the most simple movements — it does not take very high doses of the drug to cause the incoordination. Accompanying the loss of motor coordination are other motor and sensory impairments that also affect an individual's ability to perform satisfactorily .... Stimulants — especially amphetamines — are widely touted for their ability to combat fatigue and are used commonly by truck drivers, athletes, students, and executives performing under job stress. While these drugs do mask the effects of fatigue, they do *not* correct the effects of fatigue on visual discrimination, attention, concentration, and other factors critical to proper psychomotor functioning.

The critical need for proper mental and physical coordination in all forms of aquatic activities such as swimming, diving, or operating a powerboat (especially at night at high speed) has been extensively discussed. Therefore it takes little imagination to appreciate how the foregoing might be applied to individuals at risk in or on the water.

Another aspect of drug use is the potential for increased physiological stress or overload when an already drug-debilitated individual is suddenly and unintentionally immersed. A growing body of studies indicates the potential for heart arrest from high dosages used among new and/or inexperienced users of cocaine and its "crack" derivatives.[4] Panic, struggling, and the shock of cold water entry may overload the cardiovascular system of some victims, including otherwise healthy, younger persons affected by certain drugs.

One final concern involves what may happen when drugs are combined, even in relatively small amounts, by a person involved in water activities. Drug-alcohol interactions fall under three general categories, classified as follows[23]:

- The disulfiram reaction, leading to vasodilation, flushing, headache, and rapid or elevated heart rate (tachycardia)
- CNS depression, possibly leading to excessive sedation and respiratory depression
- Numerous, miscellaneous, organ-specific interactions

In the disulfiram reaction, apparently nonlethal dosage levels of drugs and alcohol combine to form a third substance, which may be lethal. Moreover, if consideration is given to the physiological impact and outcomes of unexpected immersion, especially those of cold water and hypothermia, the effect of the three categories may be greatly magnified. (Specific characteristics of hypothermia are examined in Chapters 8 and 12.) In addition to the foregoing, research has shown that the liver processes or oxidizes only one drug at a time. Hence the total effect of the combined drugs remains in place much longer.[24]

CHAPTER SUMMARY

In this chapter information has been introduced to explain how and why alcohol has a significant impact on aquatic accidents. This presentation included:

- Statistical reviews and insights into the difficulties involved in generating precise alcohol and water accident statistics.
- Explanation of alcohol's influencing balance, vision, sensory integration, and judgment and why these factors are so critical in aquatics.

- Scenarios describing specific alcohol-related causative factors in water accidents.
- Other potential drug effects, either from drugs by themselves or when combined with ethanol.

PRETEST ANSWERS

1. True
2. c
3. e
4. True

REFERENCES

1. Accident Facts, 1989, Chicago, 1989, National Safety Council, p 21.
2. Alcohol, vision and driving, Falls Church, Va, 1978, American Automobile Association Traffic Engineering Division, p 69.
3. Better think twice . . . A look at alcohol use while boating, Delaware, Ohio, 1985, FlowGraphics Photography (slide/tape).
4. Braude M: Interactions of alcohol and drugs of abuse, Psychopharm Bull 22:3, 1986, pp 717-721.
5. Burns M: Alcohol effects on skills performance, Report of Tenth Annual Education Seminar, Tampa, Fla, 1985, National Safe Boating Council, p 3.
6. Burns M: The effects of alcohol on performance, Proceedings from the 1984 Conference on Alcohol and Recreational Boating Safety, Columbus, Ohio, 1984, Ohio Division of Watercraft, p 7.
7. Conway P: Marijuana—Its highs and lows, St Louis Riverfront Times, Jan 8-14, 1986, p 4.
8. Do you know the facts about drugs? Hollywood, Fla, 1981, Health Communications, p 3.
9. Egstrom G et al.: Alcohol and diving performance, Los Angeles, 1988, University of California Los Angeles, Department of Kinesiology, pp 16-17, 41.
10. Erwin R: Defense of drunk driver cases, New York, 1981, Mathew Bender, Chapter 15.
11. Haddon W and Baker S: Injury control, Washington, DC, March 1981, Insurance Institute for Highway Safety, p 16.
12. Hafen B and Frandsen K: Drug and alcohol emergencies, Center City, Minn, 1980, Hazelden Foundation, pp 48-49.
12a. Kotulak R, Donosky L: Hypothermia: new risks of living death, San Francisco Sunday Examiner and Chronicle, May, 1983.
13. Leonard G: The silent pulse, New York, 1981, Bantam Books, pp 35-45.
14. Miller J et al.: The visual behavior of recreational boat operators, Rep CG-D-31-77, Springfield, Va, 1977, National Technical Information Service, p 69.

15. Moessuer H: Accidents as a symptom of alcohol abuse, J Fam Pract 8:6, 1979, pp 1143-1146.
16. National boating survey, final report, Washington, DC, March 1978, United States Coast Guard, p 121.
16a. National Transportation Safety Board: Recreational Boating Safety, Safety Study ntsd/ss-93/01, 1993, Washington, DC.
17. Pia F: Drowning facts and Myths, Larchmont, NY, 1976, Water Safety Films (videotape).
18. Ray O: Drugs, society and human behavior, St Louis, 1990, Mosby–Year Book, pp 68-69.
19. Ray O: Drugs, society and human behavior, St Louis, 1990, Mosby–Year Book, p 165.
20. Recreational boating and alcohol safety information kit, Rockville, Md, March 1985, National Clearinghouse for Alcohol Information, p 9.
21. Recreational boating safety and alcohol, Washington, DC, 1983, National Transportation Safety Board, p 4.
22. Report of alcohol use and recreational boating safety conference, Cleveland, June 1984, Ohio Division of Watercraft, p 6.
23. Saxe T: Drug alcohol interactions, Am Fam Physician 33:4, 1986, pp 159-162.
24. Saxe T: Drug alcohol interactions, Am Fam Physician 33:4, 1986, p 160.
25. Smith D and Smith S: Waterwise, Imperial, Mo, 1984, Smith Aquatic Safety Services, p 61.
26. Stiehl C: Alcohol and pleasure boat operators, Rep CG-D-1134-75, Springfield, Va, 1975, National Technical Information Service, p 6.

P A R T · T W O

Protecting and Rescuing Yourself

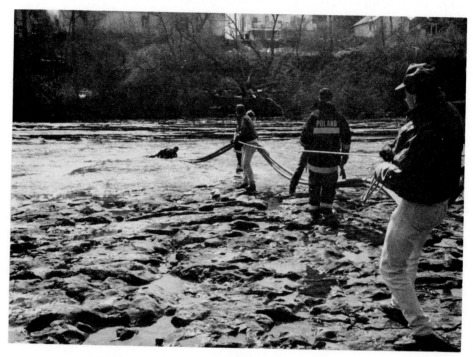

Water rescue practice in your environment.

OVERVIEW

The chapters in Part Two provide information about protecting yourself and others from water hazards and introduce the basics of self-rescue. They will help you do the following:

- Design individual defenses
- Prevent foolish drownings
- Understand basic water survival and rescue principles
- Appreciate environmental and climatic effects on rescuers

DISCUSSION

Conventional thinking would indicate that water rescues should be the responsibility of lifeguards and other specialists specifically trained in water rescue techniques. This makes sense until examining when and where most water accidents occur. As the previous chapters have indicated, only 10% of all serious or fatal water incidents happen in guarded or supervised settings such as public pools and beaches. Thus 90% of the time responsibility for water rescue or intervention principally and/or initially involves emergency services providers.

The preceding chapters also indicated that until very recently almost all water safety and rescue training was primarily oriented toward the guarded pool and beach environment, which meant that if an emergency responder was exposed to water safety information, it generally had little application for the situations that he or she might encounter. In other words, learning how to pull someone off the bottom of a sunlit, summertime swimming pool is not adequate preparation for an underwater search in turbid, swirling floodwaters or in an icy lake at midnight. In fact, a great deal of the information and procedures applicable to a swimming pool are useless, if not lethal, in other situations. Since relatively little past attention was given to training for the most likely types of aquatic emergencies, water rescue equipment for emergency services personnel was next to nonexistent.

Since the mid-1970s progress has been made in dealing with these deficiencies. However, just as aquatic accidents are spread throughout rural and urban areas, many potential responders and rescuers remain uninformed about modern equipment and procedures. Unfortunately, in far too many instances interest in gaining such information still develops only after a drowning or near miss teaches would-be rescuers what they *do not know*. Even then, when fire, emergency medical services (EMS), and police personnel realize that they need aquatic knowledge, they are not sure where to look or what to look for.

This part of the text presents basic procedures and equipment that may prevent a potential rescuer from becoming a victim during the rescue process. In particular, an extensive array of different types of flotation devices is described, many of which can be used in family recreational pursuits and as an indispensable element of the personal, on-the-job, aquatic protection package.

Learning the essentials of personal water protection provides a basis for exploring simple one-on-one rescue and extrication techniques. The text also expands the information dealing with protection from climatic and environmental hazards frequently affecting water rescuers.

5 Designing Individual Defenses

OVERVIEW

This chapter deals with basic self-protection in the water. A simple listing of priorities indicates what an individual might best do to aid himself before, during, and after an aquatic accident or emergency occurrence. Particular emphasis is placed on ensuring that a potential rescuer does *not* become another victim.

OBJECTIVES

After studying this chapter and trying these suggestions under safe, supervised conditions—initially in shallow water—the reader should understand:
1. Waterproofing himself or herself
2. Tactics for reducing in-water panic
3. Relaxing, floating, and swimming basics
4. Backyard, boating, and beach water safety principles
5. Surviving sudden, unintended submersion
6. Water currents and how to use them
7. Proper self-extrication procedures

PRETEST

1. Just about anyone can learn to back float motionlessly if he or she can relax and fully inflate his or her lungs. (True or false?)
2. A fearful nonswimmer can be aided in learning basic swimming skills by (a) blowing bubbles; (b) saying his or her name underwater; (c) bending over in shallow water and grasping his or her ankles; (d) all of the above; or (e) none of the above.

3. If your small boat capsizes, (a) personal flotation devices and occupants will be ejected; (b) the rotating gunwale might hit your head; (c) swim away from it so you will not be pulled underwater; or (d) stay on its upstream end in a current. Which *two* are most correct?
4. Strainers aid your exiting the water by pushing you into slow-moving shallows. (True or false?)
   Pretest answers are at the end of the chapter.

PRINCIPLES OF PERSONAL WATERPROOFING

Can you float? Knowing the answer to this question may be a matter of life or death. This question may seem strange compared to the more normal question, "Can you swim?" But in a potential water rescue environment, you might not be able to swim normally, and motionless floating could be a key to survival.

As indicated in Chapter 1, almost everyone is buoyant. However, many swimmers and nonswimmers may not know this, and even swimmers may lack the skill and experience to back float motionlessly.

Moreover, back floating while not moving is actually the first step in waterproofing yourself. If you learn to do this, your ability to perform all other in-water rescue tasks will be enhanced. Basically, this enhancement stems from your being able to relax and feel confident in the water; otherwise you would not be able to back float.

Flotation essentially depends on two body-related actions—relaxation and lung inflation—that are controllable once they are understood. The more you relax your muscles, the more your body expands in the water, and the lighter you become. Your specific gravity, or the comparison of your immersed body weight to the weight of the water you displace, can be favorably altered by spreading slightly more body area while not increasing weight. Try this in a pool by flexing (i.e., contracting, actually shrinking) all your muscles while attempting to float. You probably will sink. Then try relaxing as much as possible. You should notice an immediate increase in flotation. Also notice that the more familiar and adapted an individual feels in the water, the better he or she floats.

Lung expansion is directly connected to relaxation. A fearful person who has constricted his or her muscles cannot fully expand their lungs. He or she therefore is far less buoyant.

Similarly, most people who do not have much in-water experience react to the relative coldness of the water by breathing shallowly. This, in turn, impedes total lung inflation. Additionally, some learners seldom fully inflate their lungs, at least not to the point of being buoyant. Relaxation helps them overcome these initial difficulties, especially if they have good support and sustained coaching.

Remember it is essential always to *wear* your personal flotation device (PFD) around the water or at least when engaged in aquatic rescues. But suppose you find yourself suddenly and unexpectedly immersed without your PFD, possibly when wearing heavy clothing or equipment such as fire fighters' turnout gear or police body armor. Or suppose the water is very cold and moving. You know that you must swim to safety, but you also know that swimming any distance in cold water can quickly stiffen your muscles and that heavy clothing is extremely hard to move in the water as you attempt to stroke or to kick. What do you do then? The best answer may be to do nothing, thus reducing your heat loss as much as possible by minimizing or totally negating your movements.

If in still water, stabilize your position by back floating; then determine the best route to leave the water. If in a current, get on your back with your feet pointing ahead of you—downstream; ride the current and look for a shallow *inside* curve, which is the best place to paddle toward; then get out. However, to do all this you must be able to answer in the affirmative that you can back float motionlessly.

Learning how to back float in a nonpanicked, relaxed mode is *the* basic ingredient for waterproofing yourself. It is also the second step in learning how to swim. So how do you do it? To discover your own basic flotation capacity, do the following in a safe, shallow setting, preferably with a friend or assistant to aid you.

Skill Drill 1. Take as big a single breath as possible, bend over at the hips, and grab your ankles. Hold on for as long as possible. Your feet (and the rest of you) should lift off the bottom (Fig. 5-1). Have your companion tell you if your back appears above the water surface. If it does, you are positively buoyant.

With a little practice, principally on expanding your lungs, relaxing, and holding your breath, a swimmer should be able to back float without moving with at least his or her face out of the water. Try the face-down ankle grab and the back float several times. If after a number of repeated tries you continue to sink, you are probably a "sinker" and must *always* wear, or at least know the location of, the nearest PFD.

If you fail to pass the flotation test at a younger age, try it as you grow older. One of the positive aspects of gaining a middle-aged spread is that you float better and stay warmer in the water.

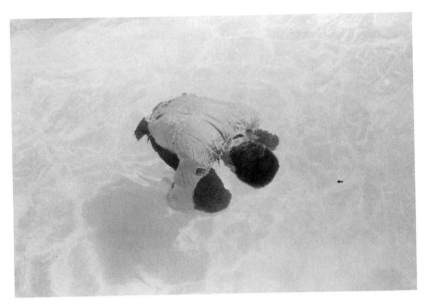

Fig. 5-1 Floating face down while grasping ankles. Notice the floating person's back is above the surface.

Back Floating for Nonswimmers

> The primary reason for the inability to swim and/or fear of the water is inability or reluctance to immerse the face.

Once a nonswimmer learns to place his or her face in the water fearlessly and to keep it there for a reasonable period, he or she is prepared to learn how to swim and to back float. This is the *first* action a nonswimmer must master. Back floating is the *second*.

The simplest way to become adjusted to facial immersion is to blow bubbles into a small bowl of warm water. If you are not a swimmer, practice until you feel comfortable doing this. Once the bubble-blowing task is mastered, the learner is ready for safe, shallow, supervised, in-water experiences. (Note that this procedure can also be used for family members or friends who are nonswimmers.)

Skill Drill 2. Have the learner, in waist-deep water, gently bend from the hips, placing the face in the water. He or she may prefer to hold a friend's hand to gain confidence while doing this step. After trying this move, the nonswimmer should be encouraged to take a deep breath,

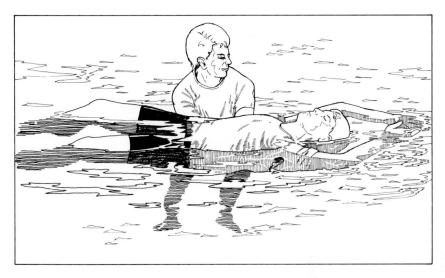

Fig. 5-2 Learner and assistant practicing back floating.

again place his or her face in the water, and say his or her full name a number of times under water.

If the individual seems comfortable with these actions, proceed to taking a deep breath, bending from the hips, and grasping and holding the knees as long as possible. If this works, move to the forward ankle-grabbing–floating-off-the-bottom maneuver. When comfortable with face-down floating, the individual is ready to try back floating.

Skill Drill 3. The learner gently lies backward across and in front of an assistant. The assistant, standing on the bottom, puts one hand under the learner's back and the other under his or her hips. The assistant then tells the learner to relax; to breath hold; to shut the mouth; to arch the back; and to keep the posterior up and head back as far as possible (Fig. 5-2). Nonswimmers often complain that water enters their nose. This will be compensated for quickly as the body adjusts to immersion. Try to persuade the learner not to hold his or her nose while in this position. (Any part of the body raised above the surface tends to submerge the remainder.) To aid back arching, have the learner's arms loosely extending in the water as far away from the head as possible while keeping his or her thumbs locked around each other. The assistant's hands are slowly withdrawn as the learner relaxes, finally leaving the learner floating on his or her own. If the water is too shallow, most men and most women with heavily muscled legs will float with their heels on the bottom. If so, keep repeating the task in gradually deeper (but safe) water, continually emphasizing the arching of the back and total lung inflation. Note that this procedure may also be used to teach a less than totally buoyant *swimmer* the basics of back floating.

> Another means of helping new water participants is to have them wear a layer of clothing anytime they are in the water. The clothing helps keep them warm while aiding their buoyancy.

Additionally, since most people in serious trouble in the water are fully clothed, practicing while wearing an outer layer helps to defuse panicked, incorrect instincts to remove "heavy" clothing rapidly.

Fully Clothed Floating

If the learners can otherwise swim but cannot back float or are relaxed but nonfloatable nonswimmers, have them put on several layers of clothing (coveralls or snowmobile suits usually work well). Then try again. The extra layers of clothing should support them enough to produce adequate flotation (while once more clearly demonstrating that clothing *does not* pull a person underwater). After they experiment with the heavy clothing, take it off a layer at a time and see if they can still float. One reason some individuals cannot back float motionlessly is that they have never experienced it and simply do not know how it feels.

Panicked and otherwise uncontrollable nonswimmers should don a PFD and follow the same procedure as that for sinking swimmers until the nonswimmers can relax to the point of trying to float (in shallow water) without the PFD.

When the nonswimmers can satisfactorily back float, they are ready to learn how to swim, starting with a basic, elementary back stroke and simple flutter kicking. (Pointing the toes while kicking helps.) By starting to swim this way, the beginners realize that if they have any difficulty, they can get on their back and motionlessly float to survive. Similarly, everyone soon realizes that staying on the back with nose and mouth as far away from the water surface, rather than repeatedly immersed beneath it, aids survival. Likewise, by remaining on the back, the individual can yell for help while being able to see above the surface.

The next step in this first learning progression is to practice breathing.

Skill Drill 4. From the relaxed back floating position, the learners simply push down with their hands so that their mouth is elevated. Then they exhale, take in another lungful of air, and gently ease into continued back floating. They should do this as slowly as possible at first since moving too rapidly may push a person's face under water.

Deep-Water Progression

The final progression is to take the learner into deep water. (Initial nonswimmers should *not* attempt this step until they have demonstrated that they will not panic and can swim a pool width, roughly 25 to 30 feet, in chest-deep water. Otherwise, the following is a good drill for them, *provided they are properly wearing a PFD* and a PFD-equipped safety swimmer is in the water with them.) Because most younger men do not have sufficient fat content to float in a horizontal position, their legs will drop, and they may find themselves in a head-back, vertical position, with only their face breaking the surface (Fig. 5-3). But they are floating motionlessly!

Skill Drill 5. An easy way to learn how to float in deep water is to have the learners grasp the pool edge with both arms extended, their feet pointing straight down, and one hand pointing across the pool. Have them take as deep a breath as possible, tilt their head back, and slowly release the pool edge. Have first floaters who can float face down but cannot manage a face-up attitude reach backward and try to grasp their

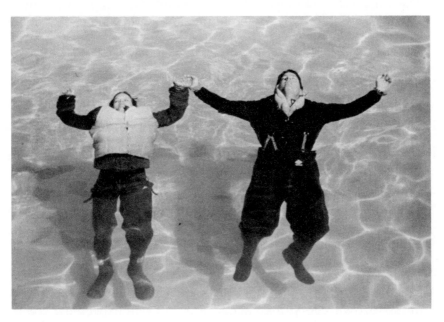

Fig. 5-3 Deep-water, feet-down float. NOTE: A backup safety swimmer, *wearing a PFD*, should always be standing by if needed.

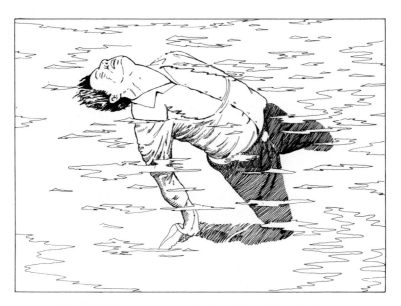

Fig. 5-4 Deep-water ankle grab and back float.

ankles (Fig. 5-4). This maneuver may help them manage a face-up float. If all else fails, have them wear layered clothing in deep water but with a PFD-equipped safety swimmer alongside, at least for the first few attempts (Fig. 5-4).

For safety, teaching these deep water techniques should be done only in a pool.

In a pool safety observers can see participants clearly and can reach them quickly from poolside. Turbid, cloudy, or murky lake water decreases this safety option. Additionally, some lake and beach settings require learners to walk an appreciable distance in the water before it becomes waist deep. These distances increase supervisory and rescue difficulties.

The Graceful Art of Falling In

A large number of individuals, even those who are competent swimmers, drown every year because as they unexpectedly (or even expectedly in some cases) fall, they hit the water with their mouths open. This position leads to torso reflex and immediate drowning. To defeat torso reflex, anyone potentially subject to suddenly landing in the water should learn to cover his or her nose and mouth instinctively until he or she regains the surface. Additionally, all potential water rescuers should learn to fall in backward, with their toes entering the water last. This allows trapped air in their boots or heavy footwear to keep their feet and legs afloat, thereby aiding back floating. A vertical position in the water speeds heat loss and drives remaining air (which functions both as a flotation aid *and* insulation) up and out of the clothing. Being as close as possible to a horizontal position in warmer surface water may make an important survival difference.

To learn how to respond to sudden immersion, again begin (with an assistant) usually at a swimming pool or a dock slightly higher than the water surface.

Skill Drill 6. The assistant stands in the water, which should be a bit deeper than his or her waist. The learner places his or her back to the water while standing on the edge of the pool or dock. The learner next checks to ensure the immediate water area is clear, then takes a breath, covers the nose and mouth with one hand, and sits or slowly falls backward into the water. The assistant should instruct the learner *not* to throw himself or herself backward into the water because this may result in a dangerous back dive into shallow water. The assistant then helps achieve a back float, telling the learner to uncover the nose and mouth when the learner's face is above the surface. The assistant should not catch the learner but should be ready to assist, especially in the case of someone who has not previously tried this step.

After doing this maneuver a couple of times, almost everyone instinctively learns to cover the nose and mouth when threatened by sudden immersion. This tactic can then be added to sudden water entry while encumbered with heavy clothing as discussed in Chapter 7. It should also be practiced while wearing a PFD because the unexpected buoyancy of the PFD rapidly returning the individual to the surface can be a surprise.

By understanding and practicing these few simple techniques, the potential for panic, especially in suddenly immersed poor swimmers, can be reduced. From this background we can initiate additional self-survival or rescue tactics.

THE POOL AS A WATER SAFETY TOOL

We have indicated that the increase in the number of family and community pools may have a positive effect on reducing drownings. The reason: as more people become accustomed from an early age to being relaxed and responsible around aquatic situations, the potential for accidents is reduced. (REMEMBER: Most drowning victims cannot swim and are usually terrified of the water.) As a potential water rescuer, there are steps you can do and can learn in your own backyard or community pool to aid your rescue potential.

Take a quick look around the pool or possible beach or lake area that will be used for self-training. Since in some states backyard swimming pools are becoming major sources of child-drowning incidents, have you "kid proofed" your pool?[4]

- Have you installed fencing around the swimming area sufficiently high to prevent small children from climbing into the pool? Fences 4 feet high with no more than 4-inch openings are the basic standard, but more height provides an even greater safety margin.
- Do you have childproof, self-activating closures on all gates (Fig. 5-5)?
- Can you be sure that children cannot gain entrance to your pool (or hot tub) from your house without your awareness? An increasing number of child drownings occur when parents believe their children are sleeping or playing away from the pool, but the youngsters manage to slip unseen into the danger area. Is your pool *completely* fenced off from your house?[5]

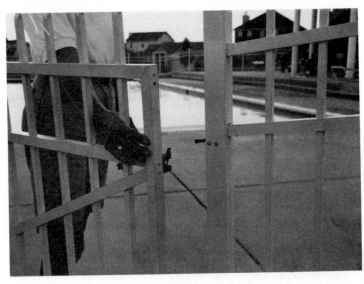

Fig. 5-5 Guarding a pool from needless child drownings: fencing *completely* around the pool; self-closing gates; childproof latches.

- Do you *always* ensure that children are *continually* supervised around any water setting?
- Even in the winter or when the pool is closed, can you ensure that children cannot fall into a water-filled pool cover?
- Do you have a telephone near enough to the pool area that anyone can call 911 or similar assistance sources? Does everyone know how to do this?
- How many of the people who gather at your water facility are cardiopulmonary resuscitation (CPR) qualified?
- Have you taken the time to mark shallow water and hazardous diving areas clearly? Similarly, have you talked with your family's "hotdogging" divers, usually younger teenage males, to determine their knowledge of diving safety (especially as their height and weight increases)?
- If your family pool or beach has a deep end or drop off, have you marked it with a buoy line? (Your family members may know where the water is deeper, but does the casual visitor?)
- Is your pool water clear? Can you easily see all bottom areas? Have all poolside tripping hazards been removed or at least been well marked? Is the bottom contour clearly visible? A number of accidents have happened because the pool-liner pattern or bottom coloring actually camouflaged changes from deep to shallow areas.
- If used at night, are the pool and the deck area sufficiently lighted?
- Do all electrical circuits have ground-fault interrupters (GFIs)?
- If yours is a beach or lakeside setting, are there any sudden drop-offs? Is the bottom level? Are there any underwater obstructions that a person diving into shallow water from a standing start on the bottom might hit? Do you make it a standard practice to warn guests about these hazards?[1]
- Do you have a reach pole or throw line nearby, and has everybody had some practice in using it? (A pool sweeper pole is good here.)
- Has what alcohol does to normally excellent diving (and swimming) prowess been discussed (Table 5-1)?

Even if you do not own a swimming pool, you should, as a potential water rescuer, be aware of the foregoing. Again, the key thought is to prevent accidents rather than respond to them.

Table 5-1 Easy-to-Learn Pool Safety

EASY TO

L Learn the causes of water fatalities:
- Inability to swim
- Cold water
- Alcohol
- No personal flotation devices (PFDs)

E Educate family members about:
- Water dangers
- Simple safety procedures
- Protective equipment
- Dangers of alcohol

A Always:
- Supervise children
- Enforce PFD use by nonswimmers

R Register in a cardiopulmonary resuscitation (CPR) class (call, for example, local Red Cross, Heart Association, Community colleges to enroll)

N
- Never dive in shallow (or unknown) water
- Never swim during storms

P Practice protection:
- Use your pool to learn universal safety procedures effective anywhere
- Practice *before* you need them
- Learn survival skills:
  Back float
  HELP
  Huddle

O Organize your own pool's rescue aids and first aid equipment:
- Reach pole
- Ring buoy
- Throw line
- Familiarize yourself and family with use of PFDs

O Observe and recognize drowning signs:
- Mouth open
- Head back
- Arm movements
- Bobbing
- MAKING NO SOUND!!!

L List telephone numbers prominently:
- Rescue squad
- Doctor
- Hospital

S Swim safely:
- Never swim alone
- Always know water depth
- Do not overestimate your swimming skills

A Adequately mark pool depths:
- Check the depth before diving (hitting the bottom is a pain in the neck!)

F Fence your pool:
- Secure and lock gates (especially when not home or *in winter*)
- Make sure the toddler from next door or down the street cannot accidentally fall in your pool (summer or *winter*)

E Educate your family about dangers of alcohol and drugs around water:
- 50% of drownings involve drinking

T Teach your family to swim:
- You do not have to be a trained instructor to teach basic swimming skills

Y Your family's safety begins with YOU!

Modified from Smith D and Smith S: Waterwise, Imperial, Mo, 1984, Smith Aquatic Safety Services, p 109.

Self-Teaching in Your Home Pool

Having completed a pool (beach and lake) anti-accident audit, check into using the facility to teach basic aquatic safety. One of your first drills would be to learn how to back float using the procedures presented previously. Any other family members available and/or interested could be included. You can practice your teaching technique at home in preparation for "taking it on the road" to your department or community.

Next, especially if your family and friends ardently enjoy fishing and hunting, you might try everyone's PFDs in actual water practice. This practice could also include the heat escape lessening position (HELP) and huddle maneuvers explained in Chapter 7. Immersion while wearing "heavy" out-of-door hunting, fishing, and snowmobiling outfits (cleaned before pool entry) also is helpful. In fact, the best possible time to learn winter water emergency skills is during the summer. All this practice should be accomplished under safe, supervised conditions.

Another key concept, especially if you have or supervise toddlers, is to have them become as adjusted to wearing child-sized PFDs as possible (Fig. 5-6). *Never* think that you can quickly place a PFD on a terrified, struggling child in an in extremis situation. *Always* have your children

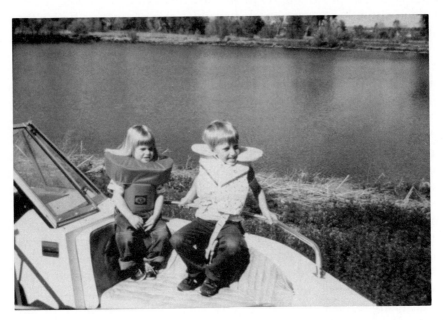

Fig. 5-6 Different styles of child-sized PFDs (From Dive Rescue International: *Waterproof your family* [slide/tape presentation].)

learn to wear properly sized flotation devices (including in-water practice) under safe conditions as soon as it looks as though they will be anywhere near the water.

Depending on the size and capacity of your facility, include the family small craft in your practice. If you have a canoe or small craft such as a johnboat, you might even consider putting it into the pool and having the family learn how to use it as a survival tool.

Skill Drill 7. As a simple drill, show everyone how to enter the craft properly and sit in a swamped (upright) small craft. You can determine whether the (clean) family canoe or johnboat really will float full of water and people as it is supposed to do.

As a final exercise, demonstrate to (or practice on) family members the techniques for simple in-water stabilization of cervical spine injury cases (see Chapter 12).

OCEAN CURRENTS

Since ocean, beach, and tidal currents are frequently misunderstood, they should be explored from a survival standpoint. In addition, because there always is a chance that a water rescuer unintentionally will suddenly be swept downstream in moving water, basic safety considerations should be examined for this environment. Even though relatively few people perish in ocean-side situations, being pulled seaward by undertow can be frightening.

Ocean water moving onto or along a beach is put, and sometimes held, there by two forces: one is tidal, and the other is wind. Wind, acting either by itself or in concert with a changing tide, can create waves. Beach waves generally result from water being forced onto increasingly shallower areas until it piles up, then falls over. The wind, or possibly storm forces, propelling this piling water may actually be located many miles distant from the beach. The more quickly the beach shoals, or the steeper the angle at which it rises from the ocean bottom, the higher and more dynamic will be the waves it creates. Beach and ocean wave power can usually be judged from a safe distance, although in some surf settings wave-generating forces can combine to create periodic breakers much larger than their predecessors. Paying attention to local information can generally warn visitors about this possibility. A person can and should closely study wave action before putting himself or herself at risk by venturing out on an exposed jetty, rock face, breakwater, or similar potentially dangerous location (Fig. 5-7).

Although some individuals are swept out to sea or into large lakes by

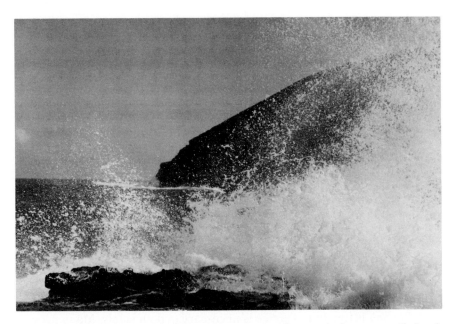

Fig. 5-7 A *very* dangerous situation. A person can be carried away easily by these breaking waves.

waves, the primary problem is the tremendous weight of water dumped on unsuspecting, potential victims when a wave breaks on a fast **shoaling** beach. Similarly, inviting body surfing scenes frequently are underlaid with hazard if the swimmer does not know how to gauge and to use and dodge the wave's action properly (Fig. 5-8). High surf in vacation areas normally generates an increase in neck, arm, and shoulder injuries.

When large amounts of water are transported onto a beach by rising tides and wind, gravity acts to return the fluids to the sea. This process may be drastically altered as tides change, and water pooled or held against a beach has an even stronger pull of gravity acting to move it seaward. In certain normally narrow areas of a beach, seaward-flowing water can create a strong undertow; however, these areas usually measure only a few yards, with the water movement rapidly diminishing as the depth increases. The basic survival ploy, if caught in such a situation, is not to panic, but to proceed as much as possible *across* the primary flow, usually parallel to the beach, to calmer, more static water on the periphery.

The "under" in *undertow* is actually inaccurate. Outward rushing water from a beach moves as a more-or-less homogeneous body, with the

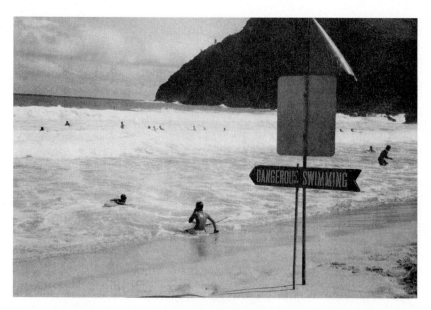

Fig. 5-8 Surfing is fun, but practice is necessary to do it safely. Many people are seriously injured at locations like this every year.

upper layers generally proceeding as fast as the lower segments. Unless an unusual, bottom contour–induced, downward thrust is present, a surface swimmer is not automatically pulled under.[6,7]

INLAND CURRENTS

The largest difference between waves in oceans and lakes compared to those in rivers and streams is that in the ocean, waves or surface components move while the water actually stays in more or less one place; conversely, in river situations the waves normally remain stationary while the water itself moves. The greatest danger from ocean waves resides in being pummeled and/or ground into the bottom by massive weights of breaking or falling water. Inland, the primary hazard is having that same momentum propel an individual into immovable objects.

The unbelievably short amount of time required for a babbling, placid stream to turn into a malevolent torrent is nearly incomprehensible, especially when upstream downpours can send walls of water down narrow, confined stream beds.[2]

If you are ever caught in such a situation, do not, repeat, do *not* attempt to stand. Attempting to place your feet under you may actually

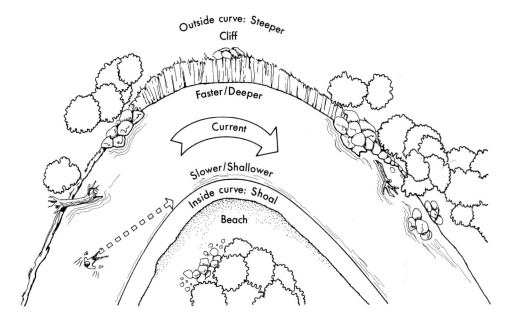

Fig. 5-9 A downstream floater aiming for shallow water at the inside of a curve.

jam one or both of your feet and legs into a hole or similar entrapment on the bottom. The water force will quickly fold you over, either backward or forward, and you may quickly drown. Hence the warning always to attempt to float on your back, feet up and pointing downstream. Your feet point downstream to ensure that if you crash into an object, your feet and legs, not neck and head, absorb the impact.[3,8]

Another normally appropriate suggestion is to try not to fight the flow. Just as swimming across the tide- or wind-created undertow allows you to escape from dangerous beach situations, going with a river's flow until you approach a bend is usually the best policy (Fig. 5-9). This suggestion is underscored by comments in Chapter 3 about cooling rates. You actually may be safer by taking your chances in floating downstream if a large portion of your body is immersed than in hanging on to a stationary object in flowing water. The heat loss rate to still water (or more properly, water that is not markedly moving relative to you) is 25 times that of air temperature at the same level; but if you are stationary, water tearing past and around you might cause 10 times more heat loss. By hanging onto a tree until torn from it, a person might actually worsen his or her predicament because of increased heat loss. Attempting to float to a calmer, downstream location could be a better choice.

If you are aboard a boat — especially in a moving water situation — and are subject to capsizing or being thrown out, understand and practice the following points: (1) in moving water rescue situations, regardless of the size of the boat, always wear your PFD; (2) if you are going overboard, regardless of the situation, attempt to cover your nose and mouth, protecting yourself from torso and inhalation responses; and (3) immediately get to the *upstream* end of a swamped craft moving in a current (otherwise you might be pinned between an obstacle and the downstream end or side of your craft and possibly crushed by a ton of moving, water-filled canoe).

As with most of the information delivered in this text, these are basic safety and survival principles that must be weighed and used according to the prevailing on-scene conditions and situations. However, the better understood the principles, the more aware a rescuer becomes of usable, useful alternatives and appropriate survival techniques.

CURRENT PATTERNS

Also of assistance in moving or white-water work is understanding the elementary dynamics involved in fluid flow. The two basic concepts are laminar and helical flow. In the former, a stream continuously moving over a fairly uniform bottom can be visualized as separated into horizontal layers, or laminar sheets. These consistent layers usually are divided by temperature, with the lowest temperature sheets nearest the bottom. When this division happens in still water, generally there is a highly marked boundary between a more-or-less uniform layer of warm surface water and a much colder underlying stratus. The boundary is called a *thermocline*.[6] It is involved with immediate drowning syndrome.

With laminar flow in moving water, each sheet moves at a speed slightly different from that of its neighbors. Because of bottom drag, the lowest layer moves the slowest, with each higher layer moving at the speed of the layer underneath it plus an increased speed of its own. However, the fastest moving layer is not the highest surface sheet, for it is slowed slightly by air drag. Thus the layer directly below it probably moves fastest (Fig. 5-10). As a result, an object, or human, settling into moving water does not sink downward at a 45-degree angle to flow. Rather its descending underwater track is a curve, with the curve becoming more vertical as the bottom is approached. This fact may help find items or people under moving water.

The concept of helical flow is similar to that of laminar flow but is

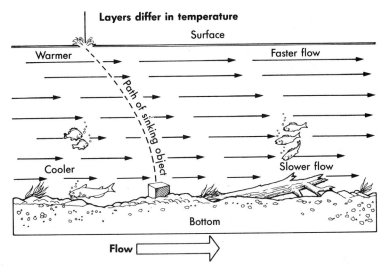

Fig. 5-10 Laminar, or layered, flow. Note that an object sinking downward moves in a curve, not a straight line, as it descends toward the bottom.

much more important from a survival standpoint. In helical flow water moving rapidly along a fairly well-defined and normally steep-sloped channel takes a twisting, screwlike course. Bottom drag again affects the lowest layer but actually causes it to rise at an angle along the bank. This rising bottom water reaches the surface, moves out toward mid-stream, then plunges under again, with components from both sides combining in the center and then twisting back toward the bottom (Fig. 5-11). This model infers two very important survival considerations. First, the rising bottom water is cold. Second, someone falling into water that is turning over in this twin screwlike fashion will be carried rapidly toward the middle of the stream. A person's best option in this situation is not to strike out directly for the shore but to angle across the helical current as with the undertow model. If you have ever watched water **upwelling** as it "blossoms" on the surface of a moving stream, you have witnessed helical flow.

In addition to understanding moving water's flow patterns, you should be aware of dangers from dynamic water pressure. As indicated in the "Inland Currents" section, a swamped small craft (e.g., a 16- to 18-foot canoe) can become an awesome battering ram. This happens when the weight of water inside the swamped craft is put into motion by current. This momentum relationship can imperil you in other ways. For instance, even your relatively smaller momentum can cause you to fetch up on and become entangled with a **strainer.**

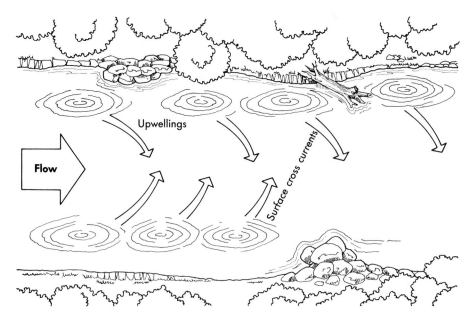

Fig. 5-11 Helical, or twisting, flow. "Blossoming" water flow represents an upwelling, helical movement. The current-driven water rises on the channel side, moves diagonally across the surface to the center, then plunges downward. A person or object falling into this type of flow is pushed toward the center.

A strainer is a porous or sievelike obstacle that allows water, but not larger objects, to pass through it. Downed tree limbs generally represent the principle type of strainer, but barbed wire fences and various types of gratings do the same thing.

If you are being carried downstream, avoid possible strainers. They can trap and force you underwater. Strainers can also catch on your clothing and PFD, thereby greatly complicating extrication. If you are being carried toward one, attempt immediately to get as much of your body *above* it as you can. If possible, attempt to roll *over* the obstruction. (This means shifting from a feet-first to a sideways or head-first position and does require practice.) The more of your body in the water, the greater the suction or force attempting to push you under and pin you against the strainer. If the object forming the strainer is attached to the shore, climbing on top of it may provide an escape route from the river.

Bridge piers present another dynamic danger. Just as with large rocks protruding from a stream's bottom, a small craft being carried sideways by the flow can actually be bent around the piers, pinning the occupants—possibly underwater. Even a person not in a boat can be endangered by bridge piers, since the piers may have large piles of flood-borne debris collected on their upstream sides. This debris then forms a hard-to-dodge series of strainers. Conversely, bridge piers offer the potential of possible rescue from above. For this reason, they should always be noted in the area of responsibility and hazard inspections outlined in latter parts of the text.

Upstream and downstream "Vs" are another facet of river or fast water knowledge. Water flowing between underwater obstacles forms a V on the surface pointing downstream. This generally indicates a safe place to pass. Conversely, a V pointing upstream should be avoided because a submerged object lies below it.

SIMPLE SELF-EXTRICATION

Removing one's self from either moving or still water has both similar and differing aspects. In both situations the forces at work in the water should be used to your best benefit and should not be fought.

The principle force to use in the case of still water is buoyancy itself. As is explained more fully in Chapter 7, a fully clothed person in the water weighs nothing. In fact, if floating, he or she is positively buoyant. But as soon as the individual leaves the stream or pond, he or she not only gains back normal weight but also must bear the load of all the water in the clothing. In a winter or cold water scenario, especially after an individual has been debilitated by the effects of heat loss, he or she will have a limited amount of remaining energy for weight lifting. Also, if the immersed individual has become considerably colder in the water, sudden, sustained exertion may markedly increase interior chilling to the point of possible cardiac malfunctions. In very cold water (i.e., icy water), the extra weight suddenly tossed on a too-thin solid surface may break it, thereby plunging the person back in the water in worse shape than when he or she started. To make the best of a bad situation, a trained and practiced person should use the effect of water's buoyancy on his or her clothing.

Skill Drill 8. By gently bobbing and gaining up-and-down momentum, a fully clothed rescuer may be able to bounce high enough to bend across the surface he or she is attempting to climb (Fig. 5-12). Once this position is achieved, the next thing is to let exposed clothing drain, then slowly wriggle higher out of the water. When enough body mass is out, slowly roll away from the edge (Fig. 5-13). Especially on ice, attempt to spread and to distribute as much body weight as possible. Again, the primary focus is to move slowly and to minimize movement and energy expenditure.

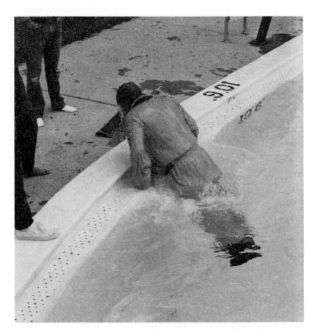

Fig. 5-12 "Bobbing" out—using the buoyancy of clothing as an aid in getting out of the water. This must be done *gently* in cold water situations.

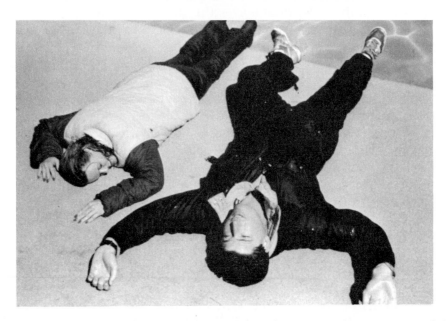

Fig. 5-13 Rolling away from the edge and distributing weight over more of the surface—good practice for *not* breaking back through ice. (From Dive Rescue International: Waterproof your family [slide/tape presentation].)

To exit from moving water, a different plan is followed. There are two locations for easiest exit in a swiftly flowing stream or river. One is a curve or bend. Depending on flow rate, water actually heaps up on the *outside* of a curve; thus there is relatively little current on the inside, and the bottom slope is much more gradual. If you find yourself rapidly being carried downstream, steer (by aiming your feet) for the *inside* of the next or nearest curve.

The second technique involves a moving water phenomenon known as an **eddy,** or back current. When flowing water rushes around an object, part of the current closest to the impediment turns back upstream.

> Depending on flow rate, depth, location, and size of the blocking object, eddy currents may sweep you toward the beach.

On the other hand, if the object is toward the center of the stream, you might be able to climb up on it; however, you could still be stranded, but you at least would be clear of the water — until the stream rose (Fig. 5-14).

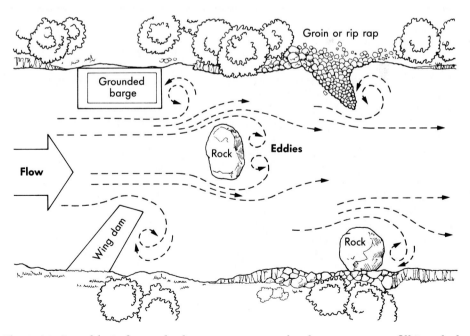

Fig. 5-14 An eddy is formed when water moves back *up-stream* to fill in a hole or depression on the *downstream* side of an obstruction.

CHAPTER SUMMARY

This chapter presented:

- Techniques for self-learning and for teaching others how to float.
- Basic concepts for helping a nonswimmer become comfortable in the water.
- Safety considerations to prevent accidents in home pools.
- Ideas for using a swimming pool, lake, or beach area as a water safety teaching point.
- Elementary considerations for surviving in various types of moving water.
- Simple procedures for safely exiting and entering the water.

PRETEST ANSWERS

1. True
2. d
3. b, d
4. False

REFERENCES

1. Awesome power, Washington, DC, 1987, National Oceanographic and Atmospheric Administration (videotape).
2. Bechdel L and Ray S: River rescue, Boston, 1985, Appalachian Mountain Club Books, p 9.
3. BSA lifeguard counselor guide, Irving, Tex, 1989, Boy Scouts of America, p 2.
4. Children and pool safety checklist, Pub No 357, Washington, DC, Spring 1988, US Consumer Product Safety Commission, p 4.
5. Consumer Products Safety Commission proposes pool barriers to Council of American Building Officials, Newport Beach, Calif, Spring 1989, National Drowning Prevention Network News, p 1.
6. Fawcett, W: Water the timeless compound, Wayzata, Minn, 1980, Fawcett Communications (film).
7. Survival swimming: To save a life, Chicago, 1989, Encyclopedia Britannica Educational Corp (videotape).
8. White water primer, Washington, DC, 1978, American Red Cross (film).

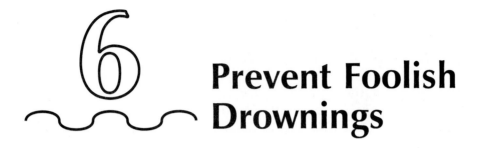

Prevent Foolish Drownings

OVERVIEW

This chapter introduces the types and performance properties of personal flotation devices (PFDs) and the procedures for their proper use. It instructs you in choosing an appropriate PFD for your situation and how to use it as an effective tool both in saving yourself and rescuing others.

OBJECTIVES

After studying this chapter, the reader should understand to the point of clearly explaining to others the following topics:
1. Background information on PFD development
2. Various categories of flotation aids
3. PFD types and applications
4. Imperatives in understanding and properly using PFDs
5. Fitting and equipping a PFD
6. Appropriate and improper use of flotation devices
7. Matching PFDs with individual, departmental, and environmental needs

---

PRETEST

1. Flotation devices can be troublesome if not properly sized and worn tightly because they can ride up on a person struggling in the water. (True or false?)
2. To be effective, PFDs must (a) in all cases turn wearers upright; (b) be easily donned; or (c) support 30 pounds in the water. (Which is most correct?)

3. PFDs can be found in the following versions: (a) soft, pliable, easily wearable vests; (b) camouflaged flotation coats with matching float pants; (c) full-length flotation coveralls; (d) none of the above; or (e) all of the above.
4. PFDs are so simple to use that a person really has no need to practice with them. (True or false?)
   Pretest answers are at the end of the chapter.

FLOTATION AIDS IN GENERAL

Prehistoric humans, especially those dependent on water resources for a livelihood, realized that a number of materials were buoyant and that this buoyancy was sufficient to float someone who was hanging onto the material. As the application of this information evolved, ships or smaller craft were designed and built for various tasks requiring large carrying and safety capacities. At the same time, others experimented with more narrowly limited buoyancy applications. For instance, in the Far East riverside dwellers discovered that sections of bamboo stalks, which are hollow, segmented, and extremely buoyant, could be used to float small or large loads. They also perceived that when increasing numbers of stalks were inserted under the object, bamboo was equally useful in raising weight off river bottoms. (Chapter 11 presents a much more modern application using an inflated fire hose.) Early Egyptians developed similar procedures using bundled reeds for personal flotation and in aggregated constructions capable of ocean crossings.

Southern European peoples developed flotation techniques using the buoyant barks of certain trees, principly cork. South Americans similarly developed the flotation properties of balsa wood. Cork and balsa were the initial flotation materials used when mass production of life vests or life jackets started in the mid-nineteenth century. The primary force driving development of these life preservers was a dynamic increase in ocean travel, which was coupled with the tremendous growth of American passenger traffic on rivers and among coastal communities. Another unfortunate factor involved the thousands of lives lost in shipwrecks, steamship boiler explosions, and resulting shipboard fires.

Part of the roots of today's U.S. Coast Guard (USCG) and the modern PFD industry is intertwined in a federal agency—the Steamship Inspection Bureau—developed to prevent such losses. One responsibility of this bureau was to test and certify lifesaving equipment. In the early 1900s it became part of the USCG, which inherited the job of overseeing life jacket generation. Although cork had long been favored as a flotation material because it was extremely light and resisted compression and water absorption, it did have two major draw backs: it was stiff and bulky, and it was flammable. Before World War II, kapok, another organic material, began to displace cork. When this lightweight vegetable fiber is suitably enclosed in a waterproof container such as an oil-sealed, painted, or plastic bag, it is very buoyant.

As with similar materials, the weight of kapok is far less than that of the volume of water it displaces or pushes aside. Hence it not only floats, but it has the capacity of floating other objects. Conversely, kapok is hygroscopic, that is, it absorbs water. If the waterproof shell containing the kapok is punctured and the interior is exposed to moisture and repeated compression, the fibers eventually become a soggy, barely buoyant mass.

Except for pneumatic (air or compressed gas) inflatable devices produced for military use during World War II, PFD manufacture was static until the mid-1950s. Then as a side product of the plastics industry, a number of floatable, closed-cell foam materials became available. Because they are filled with millions of tiny, separate air bubbles, most of these materials can be folded, twisted, compressed, cut, and scorched, but they will resume their shape and continue to provide buoyant support.

Additionally, and almost as importantly, the foam materials are excellent insulators—both in the water and out. The following pages feature many different styles of these foam rubber, or closed-cell plastic, devices. Note that they also normally are dipped in or coated with vinyl to seal them doubly. Many modern PFDs, especially float coats and coveralls, look and wear exactly like normal clothing, which is what they are (Fig. 6-1). The only exception with these items is that for interior insulation they use buoyant, pliable plastic foam, rather than wool, cotton, or similar organic materials.

Increasing numbers of potential users are discovering these improved buoyant devices. But there are many individuals and organizations who do not know about the availability and potential use of modern PFDs. Unfortunately, community rescue and emergency response groups sometimes fall into this grouping.

Part of this problem concerns the difficulty of keeping pace with developments in specific professional fields. This situation can be remedied through educational applications and informational network-

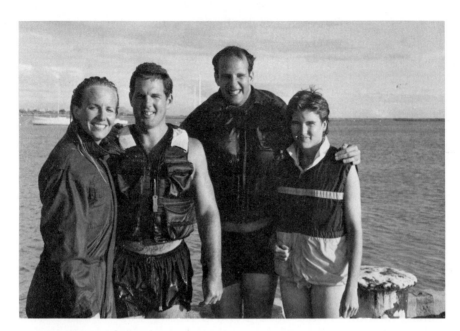

Fig. 6-1 Note the different styles of float coats and coveralls worn by individuals in this group.

ing. Not keeping up because "We've always done it this way" is dangerous and unfair to everyone involved in a rescue operation—including both fellow rescuers and the victim. The cost of one lawsuit, including monetary considerations, human elements, and jobs lost, is far more expensive than the relatively insignificant purchase price of any PFD.

Thus one of the main topics in this section of the text is how someone who begins to understand and use these devices properly—that is you—can productively encourage others in gaining the same understanding. *In the active, interventionist stages of water rescues, PFDs are the key. They must be present and used properly.* Therefore read this information and the training procedures carefully; then practice the in-water drills and protocols recommended in the text.

CATEGORIES OF FLOTATION AIDS

Devices or objects that can be used to support a person in the water fall into three broad divisions: generic floating objects, designed devices, and federally approved devices.

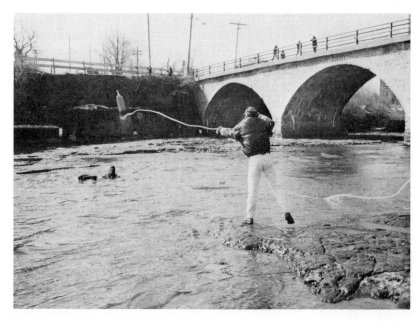

Fig. 6-2 A throwing rescue. The thrown objects float and mark the victim's position. Note that in moving water, the line or flotation object or device *must* land within the victim's grasp; otherwise the victim will not be able to reach it.

Generic Floating Objects

Generic floating objects are items or things that float that can also be used as a swimming or buoyancy aid by someone in the water. They might be as large as a tree floating downstream or as small as table tennis balls in a jacket pocket. Although not normally thought of in a formal rescue sense, such objects may be the only means of assistance available to a would-be rescuer, especially when an emergency situation is neither expected nor planned for. This category may be further subdivided into items that can be used in a reaching rescue or items that can be thrown to someone in distress. Remember that many people in trouble in the water are 10 feet or less from safety. Hence branches, oars, canoe paddles, broom or mop handles, and building timbers (e.g., 2 × 4 lumber) fit into this subcategory.

"Throwables" might also include capped bottles and jars of certain types, with large thermos or picnic coolers working best; sealed cans and boxes; and inner tubes and other inflatable objects such as larger beach and sports equipment, including basketballs, footballs, and plastic wading pool toys (but only in an emergency) (Fig. 6-2). This throwables category may be further divided into objects that can be retrieved for another toss and those that cannot. Objects that either are ropelike such as a garden hose or are in fact ropes or lines (actually, smaller diameter ropes) or have a line tied to them are all retrievable. For extemporaneous rescue, the best results are obtained by combining highly buoyant objects such as large thermos containers with a retrieving line—as long as attaching the line does not take a lot of time.

The foregoing aids are of value for two main reasons. First, the more buoyant objects placed within distressed persons' grasp, the better they can support themselves. Second, everything thrown into the water helps mark the last known position of the individuals in danger should they disappear beneath the surface. This is especially helpful in still water, although it also has some merit in moving water situations.

Designed Devices

A number of swimming aids have been designed and used in personal flotation roles. Some such as water wings have been in use a long time, whereas others such as lifeguards' **rescue tubes** represent relatively recent developments. Although many are specifically intended for use in rescues, they nevertheless are not certified as federally approved devices. A major reason many aids designed for rescues are not approved by federal law (i.e., USCG regulations) is that they are purely inflatable or pneumatic. Hence, even though the text presents a number of types of self-inflated safety equipment, you could receive a citation from a state or federal boarding officer if these devices were the only flotation gear you had on your boat.[2] Federal lawmakers do not believe that inflatables are dependable enough for everyday use in the normal boating environment.

Nevertheless, we recommend you use some forms of non-USCG–approved inflatable devices. These recommendations pertain to your professional, as opposed to recreational, use and on-the-job storage requirements. Also, federal PFD evaluations are usually based on the durability of the devices, emphasizing worse-case situations. Conversely, as a professional rescuer, the care you would give an inflatable, or any, PFD is probably much greater than that of the average boater. Therefore, even though pure inflatables are *not* USCG approved, they may have a definite application in specialized water rescue situations.

Some devices initially intended for use as flotation equipment do not work very well. A common example is waterskiing belts. These devices are not acceptable because they usually lack sufficient buoyancy. Another reason, which separates them from approved waterskiing vests, is that the belts easily come loose on impact with the water. Conversely, the approved vests have buckles that must withstand the shock of hitting

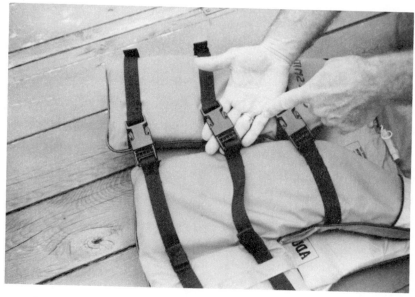

Fig. 6-3 These Type III, USCG-approved waterskiing vest buckles are high speed and water-impact resistant.

the water at 55 miles per hour (Fig. 6-3). Waterskiing belts usually are inferior safety devices, but they do make excellent boat fenders; and they can be used, when several are lashed around the perimeter of a Stokes litter, for buoyancy.

Lifeguards' rescue tubes are also unapproved by federal law for a totally different reason—they *do* require special training to don and/or use properly and thus do not meet federal criteria. Nevertheless, rescue tubes are usable in the hands of a trained and experienced person and usually have similar or greater buoyancy than approved PFDs. You might consider them for some of your department's water rescue needs.

You can wear the float coats and coveralls presented in the following sections of this chapter; but when the weather turns warm and they become uncomfortable, where do you put them in an already overly crowded rescue truck or squad car? One answer (and not that expensive an alternative) is to rotate the coats in warmer weather with readily storable, yet handy devices such as rescue tubes and self-actuating inflatable hip kits.

One final nonapproved set of useful devices, which, however, must be watched closely, are inflatable cuffs usually found as swimming aids on smaller children. They are helpful in benign, easily supervised environments such as wading ponds or portable and backyard pools.

> However, *these inflatable cuffs are not approved PFDs* and can actually become dangerous when either the child or the parents become too dependent on them.

As with all the other items discussed, inflatable cuffs have their proper application. The important thing is to know when and where it is suitable to use each device.

Federally Approved Devices

Federally approved PFDs receive this certification only after they are tested and compared against a strict set of well-examined criteria (Fig. 6-4). Some of the criteria concern the breaking strength of the thread used in sewing the device; the usable life of the flotation materials, including compressibility factors; the colors and fading potential of certain dyes used in the devices; and the breaking force required on buckles and tie straps.

The following are excerpts describing the four primary types of PFDs plus the fifth special purpose category.* Federal law requires that informational material be provided with each new PFD.

- *Offshore Life Jacket (Type I, 22 lb buoyancy).* This type PFD has the greatest required buoyancy and is designed to turn most unconscious persons in the water from a facedown position to a vertical and slightly backward position plus maintaining the person in the vertical and slightly backward position. This positioning greatly increases his or her chances of survival. The offshore life jacket is suitable for all waters, especially ones in which there is a probability of delayed rescue (e.g., on large bodies of water where it is not likely that a significant number of boats would be in close proximity). This type PFD is the most effective of all types in rough water. The offshore life jacket is easiest to don in any emergency because it is reversible. It is available in only two sizes—adult (90 lb or more) and child (<90 lb)—which are universal sizes (designed to fit all persons in the appropriate category).
- *Near-Shore Buoyant Vest (Type II, 15½ lb buoyancy).* This type PFD is designed to turn the wearer to a vertical and slightly backward position in the water. The turning action is not as pronounced as with an offshore life jacket, and the device will not turn as many persons under the same conditions as the offshore life jacket. The near-shore buoyant vest is usually more comfortable to wear than the offshore life jacket. This type PFD is normally

---

*The described types of PFDs are designed to perform as described in calm water and when the wearer is not wearing any other flotation material such as a wet suit.

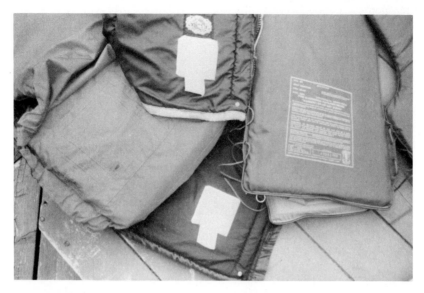

Fig. 6-4 Look for these USCG approval labels when you purchase a PFD.

sized for ease of emergency donning and is available in the following sizes: adult (>90 lb); medium child (50 to 90 lb); and two categories of small child (<50 lb or <30 lb). Additionally, some models are sized by chest circumference. Wearing the near-shore buoyant vest may be preferred where there is a probability of quick rescue. These are areas where it is common for other persons to engage in boating, fishing, and other water activities.

■ *Flotation Aid (Type III, 15½ lb buoyancy).* The flotation aid PFD is designed so that the wearer can place himself or herself in a vertical and slightly backward position, and the device will maintain the wearer in that position, having no tendency to turn the wearer face down (Fig. 6-5). A flotation aid can be very comfortable. It comes in a variety of styles that should be matched to individual use and usually is the best choice for water sports such as skiing, hunting, fishing, canoeing, and kayaking. This type PFD comes in many chest sizes and weight ranges. However, some universal sizes are available. Use the flotation aid in areas where there is a probability of quick rescue such as ones where other persons commonly are engaged in boating, fishing, and other water activities.

Throwable Device (Type IV). Fig. 6-6 demonstrates a PFD that is designed to be grasped and held by the user until rescued and to be thrown to a person who has fallen overboard. Although the throwable device is acceptable in place of a wearable device in certain instances, this type is suitable *only* if there is a probability of quick rescue in areas where other persons commonly are engaged in boating, fishing, and other water activities. It is not recommended for nonswimmers and children.

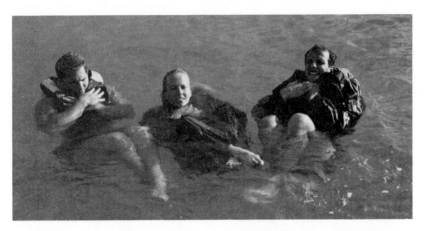

Fig. 6-5 Flotation characteristics of various types of PFDs.

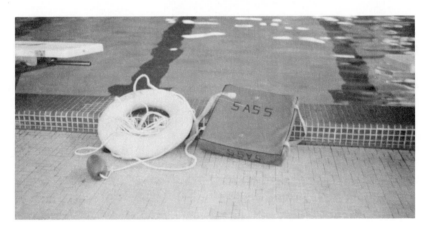

Fig. 6-6 Type IV ring buoy and cushion.

Special Use Devices (Type V). Fig. 6-7 demonstrates a PFD intended only for certain activities in which a boat is used. The label on the device shows approved uses, limitations, size, and performance types. A modified Type V device combining body armor and a PFD is available for boarding and law enforcement officers. (See list of manufacturers in Appendix I.)

Hybrid Device (Type V). Fig. 6-8 shows a device that must be worn to count as a regulation PFD. The advantages of the hybrid devices are they are the least bulky of all types; they have high flotation when inflated; and they are good for continuous wear. The disadvantages are that they may not adequately float some wearers unless partially inflated, plus their inflation chamber requires active use and care. The performance level of this type should be noted on its label (Table 6-1).

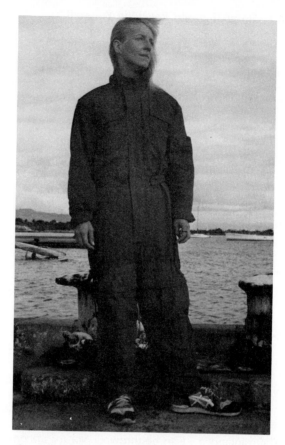

Fig. 6-7 Type V coveralls out of the water.

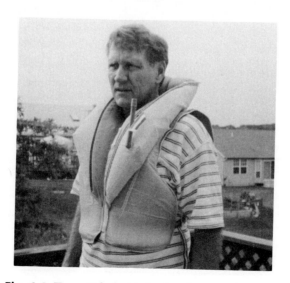

Fig. 6-8 Type V hybrid device (part inflatable).

Table 6-1 Personal Flotation Devices—Approved Types

Type	Best Use	Advantages	Disadvantages	Sizes
Offshore life jacket (Type I, 22 lb buoyancy)	Open, rough, or remote water; rescue slow in coming	Floats best; turns most unconscious wearers faceup in water; highly visible color	Bulky	Two: child and adult
Near-shore buoyant vest (Type II, 15½ lb buoyancy)	Calm, inland water; rescue fast in coming	Turns many unconscious wearers faceup in water; less bulky, more comfortable	Not for long hours in rough water; will not turn some unconscious wearers faceup in water	Four: infant; child—small; child-large; adult
Flotation aid (Type III, 15½ lb buoyancy)	Calm, inland water; rescue fast in coming	Most comfortable; freedom of movement; available in many styles (vests and coats)	Not for rough water; wearer may have to tilt head back to avoid face-down position in water	Many: from child—small to adult
Throwable device (Type IV)	Calm inland water with heavy boat traffic where help always nearby	Can be thrown to someone; good backup	*Not for unconscious persons; not for nonswimmers or children; not for rough water*	Kinds: cushions, rings, and horseshoe buoys
Special use devices (Type V, 15½-22 lb buoyancy)	Only for special uses or conditions	Made for specific activity	See label for limited use	Many varieties and sizes
Hybrid device (Type V, 22 lb fully inflated, 7½ lb deflated)	Must be worn to count as a regulation PFD	Least bulky; high flotation when inflated; good for continuous wear	May not adequately float some wearers unless partially inflated; requires active use and care of inflation chamber	Many adult sizes

Modified from Boating basics—a small craft primer, Seattle, 1989, Outdoor Empire Publishing Co. Note that most type III and V devices cover more of the body than types I and II. Thus types III and V generally provide greater hypothermia protection.

Although the offshore (Type I) and the near-shore (Type II) devices are designed for high seas and rough water uses, they do have drawbacks. They are bulky, encumbering, and difficult to work in or to wear regularly. Most experienced boaters know they can trust these devices in a storm. Accordingly, the boaters suit up only when the barometer falls. Since most drownings do not occur offshore or during inclement weather, many different flotation aids (Type III) are on the market and include vests and various kinds of coats.

Even though they usually depend on a layer of flexible closed-cell foam flotation, some of these coats or coveralls are no heavier than windbreakers or similar garments. They can be worn with comfort on all but the warmest days. They are also excellent in colder climates as outer covering for ice fishing, hunting, cruising and angling from small craft such as bass boats, snowmobiling, or watching a football game in a frigid stadium. They keep the wearer warm, dry, and comfortable out of the water. Should he or she fall in, they provide excellent flotation while simultaneously giving effective hypothermia protection (particularly if the wearer knows what to do in and with them).

The special use devices (Type V) are in part an outgrowth of the heavier, industrially designed flotation aid (Type III) coats and coveralls. Since they have a number of closures, including zippers and Velcro-held flaps, they cannot be donned rapidly. Under certain conditions, some of these devices can take the place of flotation aid (Type III) PFDs, but to meet state and federal carriage standards, they must be worn. Simply stowing them on board will not satisfy safety requirements.

When purchasing PFDs, check them for an approval stamp or decal plus a model approval number. If the device does not perform as required for its particular type, contact your nearest USCG office for corrective action.

PFD POINTERS

PFDs are designed as *aids* in your survival. In the ultimate analysis, the probability of their working properly is proportional to the *degree of knowledge and amount of practice of the user.*

Drowning tends to claim fully clothed, inebriated nonswimmers or poor swimmers suddenly immersed in relatively cold water. Conversely, governmental certification testing for standardization of results involves near-naked swimmers in fairly warm water. To date, this unavoidable bit of dichotomy opens the door to the inner workings of "Mr. Murphy's infamous law." Not only will something go wrong if it can, but the wrong will come about when and where it is least desired or expected.

In-water testing under safe conditions is valuable to make sure you know what your PFD will do to and for you. This experience is especially essential for nonswimmers and poor swimmers. A few specific examples follow to emphasize and enhance the previous statements.

Righting Moment

Offshore life jacket (Type I) and near-shore buoyant vest (Type II) PFDs are designed to turn most unconscious persons upright in the water and hold them in that position. However, since tests are *not* done using fully clothed individuals, the air trapped in the clothing of an unconscious victim thrown face first into the water may counter the PFDs righting moment (Fig. 6-9). Relatively few water accident victims, probably less than 8%, enter the water after being knocked out. Nevertheless, try a fully clothed, facedown entry in your offshore or near-shore buoyant vest under safe conditions (make sure you hold your breath) just to see what happens.

A number of magazine articles have condemned certain types of PFDs as unsafe. A large part of this condemnation stems from the writers' not completely understanding the criteria used in testing and accepting PFDs. Moreover, most of these articles provide pictures showing the PFDs being tested by bathing-suited individuals in fresh water pools.[3] In their concern about the devices' ability to turn and keep wearers upright (as applies to Types I and II), authors may forget the devices'

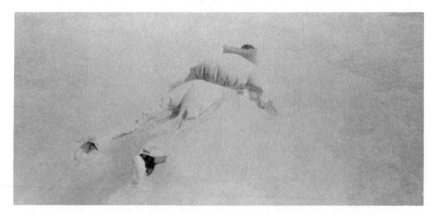

Fig. 6-9 Air trapped in heavy clothing may counter the righting moment in Type I or II PFDs.

potential, especially if Type I, for use in salty rather than fresh water. Hence buoyancy and turning moment will be increased.

Another point underscored by PFD critics is that boating accident reports indicate large numbers of victims have PFDs with them when they drown. This is not an accurate argument.

What actually occurs is that the average boating-related drowning involves a craft less than 16 feet long. Occupants of this size vessel are not required to have wearable PFDs. Since a Type IV cushion meets state and federal requirements, unsuspecting nonswimmers *think* they are safe. They believe the flotation cushion on which they are sitting (which is designed for throwing to someone in distress) can be grabbed should the boat capsize. When the boat does flip, the startled, panicked nonswimmers are usually thrown out of the boat, away from the cushion. Hence, the PFD is available – but only in a manner of speaking.

Federal reporting and classification changes started in 1991 to require more specific information about types of PFDs available in an accident and whether they were used properly. Development of this data should reduce some of the foregoing misunderstanding.

Canoes and Cushions

Repeated testing has demonstrated that a capsizing canoe or other small craft ejects the occupants but not their cushion-model PFDs. This is an elementary outcome of centrifugal force.

> Objects with greater mass and a high center of gravity (e.g., boaters, fishermen, hunters) are flung a greater distance from the center of rotation of the capsizing boat. Hence a nonswimmer who is not *wearing* a PFD is in obvious danger.

Guard against this occurrence by requiring nonswimmers always to don PFDs when using any small craft. Also, research indicates that short-term memory may be scrambled by cold water immersion.[1] Consider this: if you are not wearing a PFD and go overboard – even if it were somehow available and/or reachable – you might have a hard time remembering where you put it or how to don it.

Another aspect of Type IV cushions is that they *are* cushions and their intended use is for sitting. The intended use of other types of PFDs differs. Therefore do not use PFDs as abrasion barriers or buffers between heavy objects. Even though they will take a lot of abuse, you might inadvertently tear them or cause them to function improperly.

A final warning on Type IV cushions concerns their straps. *Do not* allow them to be worn as backpacks, for if they are, during immersion they will act to hold a person's head down. Rather, grasp them to the chest while lying on your back in the water.

Two-Sided PFDs

With some near-shore (Type II) and flotation aid (Type III) models, telling the inside from the outside, particularly when in a hurry, can be difficult, especially when you attempt to tie, zip, or belt yourself into a wrong-side-out PFD rapidly. To guard against such hindrances, be sure you know your PFD well enough to distinguish the back from the front. Do not place yourself in situations in which rapid and distracted donning may be necessary. Always wear your PFD *before* you really need it. Finally, apply retroreflective tape, obtained in sports or auto parts stores, to the outside shoulders of the device (or to the hoods of jackets) (Fig. 6-10). In addition, letter your name on the front or above a breast pocket. The retroreflective tape helps determine the outside of the device in poor lighting situations and helps others find you at night. The name marking ensures everyone has a PFD adjusted to fit properly.

For the water rescuer, other basic additions include a whistle to help in locating you easily and a securely stowed, quickly reachable sheath

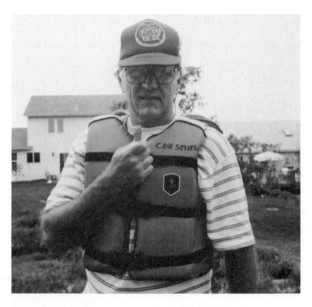

Fig. 6-10 A well-outfitted PFD. Name, retroreflective tape, and whistle are in place and ready for service.

knife, which allows you to cut yourself out of tangled lines or strainers.

Advanced rescuers often attach **prusiks** and **carabiners** to their PFDs. Prusiks are short loops of small-diameter, high-strength line. Carabiners are metal rings, usually *D* shaped, closed with a screw fitting. Both are used in rigging lines for rescues, boat moorings, and other situations in which heavy loads and strains are involved.

Kapok Versus Closed-Cell Foam

Consider the differences between flotation devices using kapok in sealed plastic bags and those using closed-cell foam. The former is less expensive, but once the bag is punctured, the kapok readily absorbs water. The final decision is the buyer's, but usage considerations compared to price are important. Although kapok absorbs water, it does not sink but floats in a soggy mass. However, a water-logged PFD is just about useless per design specifications. A number of throwable device (Type IV) closed-cell foam cushions are available. Since kapok cushions are especially susceptible to puncture, the higher priced, closed-cell foam models may prove more economical over time.

Crotch Strapping

A hold-down strap may be needed in flotation aid (Type III) vests and coats. Since these devices have much buoyancy (but a poor swimmer does not), the more he or she struggles, the higher the PFD rides on the wearer if no such strap is in place. The devices will not come off, generally settling under the armpits, but the exhausted wearer's mouth may stabilize precariously close to the water's surface. Even when the water is not moving, its pressure may squeeze a person's lower abdomen sufficiently to allow a PFD to slip upward. Once again, it is important to practice with a device before unplanned plunges and to tighten or adjust the PFD if necessary. Of note, swimming on the back results in less ride-up by the PFD.

Flotation coats intended for colder climates usually have hold-down devices built in. The devices serve two purposes: (1) securing the bottom of the coat and (2) providing hypothermia protection and insulation to the groin area. Flotation coats or windbreakers with drawstrings in their bottom seams can be tightly cinched around the posterior as a hold-down measure; to slow heat loss and the advent of hypothermia; and to trap air and increase buoyancy (Fig. 6-11). If your PFD needs but does not have a drawstring, simply insert a long, preferably heavy-duty, shoestring or bootstring into the lower seam or selvage around the device's bottom. (This may be needed on some float coats or designer-

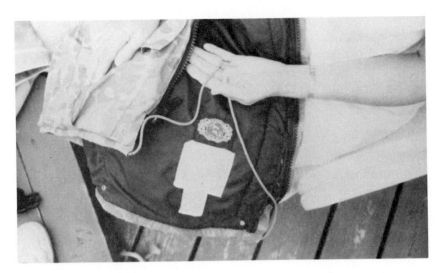

Fig. 6-11 Placing a drawstring in a Type III float coat.

style float vests — models that look as though they are filled with down.)

Children's flotation aid (Type III) devices are available with straps on both the bottom and top. The former keeps the child from slipping down in the device. The latter is an aid for quickly and surely scooping the child from the water.

Accessories

Attaching plastic or brass whistles as pull tabs on PFD zippers is an inexpensive, yet effective idea. When hands are cold, it is difficult to grasp a small zipper tab, and situations may arise that require getting out of the PFD in a hurry (e.g., its snagging an underwater obstruction in flood waters). The larger whistles are more easily grasped. In addition, the trill of the whistle can be heard much farther than a human voice. Flares, small mirrors, and strobe lights should be attached to PFDs of potential rescuers or anyone who might go overboard in large bodies of water to help spot them. Federal requirements for flares and pyrotechnics for coastal and Great Lakes boaters must be observed.

Ice fishermen or cold water anglers should carry emergency ice picks. They are easily constructed as follows: aluminum tenpenny nails can be driven down the long axis of 3-inch broom handle sections; the protruding nail tips are stuck into small plastic foam balls or corks; and shoestrings are used to tie the picks to upper pockets in the PFD or outerwear. The shoestrings can also be used to attach yourself to flotsam, an overturned and unrightable or unenterable boat, or others in the water.

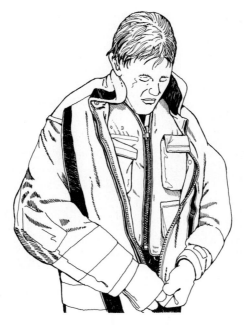

Fig. 6-12 Type III device worn *under* a fire fighter's turnout coat.

Another accessory item is flotation pants. These outerwear trousers float as well as the coats with which they are designed to be worn. They are not, however, classified as approved flotation devices per federal standards. They do make a warm, comfortable, super-buoyant outfit for the hunter and fisherman. Also, if worn by themselves, they will not turn someone upside down in the water.

PFDs As Underwear

Several flotation aid (Type III) PFDs that can be worn beneath outer clothing are on the market (Fig. 6-12). Some foam-insulated models look, wear, and feel exactly like down-filled vests. Their warmth and comfort are enhanced out of the water by wearing them under coats or windbreakers. If used in the water, the outer clothing hinders the vest's riding upward. A somewhat similar device is worn on the hips. Inner rib pads prevent its riding upward. It does not encumber arm, chest, or shoulder movement and can be worn under other clothing. Both of the foregoing styles work well under turnout gear.

Pneumatic Devices

Several manufacturers have developed compressed air or CO_2-inflated devices (Fig. 6-13). At present, they have not been approved for

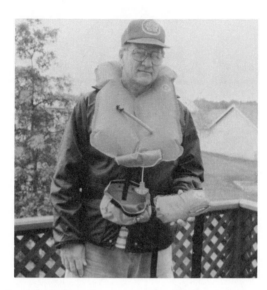

Fig. 6-13 Inflated and deflated pneumatic flotation device. This device is automatically inflated when immersed, or it can be toggled and orally inflated.

recreational use. The only type now accepted is a hybrid that combines an inflatable collar on a device similar to a lightweight flotation vest. This style of approved Type V device is light and comfortable enough for wear in very hot environments.

You might wish to review the other pneumatics in addition to the approved PFDs. Remember, however, that they do not take the place of approved models as far as governmental boating safety agencies are concerned.

Several inflatables feature automatic CO_2 mechanisms that are triggered by immersion. One model is designed to be thrown to a person in distress. When it hits the water, it begins to inflate (Fig. 6-14).

Earlier, simpler designs, which are basically yoke or "Mae West" type air bladders, can be placed inside coats and other outer clothing and are orally inflated when needed. Another concept is a small raft easily carried (when deflated) inside a flotation coat's pocket. It also is orally inflated.

Aquatic Insurance

PFDs provide a form of aquatic insurance. Attempting to understand your life insurance policy completely at the particular moment you need it most simply cannot be done. But a lot of otherwise bright rescuers find themselves in a similar precarious predicament with(out) their PFDs. If

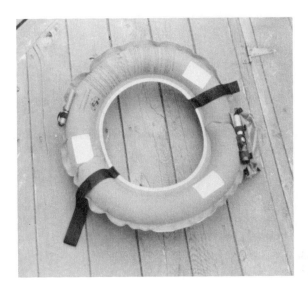

Fig. 6-14 A "man overboard" throwable, autoinflatable pneumatic device.

in the past you have been a less-than-ardent proponent or infrequent user of PFDs, take time to check what is currently available. Most larger sporting goods companies have catalogs from major PFD manufacturers if not samples of the latest gear. When you or your department decides to acquire flotation gear, review the various types of PFDs (actually try them in water if possible). Attempt to compare use against price while factoring in the weather and environmental aspects of your personnel and probability situation. (See Appendix I for PFD sources.)

This tremendously functional, protective, yet comfortable wearing apparel can be used by rescuers and by boaters, fishermen, hunters, and/or persons engaged in almost any type of outdoor pursuits. The comparatively small amount of time, money, and effort you expend updating your PFD proficiency cannot begin to match the losses these devices are designed to prevent.

CHAPTER SUMMARY

REMEMBER: PFD means *personal flotation device*. Make sure your PFD fits *you* properly and *you* have tried it out in the water while fully clothed. Otherwise, it may turn into a *probable floundering demonstration*.

PRETEST ANSWERS

1. True
2. b
3. e
4. False

REFERENCES

1. Cooper K: Respiratory and thermal responses to cold water immersions. In Proceedings of cold water symposium, Vancouver, May 1976, Canadian Red Cross.
2. Federal requirements for recreational boats, Pub No DOT 514, Washington, DC, 1986, Department of Transportation.
3. Life jackets, Consumer's Report, pp 410-412, Aug 1982.

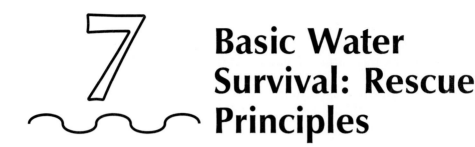

Basic Water Survival: Rescue Principles

OVERVIEW

The preceding chapters in this part of the text provided instruction on safely entering and exiting the water in emergencies plus basic information on personal flotation devices. This chapter expands the foregoing information by presenting longer term, in-water survival techniques. It also introduces simple rescue procedures.

OBJECTIVES

After studying and practicing the topics covered in this chapter, the reader should understand:
1. Appropriate use of differing survival techniques
2. Water survival in "heavy clothing"
3. Elements of in-water heat retention
4. HELP and huddle
5. Simple rescue methods
6. Basic throwing rescue devices
7. One-on-one water extrication

PRETEST

1. A fire fighter accidentally entering the water should immediately remove self-contained breathing apparatus because it will quickly drown him or her. (True or false?)
2. Clothing removal and inflation are no longer considered primary in-water defenses because (a) clothing removal makes a person colder; (b) most clothing is at least neutrally buoyant; (c)

a person must immerse his or her face to untie shoestrings; (d) none of the above; or (e) all of the above.

3. Rolling into a fetal position when immersed and wearing a personal flotation device (a procedure called *HELP*) can reduce body heat loss by (a) 30%; (b) 60%; or (c) very little.

4. When entering the water from an elevated position, always look straight out before jumping. This will (a) help you determine if rescuers are enroute; (b) allow you to gain a better vertical orientation for water entry; or (c) tell you about water currents. Choose the most appropriate reason.

Pretest answers are at the end of the chapter.

SURVIVAL ALTERNATIVES

The text has repeatedly stressed that a personal flotation device (PFD) is your primary professional in-water survival tool. Although this focus on the need for proper PFD use seems elementary and self-evident, the precedent has not always been so. Until relatively recently, major aquatic safety training programs taught other, preferred survival methods. In these courses PFD usage was encountered last *if* time allowed. Part of the reason for this widespread oversight was that aquatics instructors and institutions knew relatively little about the statistics and causes underlying water accidents. Additionally, the few types and limited styles of PFDs then available did not encourage public examination and use.

Times have changed, with water safety and rescue personnel becoming much more aware of the role of flotation devices at the head of the self-rescue and survival line. However, since older techniques still are taught, reviewing and comparing them to the concepts offered in this book are worthwhile. Principle among these now somewhat bypassed methods are clothing inflation and face-down, motionless "drown-proofing," or survival swimming.

Clothing Inflation

In clothing inflation practice, students are taught to remove their pants, knot the cuffs, then inflate them.[1] This practice grew from naval experiences in World War II. Even though sailors participating in combat engagements should be wearing life preservers, large numbers of them entered the water without flotation devices, and many subsequently drowned. To counter these losses, survival specialists developed clothing inflation procedures.

> Even though this survival alternative was basically intended for survivors of ship sinkings miles from shore in relatively *warm salt* water (primarily the equatorial areas of the South Pacific where almost anyone can float), a number of water safety programs still teach it as a standard practice.

When this practice is considered in peacetime situations in which few individuals are suddenly deposited in large offshore situations, a series of questions immediately arise. For instance:

- If this is intended as a long-term, big-water survival ploy, why is the person not already wearing a PFD?
- How many people suddenly find themselves deposited in the middle of large bodies of water without any nearby source of safety? (If it appears likely you might tumble out of a craft that conceivably could be blown or carried away from you, do not be an aquatic statistic — wear your PFD!)
- Since water is normally colder than air or the people immersed in it, what happens to body heat loss rates when clothing is removed?
- What part of the body must be repeatedly immersed to untie shoestrings before removing shoes and pants?
- How easy is it to untie knotted leather shoestrings   derwater?
- What comparative level of training, practice, and aquatic skill is needed to carry out this maneuver safely?
- Can it be accomplished while someone is carried rapidly downstream in a tumbling river?
- Can an individual who is proficient in this technique as a physically fit teenager, successfully remember and perform it in an emergency situation without immediate prior practice 20 years later?
- If an uninformed person observes clothing removal (not realizing it is being removed to be inflated), might the scene reinforce misguided thoughts of heavy clothings' dangers?
- Clothing inflation provides extra buoyancy for use in crashing seas — but is this the normal inland rescue environment?

Answering these questions, especially with an understanding of what causes most serious water accidents (i.e., cold water, alcohol, and poor swimming skills), supplies evidence to begin ruling out using clothing inflation practice as a primary survival technique.

Although some parts of the disrobing and inflation routine are usable, overall it is quite dangerous. These dangers include the following:

- Rapid cooling resulting from insulation loss and vigorous activity
- The need to immerse the head, face, nose, and mouth in an emergency situation
- Perpetuation of the myth of clothes pulling a person under

Conversely, air trapped by or blown into clothing is a definite benefit discussed later in this chapter. However, the method of inflation or air entrapment, for best possible results, should not include clothing removal. One possible exception to this rule might be extra-heavy footwear. Most shoes made of leather, rubber, plastic, or canvas either float or are at least neutrally buoyant. If a person is careful and practiced in remaining on his or her back, sufficient air may be trapped in the footwear to keep toes above the surface (Fig. 7-1). For example, the heavy clothing section of this chapter examines the potential for floating in chest and hip waders. Most relaxed swimmers can remain motionlessly afloat in flooded footwear.

> Even if water fills an object, the water inside is no heavier than the water outside. If the inner water is warmed by body heat, it is actually more buoyant than the surrounding, cooler fluid.

However, should the situation occur that boots or shoes are a deterrent to survival, they should be jettisoned with as little struggling and facial immersion as possible.

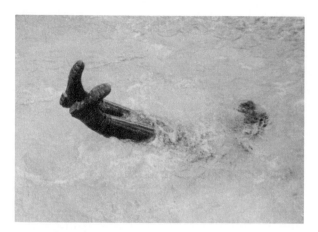

Fig. 7-1 Falling in toes last to trap more air in footwear.

Drown Proofing Comparison

Drown proofing is a survival technique that features a motionless, facedown float occasionally punctuated by pushing down with the arms while raising the head to breathe.[5] It is a good method for teaching basic relaxation to beginning swimmers, but unless it is used in water only a few degrees cooler than body temperature, far too much heat is lost from the immersed face and neck. Studies have proved that this is the fastest possible way to lose body heat, short of being anchored underwater.[3] In addition, breathing orifices are continually immersed, and there is little opportunity to see if help is coming or to yell to possible rescuers (Table 7-1).

Several factors have influenced some water safety organizations to continue emphasizing drown proofing. A primary one is that drown-proofing practitioners have not been sufficiently informed about the need to counter heat loss in long-term survival situations. Basically, they are conditioned to teaching physically adapted persons in fairly warm, controlled swimming pool surroundings—with little relationship to actual survival conditions. Also, they have not learned the potential of modern PFDs.

Drown proofing has saved lives in warm waters, and it is a helpful technique in teaching relaxed facial immersion, but as an overall emergency response, its use is limited. Knowing about and properly using approved flotation devices is a far better alternative.

Note that back floating may also suffer from some of the foregoing problems, mainly that of having the back of the head immersed so that body heat loss is increased. However, back floating is only a secondary practice. Properly wearing a PFD and practicing the heat reduction

Table 7-1 Comparison of In-Water Survival Techniques

Technique	Survival Time in 50° F Water*
HELP	4 hr 10 min
Huddle	4 hr
Floating still with PFD	2 hr 15 min
Treading water†	1 hr 45 min
Swimming	1 hr 15 min
Drown-proofing	1 hr

Modified from Hypothermia and cold water survival, Tulsa, Ok, 1980, Recreational Boating Institute.

*Approximate median lethal exposure.

†This is twice the median limit given per the 50 × 5 rule in Chapter 3 because these tables are extrapolated from data for healthy, *young* males.

ploys described in this chapter comprise the *main ways* to survive if you cannot get out of the water.

HEAVY CLOTHING FLOTATION

Common sense seems to indicate that someone falling into the water while wearing multilayered, insulated clothing would sink like the proverbial rock. This is not necessarily true. If a panicked, unknowing, unpracticed person finds himself or herself in this situation, conventional wisdom applies, with the final results predictable. Conversely, with someone who does know what to do and who is practiced, the result may be different from the expected outcome. To understand this other outcome in which the apparently "heavily" clothed, presumably doomed person survives, reinvestigating a few basic flotation facts is necessary.

Flotation essentially is based on an object's or person's displacing a volume of water that weighs more than he or she does. PFDs do this by combining a large volume with relatively little inherent weight. In fact, the more the PFD is immersed, the lighter it becomes. This is the reason a PFD will rapidly return you to the surface if you fall in the water while wearing it.

Insulation in clothing produces roughly the same result relative to heat retention. Many layers of dead air space trap heat next to the body. Again it is a volume versus density relationship. The greater the volume of dead air insulation surrounding you or the less dense the material (allowing more insulating cells) you are wearing, the warmer you remain.

> If a person enters the water wearing high-volume, low-density garments, he or she will float *unless* the wearer does something to decrease clothing volume and increase its density.

The most dangerous maneuver is struggling in the water to the point of compressing the garment and loading its pores and cells with water, thereby driving out supporting air. Secondary to struggling is positioning. As previously mentioned, if the individual remains horizontal on the surface, water pressure squeezes relatively little air from clothes. (Water is also warmest at the surface.) But when a vertical orientation is assumed, increasing pressure on submerged, lower parts of the body again drives out supporting air, and the body is in colder water.

Similarly, by not struggling, back floating, and conserving trapped air volume, a person both floats and stays warmer or at least warmer than if he or she were naked, completely immersed, and surrounded by colder water. This last point is important. Note that body-warmed layers of water keep you comfortable in a wet (diving) suit. Water held between your skin and the inner side of the suit (or clothing) is much warmer than water outside the suit.

> Similarly, warmed water inside clothing slows overall heat loss unless it (and insulating air) is pumped out by struggling or attempting to swim.

Especially in water 10° to 15° F less than body temperature, removing clothing (per the inflation routine) may be damaging if not deadly.

In this discussion, do not forget that a PFD, preferably a float coat or flotation coveralls (better), is the true survival ticket. But suppose that for some reason you do not have a PFD and you do fall in water while wearing clothes, especially heavy clothes. What do you do? Moreover, how could something like this happen? For the fire fighter, the scenario is not hard to imagine. A number of fire fighters have fallen into flooded, fire-scene basements or elevator wells. Also, with home pools more common, falling into one of them on a dark or smoke-obscured night is not an impossibility. Responding from shore side to dock fires or to manufacturing facilities or over-water warehouse alarms is another possibility.

Police and emergency medical services (EMS) responders could also find themselves unintentionally in the water in such circumstances, and flash floods can catch anyone unaware. In this regard, the more surface paving in a given area, the less ground water that will be absorbed – and that free water must go somewhere. You should prepare carefully for such possibilities and plan to use your best and most secure equipment. But if being caught without a PFD is at all possible, Murphy and his infamous law will most certainly try to have you do it!

Heavy Clothing Floating Progression

The progression used to teach floating in, for example, fire fighter turnout gear, insulated coveralls, chest or hip waders, and body armor is very similar to the initial back flotation drill outlined in Chapter 5. Before discussing it in detail, a few essential safety rules must be reviewed and underscored. When trying to float in heavy clothing, especially for the first time:

- Start in water no deeper than your chest.
- Have PFD-equipped safety swimmers in the pool, one for each learner.
- Take your time and make sure *everyone* understands what is being done.
- Move to deep water *only* after everyone demonstrates floating ability in the shallow end.
- For learners who cannot seem to float in the shallow section, provide them with a PFD (preferably worn under their coat) in the deeper water. Make a careful note of who is a nonswimmer. Ensure they wear a PFD and are closely watched by their safety assistant.
- Repeatedly lifting sodden turnout gear (and yourself) from the water is hard work. This drill is *not* recommended for grossly out-of-condition individuals or those who have cardiovascular problems or deficiencies.
- Especially in deep water, provide one safety swimmer, wearing a PFD, for each learner. All initial deep-water learning takes place close to (within reaching distance) of the side of the pool.

  Skill Drill 9. 1. The progression begins with learners wearing full fire fighter turnout gear on their hands and knees parallel to the side of the pool. Before getting into this position, learners should take off their helmets and push them under water. Test the helmets for buoyancy, for they will be used as flotation aids later. They are *not* worn during this initial immersion. (NOTE: Most helmets of any type such as used on motorcycles or snowmobiles will float and can be used as a self-rescue or throwing aid.)

  2. The learners take a deep breath, cover their nose and mouth with one hand, and while remaining in a tucked position, roll into the water (Fig. 7-2).

  3. The in-water assistants aid the learners in rolling onto their backs while the learners keep their knees up and arms crossed over their chests. The assistants may help stabilize the learners as the latter take their hands away from their faces and attempt to become motionless on their backs.

  4. The learners may grasp the collars of their clothing to keep trapped air inside, or they may actually blow in air and then trap it if the collar openings are big enough to allow doing so. (NOTE: Insulated *waterproofed* clothing floats especially well because the insulation and waterproofing combine to hold air.)

  5. When all the learners appear stable and are floating in a tucked position by themselves, have them try to back paddle gently to the side, then bounce themselves out. After allowing water to drain while they bend over the

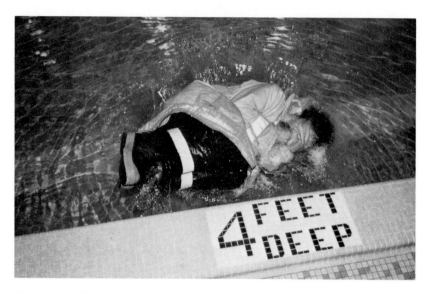

Fig. 7-2 Rolling into the water while maintaining a tucked position.

pool edge, they do a spread-eagle roll away from the side across the pool deck.

6. After draining water from clothing and boots (from the boots by lying on their backs and elevating their feet), the learners are ready to enter the water by covering the nose and mouth, then gently falling backward from a standing or sitting position. *Do not allow back dives into the shallow water.* The assistants help the learners into a tucked back float. Their legs are drawn up toward their chests to aid flotation by maximizing the amount of trapped air in their boots and to reduce heat loss. Most people float better the more they repeat the water entry because they become more relaxed and their wet outer clothing traps and holds air more efficiently than when dry.

7. After removing themselves from the water as in step 5 above, the learners don their headgear. *Do not tighten chin straps.* The learners repeat the backward fall into the pool, but they place one hand over their nose and mouth and one hand on top of their helmet. This latter move keeps the front or back of the helmet from bashing them in the nose or neck when they strike the water. After becoming stable on their backs in the water, the learners remove their helmets and place them brim down on their chests. Air trapped in the helmets will aid buoyancy (Fig. 7-3).

8. After all learners have demonstrated they can safely perform step 7 above in shallow water, move to the deep end. *Follow all deep-water precautions.* Have the learners fall in backward while wearing their helmets; properly remove them; then back paddle to the side of the pool.

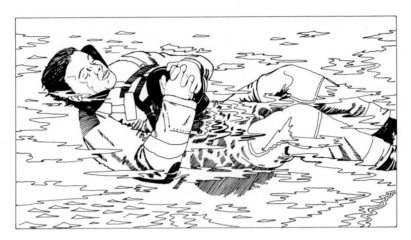

Fig. 7-3 Air trapped in the helmet aids flotation.

9. The final step is to have the learners push their feet down and completely flood their boots so that they are vertical in the water. As described in Chapter 5, have them hold onto the pool side with one hand while pointing across the pool with the other. Have them rotate their head as far back as possible while *not* moving their feet or body from the vertical, then take and hold a deep breath and *slowly* let go of the pool edge. Most should have no trouble floating with their face out of the water. To breathe, they gently press down with their hands, expel used air as their face rises, draw in fresh air, then return to the same floating level.

Through this exercise, just about everyone learns that he or she actually can float with all that (out-of-the-pool) extremely heavy clothing on. The few who cannot master the technique will appreciate more completely why they *must* wear a PFD on waterside calls. NOTE AGAIN: The purpose of this exercise is to demonstrate that "heavy clothing" will not necessarily sink a practiced wearer.

Additional Flotation Tips

An additional element is to have someone in normal fishing or hunting clothing and wearing chest or hip waders follow the same progression. There should be no difference in floating. But just as with the turnout gear, there is no rule that says PFDs and waders cannot be worn together. In fact, putting a PFD over waders should become a habit after seeing this demonstration (Fig. 7-4). The waders, even when filled with water, will float most of the time.

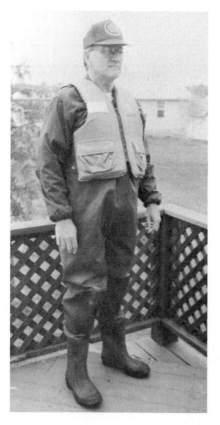

Fig. 7-4 A super water safety combination—waders *and* a PFD.

A similar learning progression may be followed for police body armor. It usually floats well as long as the outer, protective plastic cover is not punctured.

Fire fighters' self-contained breathing apparatus (SCBA) may also float and can be safely demonstrated, providing certain rules are followed:

1. *Do not* encourage the use of SCBA equipment for diving. This is strictly an emergency, self-survival technique. Also, since the SCBA control valve must be fully opened to allow free flow underwater, it is frequently damaged and may need replacement.

2. The face mask must be as tight as possible, with compressed air

Table 7-2 Flotation Potential of Self-Contained Breathing Apparatus (SCBA) Tanks*

Type of Tank	Capacity	Buoyancy
Steel	100% full	Negative (sinks)
	50% full	Positive (barely)
Aluminum	100% full	Neutral
	50% full	Positive (floats)
Fiberglass	100% full	Positive
	50% full	Positive

*NOTE: Individual tanks may vary. Test their buoyancy *only* in safe, supervised, shallow conditions.

pressure from within the mask, along with the tightened face straps, keeping water out of the mask.

3. Under certain conditions, specific types of SCBA tanks are heavier than water, with the wearer unable to float unless his or her buoyancy and that of his or her clothing will support the weight of the tank. Generally half to completely filled steel tanks are heavier than water; half to completely filled aluminum tanks are neutrally buoyant; and fiberglass tanks with any loading, full or empty, *probably* will float (Table 7-2).

4. When demonstrating floating with SCBA tanks, be sure the participants have completed Skill Drill 9. Also, follow all safety procedures used in Skill Drill 9 and attach a safety line to the student. Note that the SCBA tanks usualy do not roll a wearer on to the stomach.

RETAINING BODY HEAT

As the foregoing rules have emphasized, in-water survival techniques must be designed to reduce the loss of heat to the water.

Heat is lost through three principle body areas: the head, neck, and face; armpits and chest sides; and groin.

Most of these areas are more susceptible to heat loss because they have relatively little covering by body fat. More importantly, large-bore blood vessels carrying substantial amounts of warm blood are positioned close to the surface in each of these areas. Nature and evolution have attempted to protect these blood vessels by providing a covering of hair over most of the exposed surfaces. This hair insulates from cold and also works as a heat exchanger in warm climates. In warm areas perspiration trapped in hair over warm blood vessels evaporates, thereby reducing the temperature of the skin, blood vessels, and the blood within them.

Humans have been conditioned to reduce heat loss through their posture. For instance, a small baby, who is highly subject to hypothermia because of a lack of hair, skin fat, and shivering ability, automatically will roll into a fetal position. By doing this, he or she covers the groin and usually keep the arms tightly placed over the armpits.

Heat loss from the area above the collar bone to the top of the skull represents 40% to 50% of the body total. To combat this heat loss, all of us are encouraged from the time we are small children to wear hats or suitable head covering.

Survival in the water follows similar rules. Reducing heat loss from the head is the highest priority, followed by loss from the armpits and groin. The fetal tuck described in learning to float while fully clothed in heavy footwear is a major contributor to a ploy called *h*eat *e*scape *l*essening *p*osition (or *p*osture) (HELP), which was developed by the Canadian researcher, Dr. John Hayward.[2] HELP is an in-water tuck or head-up fetal position.

Through HELP, a practiced person can reduce his or her heat loss by as much as 60% compared to the loss from moving while swimming or treading water (Fig. 7-5).

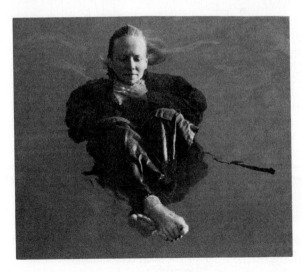

Fig. 7-5 Heat escape lessening position (HELP). Notice the hands insulating the HELPer's throat while keeping the fingers pliable. Also note the excellent buoyancy of Type V coveralls.

Skill Drill 10. To get into HELP, a back floating person crosses the ankles (thereby helping to cover the groin); pulls the knees to the chest; and crosses the arms across the chest while clamping the upper arms on the sides. Although a few very buoyant persons can do this without a flotation device in fresh water (many can do it unaided in salt water), a PFD must almost always be worn for best results. Since heat loss from the immersed back of the head can be a problem, the head is tilted forward and out of the water. Maintaining this position while wearing a PFD normally can triple survival times.

There is a problem, however. Some persons, depending on the type of PFD they are wearing, either roll from side to side or pitch forward while doing HELP. To counteract rolling, move the head sideways opposite to the direction of the roll. Extending the feet in front of the body until a stable position is achieved also stops forward pitching.

In spite of these corrective moves, some people are unable to remain still. If you are in this category, try several different styles of PFDs worn over the type of clothing you normally use in or near the water. After a few experiments, you should discover which device works best for you.

To aid HELP, cross your hands around your throat, almost as if you were choking yourself. This will insulate your **carotid** artery further while keeping your fingers above the water, potentially keeping them warm and flexible enough to grasp a line if one is tossed to you.

In heavy seas HELP frequently results in a person's being turned into the waves. To combat this and the potential for forcing water into your nose and mouth, move one hand up and over your face.

The text has encouraged your covering your nose and mouth when suddenly and unexpectedly entering the water. Now add automatically doing HELP to allow you to stabilize your situation, find your bearings, and determine what must be done next.

HUDDLE

In an emergency most approved PFDs will support two people.

HELP is intended as the first, stabilizing response for one person suddenly finding himself or herself in the water. If more people are near and at least half are wearing PFDs, huddle is in order. Huddle is similar to HELP in that it reduces heat loss, again by approximately 60%.

Skill Drill 11. Two or more persons who are in the water wearing

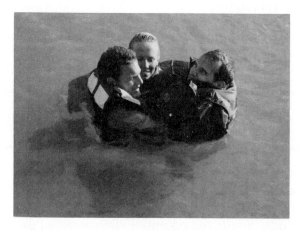

Fig. 7-6 Huddling in a close group conserves body heat, makes a better visual target, and aids group and individual morale.

PFDs wrap their arms around each other's waist. (Draping wet arms around someone's neck *above* the surface will push him or her under the water.) The persons doing huddle also wrap their legs around each other.[4] They may also put their hands inside each others' clothing to keep their hands and fingers warm. Smaller or injured people can be placed inside the huddle to provide them with the greatest warmth (Fig. 7-6).

Huddling provides three essential services:

- It reduces heat loss.
- It aids rescuers in finding persons in the water. Single heads spread out over a large area are difficult to find. Getting them together makes a much larger, more easily perceived visual target.
- It aids morale by allowing and assisting people to talk and to support each other.

When learning huddle, a good procedure is to assume that a number of people are suddenly placed in the water at night. The group members, while keeping their eyes shut, are encouraged to find each other through voice alone. Another method of having everyone appreciate the heat-retention properties of these procedures is to have both HELP and huddling motionlessly performed for a minute or so. Then have the participants slowly move apart. They should quickly appreciate the relative warmth of the still, warmed water next to them. When doing this in an indoor heated pool, it helps to remind everyone of the actual, relatively elevated indoor water temperature, especially when they perceive how much warmer HELP and huddle make them in this comparatively benign setting.

SIMPLE RESCUE METHODS

Part III discusses *team* rescue tactics, which use three main approaches: shore based, boat based, and water based. This section presents *one-on-one* rescue procedures from the same initial approaches.

In simplest terms the foregoing rescue types can be expressed using the Boy Scouts' rhyming rescue rule: "Reach; throw; row; go."[6]

Even in a basic single rescuer mode, the progression from least to most dangerous rescue tactics is the same:

- Shore based is the safest for the rescuers since they stay on land. (This may also include *talking* the potential victims out of the water, thereby allowing them to rescue themselves). In the rhyming mode, rescuers reach or throw.
- Boat based is the next most dangerous because the rescuers may end up in the water. In the rhyming mode, they row.
- Water based is potentially the most dangerous for both rescuers and victim since they are subject to unseen and often unpredictable water factors. In the rhyming mode, rescuers go. Make sure you know (what to do) before you go. The last thing you want to do is enter the water. If there is no alternative, at least take an extension or reaching device with you.

A number of elementary reaching and throwing concepts already have been introduced. Even though they are quite basic, they should not be ignored because most people in serious trouble in the water are only 10 feet (or less) from safety. Potential rescuers should always be alert to anything in or near a potential accident scene that would make a rescue easier. The following are basic suggestions to incorporate into the reaching and throwing techniques:

- Try to position yourself so that the victims will not pull you in. Attempt to work toward them from a stable, dry, elevated area if possible, and lean away from the victims with one side facing them.
- If others are present, have them do the following:
  Continually point at the victims so if the victims disappears, a search point can be established rapidly.
  Send someone to get more help.
  Have one or more persons back you (e.g., by holding onto the rear of your clothing or belt or possibly your legs if you must assume a risky near- or over-water position).
- If throwing a line, stand on the end nearest you. *Do not tie or wrap the*

line around any part of your body. If you do tie the line to yourself, either the victims or the current or both may pull you in. After you have thrown the line, quickly pick it up either to work the victim into shore or to haul it in for another toss. (You may have to modify this step if standing on an uneven, crumbly surface that would interfere with your picking up the line after throwing it.)

- Practice throwing rescues by using a line attached to a flotation device object and having a moving target. Try doing so without any pressure. In almost all initial practice sessions the line(s) is far more likely to land in the nearest trees rather than close to the target. Accurately throwing a line to a moving target under stress takes a lot of practice.
- Resist any urges to jump in to assist the victim *unless* there is no other alternative.
- Have extra throwing lines readily available as a backup.

SIMPLE BOAT RESCUES

> If you are attempting a rescue by yourself from a boat, do not place yourself in a position of danger by focusing solely on the victim. You must watch the victim, but you must also know what is happening around you.

If rowing, do not leave the oars. Get as close as possible with the boat; then extend an oar and pull the victim alongside the boat. Initially do not attempt to pull the victim into the craft because he or she may pull you out or capsize the boat. If possible, have the victim hang onto the stern as you slowly row stern first toward shallow water. If you must bring him or her aboard, do so over the stern because this is usually the most stable part of a rowboat.

If in a canoe, beware. Canoes are second only to logs for instability. If you rescue someone, the preferred technique is again to initially have them grasp an extended paddle and then hang onto the side until you get to safe, shallow water. Do not attempt to bring anyone into a canoe unless you are practiced in proper canoe-based rescue procedures.

Even when dealing with someone outside a canoe, keep your weight as low as possible. Sit on the bottom of the canoe rather than on a more elevated seat or thwart. Always try to reach the person with a paddle or pole first rather than allowing him or her to grab you and upset the canoe.

Do not leave the controls of a motorboat until you have either extended an oar, paddle, or similar object to the victim who has firmly grasped it or the victim has a firm hold on the boat itself. Otherwise you might simultaneously lose control of the boat and the victim. If possible, attempt to throw one or more lines to the victim but ensure that the lines will not foul the boat propeller. Depending on the size of the boat, have the victim hang onto the front of the craft until you slowly ease it into shallow water. If this is not possible, have the victim work around to the stern and climb aboard using the nonrunning engine as a hand and foot hold.

Any time a conscious, moving victim is alongside in the water, hang onto him or her and help the victim into a PFD *before* you try anything else.

If the victim is unconscious or cannot help himself or herself either because of the cold or exhaustion, you must consider bringing the victim aboard. Again attempt to put a PFD on the victim. If safety is located relatively close, the best action probably is to pass a line several times around the victim and secure him or her to the boat with his or her head and face out of the water while moving *slowly* toward safety. If you decide to bring the victim aboard, move to the stern and follow *Skill Drill 12:*

- Turn the victim so he or she faces you.
- Place his or her hands on top of each other, with your hands grasping both of his or hers. (If you only held one hand of a victim in one of yours, a slipping grip might result in totally losing the victim. By holding both hands in both of yours, you have much better control.)
- Gently bounce the victim up and down. When he or she is high enough, step or fall backward (not letting go of the victim) so he or she is bent over the side of the boat. Slowly, and again without letting go, slide your hands down his or her clothing until you can get a secure grip, then pull the victim further into the boat. (NOTE: This technique also can be used ashore to land a victim.)
- Practice this method with different-sized persons until you can do it with relative ease. The idea is to let the water provide most of the upward force rather than depending on brute strength. If carried out properly, a smaller person can land someone much larger. Be aware, however, of potential neck and back injuries. If you even slightly suspect the victim has sustained this type of injury, he or she is best left in the water until he or she can be properly stabilized and placed on

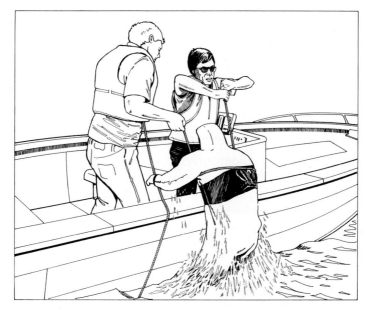

Fig. 7-7 Two-on-one lift practice.

a backboard. Also protect your back. Remember to bounce/lift using your legs, not your back.

- *Skill Drill 13*. If two rescuers are present, the same principles can be expanded by first having the victim face the boat. Pass a line *under* the victim's armpits and around his or her back. Each rescuer holds one end of the line approximately a foot above the point where it emerges from under the victim's armpits. Both rescuers *gently* and jointly bounce the victim into the boat. With practice, this is a very simple, rapid method for assisting people into boats. Again, however, before using it, be sure the victim does *not* have an injury to the neck or back (Fig. 7-7). NOTE: Small diameter line might cut or burn the victim's skin. Either double smaller line or ensure that the victim (in practice or in actual rescue) is wearing heavy clothing.

GO CONSIDERATIONS

If you have no other alternative but to enter the water, keep these principles uppermost in your thinking:

- Drowning humans cannot see, hear, or reason. They have only one driving need and that is for air. They will kill you to get it.[7]

- Even a small child can pull an adult under the surface. This happens when a would-be rescuer allows the child to grab the rescuer about the shoulders or head. The drowning person will use a rescuer as a ladder to climb out of the water.

> As you enter the water and approach, do not lose sight of the victim. He or she may go under the water and you will have to decide where they disappeared or in the worst case you will swim into them.

- Take something that can be extended to the victim with you as you enter the water. Do not get close enough to the victim to allow him or her to grip any part of your body. The object extended or flipped (as you hold one end of it) to the victim can be as simple as a towel, a PFD, or a piece of clothing. If nothing else is available, use your bathing suit.
- In rare instances the victim may actually be keeping himself or herself afloat. If so, try to talk the victim into following you to safety. Similarly, if the person has stopped struggling and has remained on the surface, it probably is safe to get close enough to grab him or her. But try extending a reaching device to the victim first.
- Since the victim may not know you are there (unless you unintentionally rush into them), you may have to touch the victim's head or chest with the extended or flipped object, or you might be able to place it under an outstretched arm.
- Once the victim grasps the extended object, start pulling him or her to safety. Begin talking to calm the victim if you can.
- If the victim should manage to collar you, tuck in your chin, then push yourself straight underwater while grabbing his or her elbows. Place your thumbs on the inside aspect of the joint, dig as hard as possible with your thumbs, and push the victim's arms up and away (Fig. 7-8).

There are two major exceptions to the foregoing: (1) if you are wearing a rescue (dry) suit, or tethered to a rescuer on shore, and are floating horizontally, you may allow and encourage the victim to grasp your feet; and (2) if you are qualified as a lifeguard by the major national water safety organizations, you are entitled to grapple with the victim as you see fit. However, a few words of caution are needed. If you were a lifeguard at age 18 but have not tried a rescue in 20 years, discretion and subscribing to the above procedures are recommended. Also remember that formal water safety classes are primarily oriented toward relatively benign swimming pools. That is *not* your environment.

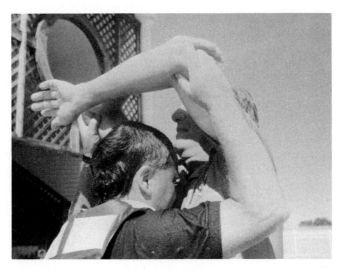

Fig. 7-8 Basic self-protective push away. Note that the rescuer's head is tucked and he is pushing up on the victim's elbows while gouging them with his thumbs.

The previous information is offered as the best procedure in a worse-case situation, which is typical of your actual working conditions.

ELEVATED WATER ENTRY

One final technique is needed. Entering the water backward from a low level, placing emphasis on covering the nose and mouth to defeat torso reflex, has been discussed. But if an elevated emergency entry is required, what procedures are followed?

The first concern in elevated entry is not to land on anything beneath you. The second concern is to land as cleanly and as close to vertical as possible. Hitting sideways or head first could cause you big trouble. Third, guard against torso reflex; but when you enter from a height, your hands may be knocked away from your face.

To deal with these problems, follow *Skill Drill 14:*

- Before entering from a height, look down to ensure nothing is beneath your potential point of entry into the water.
- Look ahead to make sure you are initially stable on a horizontal and vertical axis. In other words, be sure you are straight up and down.
- Take a breath; then place one hand over your nose and mouth. Reach across with the other hand, firmly gripping clothing on your shoulder

or your PFD strap. The hand on your face should be locked in place by the outer arm across your body.

- Step off, crossing your ankles in midair. This position prevents your landing astraddle an unseen object in the water (Fig. 7-9).

In the best of circumstances you should be wearing a PFD when attempting this entry. However, even if you are not, air initially trapped and compressed in several layers of clothing should return you rapidly to the surface.

If an elevated, as opposed to wading, entry is needed to assist a victim in immediate danger, first consider reach, throw, row, then go. If your only alternative is in-water rescue, you have two priorities: (1) not losing sight of the victim and (2) not injuring yourself in an elevated entry.

Skill Drill 15. If you *know* there are no underwater dangers, lean forward; jump with arms spread to the side; and spread your legs, one in front, one in back. Attempt to bring your arms down and forward and your legs together as you enter the water.

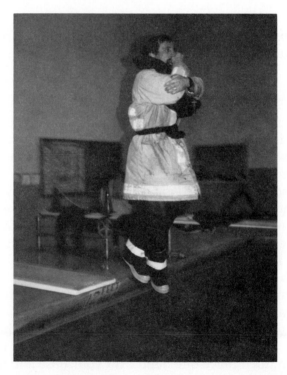

Fig. 7-9 Deep water entry: hand locked over nose and mouth after checking below and straight ahead, then crossing ankles after stepping off.

This *practiced* rescue jump will give you the best chance of maintaining visual contact with the victim. Wear your PFD, and take something with you to extend to the victim. If you are not sure what is under the surface, jumping from a height is a last alternative. If it must be done, use the closed position as initially discussed.

CHAPTER SUMMARY

This chapter has explained:
- The differences between several water survival methods.
- How to learn to float in heavy clothing.
- How to protect yourself from heat loss in the water.
- HELP and huddle.
- The basics of simple one-on-one water rescues and extrication.
- The underlying principles of boat and moving water operations such as the reminder contained in Fig. 7-10.

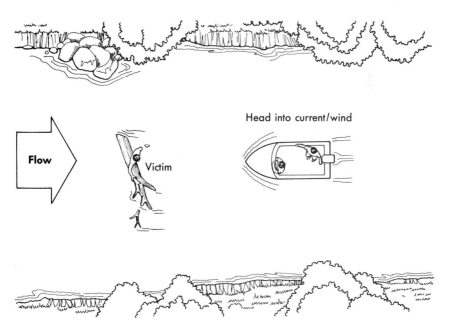

Fig. 7-10 The best method for approaching the victim is to come up into the wind or current, whichever is greater.

PRETEST ANSWERS

1. False — *if* a fire fighter knows what to do and has practiced for this situation
2. e
3. b
4. b

REFERENCES

1. Basic rescue and water safety, ed 2, Washington, DC, 1980, American Red Cross, pp 34-37.
2. Bernhartsen J: Cold water primer, Phys Health Educ Recreat Dance May, 1980.
3. Hayward J et al: Effects of behavior variables on cooling rate of man in cold water, J Appl Physiol 38:6, 1975, pp 1073-1077.
4. Hypothermia and cold water survival, Tulsa, Ok, 1980, Recreational Boating Institute (slide/tape).
5. Lanoe F: Drownproofing, a new technique for water safety, Englewood Cliffs, NJ, 1963, Prentice-Hall.
6. Lifesaving merit badge pamphlet, Irving, Tex, 1992, Boy Scouts of America, p 21.
7. Pia F: The reasons people drown, Larchmont, NY, 1987, Water Safety Films (videotape).

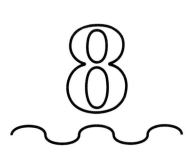

Environmental and Climatic Effects on Rescuers

OVERVIEW

This chapter examines the effects of weather and situation on the individual rescuer. A simple psychological profile of an average rescuer is developed. The "one-hand-for-yourself—one-hand-for-the-victim" rule is defined and applied to different rescue scenes. Basics in avoiding environmental injury to the water rescuer are explained.

OBJECTIVES

After studying this chapter, the reader should gain valuable insights into himself or herself as a rescuer (in *any* environment). In addition, he or she should understand:
1. The rescuer's overall mental status and focus
2. The need to think before reacting
3. Environmental and situational effects on water rescue operations
4. The need for understanding stressors
5. Importance of rest breaks, nutrition, and proper clothing
6. The acronym COLD
7. Adaptive, in-water drill routines

PRETEST

1. Most persons involved in rescue and emergency services can be described as (a) others oriented; (b) altruistic; (c) action oriented; (d) none of the above; or (e) all of the above.
2. For safety and success in the rescue business, a good on-scene

rule is to spend as much time thinking about yourself as about the victim. (True or false?)

3. Environmental stressors can double your reaction time after how many hours of boat operation: (a) 2 hours; (b) 4 hours; or (c) 6 hours. Choose the most correct answer.

4. The heavier and more dense the clothing you wear, the warmer you remain. (True or false?)

Pretest answers are at the end of the chapter.

FOCUS ON THE RESCUER

As might be expected, most rescue texts specifically focus on the victim's needs, especially what must be accomplished to move the endangered person to safety; treat any injuries; and then transport the victim(s) to higher levels of assistance. In this chapter the viewpoint shifts from the victim to the rescuer for three essential reasons, with all three reflecting different properties of water that definitely affect the rescuer:

- The potentially injurious effects of cold water
- The variable dynamics of moving water
- The unexpected, unpredictable force of water

To understand the impact of the foregoing factors, consider the average person involved in water rescue. At the present time, there are comparatively few professional water rescuers spread throughout North America. Even though there are many trained and experienced (but generally part-time) lifeguards, most have not received a comprehensive exposure to all of the facets of water safety presented in this text. In contrast, coastal and surf lifeguarding organizations do have expanded water understanding and competencies; but their organizations are rather small and highly specialized and are located in narrowly limited geographical areas. The same also holds for similar military rescue personnel.

Conversely, a small but growing number of participants have been trained in extended surface and underwater safety and rescue operations by several private and state sponsored schools, primarily in Ohio, Indiana, and Pennsylvania (state) and in California, Colorado, and North Carolina (private) (see Appendix I). However, the number of these specialists becomes insignificant when compared to the fact that half the total population of North America is involved at least once a year in some form of recreational water activity, thereby representing an extremely large body of potential water accident victims.

What this comes down to, especially when considering the statistical, rural input of most aquatic emergencies, is:

- The average rescuer initially responding to a water call probably will *not* have either a great deal of understanding or comparative experience and practice in this field.
- The rescuers will, with the greatest probability, be volunteer fire or emergency medical services (EMS) providers or municipal, county, or state police officers.
- They will not have access to or funding for resources allowing extensive or expensive equipment and resources.

The picture presented above is a worse-case overview. A number of departments and individuals are well beyond this level. However, the point is that for the best results, all procedures should be made as simple, as self-explanatory, and as immediately acceptable as possible.

While holding onto the supposition that the majority of individuals likely to be involved in a water rescue are relatively inexperienced (in aquatics), consider two other facets of this equation: rescuer orientation and the old sailor's rule.

Rescuer Orientation

Most people involved in rescue operations are what psychologists term *others oriented.* Another psychological-philosophical term is *altruistic.*

Most of the wonderful, selfless, people in rescue organizations fit a more or less standard behavioral profile: strongly inclined to help others and just as strongly geared to have a practical, hands-on, action-oriented outlook. In other words, they would rather do something as opposed to analyzing or talking about it.

The effect of water on rescuers must be considered. It is cold; it may be highly unpredictable; and it has great force. In particular, the coldness can be very damaging to a rescuer because, the colder he or she becomes:

- The less clearly the rescuer thinks
- The less rapidly and adequately he or she can respond to the fickle alterations of current
- The less strength he or she has to work against moving water's truly awesome force

Stirring all these factors together may result in relatively inexperienced, action-oriented individuals so intent on doing good things for the person in jeopardy that they totally forget about themselves. When this point is reached, the situation becomes even more complicated because the rescuers' focus, affected by their reduced brain temperatures and their normally driving concern to do something, is *only* on the victim. However, for rescuers in any environment to be effective, they must think clearly and rationally about what they are doing. Doing without thinking, especially in something as possibly life threatening as water, simply cannot be allowed.

Multiple drownings are characterized by this reacting-without-thinking urge. A family member, forgetting he or she cannot swim, will jump into the water to assist a struggling child. Or a series of otherwise trained, professional rescue personnel will run out on unsafe ice, without personal flotation devices (PFDs), and sequentially break through while attempting to aid a victim.

The Old Sailor's Rule

To counter the highly dangerous, potentially deadly progression that might be a plausible result of the foregoing interactions requires calling on a trait not usually found in most rescuers: *being selfish up to a certain point*. This point is best epitomized by an old sailor's saying, coming from the "wooden ships, iron men" days: *one hand for the ship; one hand for yourself!*

> In other words, you must spend as much effort thinking about aiding yourself as you do in assisting the victim.

This can also be taken to mean that you and someone who is designated as a safety observer, both in drills and in on-scene operations, must observe the participants closely. Losing the victim and the rescuer is not your intention. By closely and continually paying attention to what you are doing, rather than totally and exclusively focusing on the victim, you are much more likely to save both.

PREPLANNING FOR THE INDIVIDUAL

The normal environment for the water rescuer is, in at least one way, highly predictable in that it is guaranteed to be wet. *Wet* translates into a several advanced considerations for the individual. Water rescuers must protect themselves from cold, with both exterior and interior protection. *Exterior* refers to how a person envelops, or wraps, himself or herself to keep warm and functioning in a potential or actually hostile environment. The wrapping connotation can also be expanded to include the type of water craft used in rescues and protective clothing, including PFDs.

Exterior protection may also include what is done physically to keep warm. Most people believe exercising or speeding up the heart and respiratory rate is a good way to increase internal heat production, thereby staying warm. It is, *except* in certain long-term survival situations. The relationship of minimized movement in the water and heat retention has already been discussed.

Similarly, on land if you know or at least strongly suspect you will be in a cold situation or environment for a while before someone finds or gets to you, *conserve* energy. Imitate the hibernating bear. Get out of the wind and up off the ground; cover or insulate your primary heat loss area—your head; place as much insulation as possible between you and the nearest, greatest heat loss source (e.g., under you to reduce conduction); roll into a ball (or fetal position); and hope someone finds you soon.

Interior considerations are divided into two primary groupings: (1) what you are thinking and (2) what you are eating. The thinking aspects are addressed later in this chapter in an analysis of simple in-water drill routines (actually teaching you how *not* to think). The following discussion concerns what you should or should not eat (ingest) to fuel yourself efficiently in an aquatic incident (Table 8-1).

Fueling Procedures

Chapter 2 stated that warnings about swimming too soon after eating are somewhat misplaced. People who get into aquatic trouble after eating usually have difficulties because they regurgitate, then aspirate

Table 8-1 Voluntary Responses to Cold

Eating	Exercising	Enveloping
Three square meals and four main food groups daily **Dangerous to ingest:** **Alcohol** **Nicotine** **Caffeine**	Exercise *when appropriate* to stay warm. Do **not** waste energy and heat reserves by exercising in a long-term survival situation!	Rules for dressing: **Loose** **Light** **Layered** Remember COLD (see Table 8-3)

stomach contents. The major problem is not cramps. It more likely is rooted in overeating (and drinking) and then overexercising.

> Working in and around the water burns off large amounts of energy. If internal energy stores are too depleted, the water rescuer may become an unknowing, poorly thinking target of hypothermia. Therefore to protect yourself from energy depletion, you must increase your food intake.

Basically the question is: What should I eat to stay warm best in an aquatic environment? The answer: almost anything! To put it another way, eat three square meals daily, including the four major food groups. However, remember that overeating can cause trouble in the water. During an aquatic encounter, if you are or can become a compulsive nibbler, snacking on small, fairly well-spaced portions of easily digested food, internally you should be all right.

The real question, particularly in view of the larger overall background of hypothermia, concerns what you should *not* ingest. Two substances especially should be avoided: alcohol and nicotine. Alcohol is risky around the water for any number of previously discussed reasons.

One of alcohol's primary effects is that it causes blood vessels that should close to open and vice versa. This mainly results in increased heat loss through the skin as a result of conduction (heat flow from a warmer to cooler, contacting object), evaporation (heat lost in warming water vapor), and radiation (heat projected outward to cooler surroundings) (Table 8-2). Heavy caffeine usage may produce a somewhat similar effect.

Some individuals also have problems with nicotine in a cold environment. As opposed to alcohol, nicotine causes peripheral blood

Table 8-2 Means and Mechanisms of Heat Loss

Type of Heat Loss	Mechanism
Conduction	Direct transfer by surface-to-surface contact
Convection	Heat carried from surface by air currents
Radiation	Transfer through a medium (usually air or water) to a cooler object
Evaporation	Heat used to vaporize fluid on surface
Respiration	Warmed air exhaled from lungs
Elimination	Hypothermia-induced increase in urination

vessels to "overly" constrict. This effect can decrease an individual's ability to deal with cold or at least to function effectively in a colder environment.

Research has shown that in conjunction with normal cold-related constriction of outer blood vessels, circulation in the hands of heavy smokers is even further impeded. This additive constrictive effect can impair manual dexterity. "Tobacco causes vasoconstriction, which reduces blood flow to the skin, hands and feet. There is a resultant stress on the heart and an increased risk of frostbite."[4]

Smoking reduces lung capacity. Thus a person who smokes cannot swim as effectively, especially if called on to swim under water, as he or she would if not a smoker. (NOTE: This last point is doubly important when normal oxygen usage is already reduced by increased situational excitement and adrenaline-based heart and respiratory factors.)

Understanding Stressors

An interesting, partially unexpected, and highly usable aspect of research into boating accidents involves stressors. *Stressors* are internal or external factors that influence an individual's behavior and physical (motor or muscular) performance. The definition can be further subdivided by examining the internal factors on a chemical (drug) or behavioral (e.g., perceptions, outlooks, prejudice or bias) basis. The external stressors are those induced by exposure to environmental factors such as wind, sunlight, noise, vibration, rain or snow, and heat or cold.

The interesting, readily usable results of studying the foregoing concern deteriorations in mental processing, alertness, and reaction time, which develop after exposure to environmental stressors over certain specified time periods.

It was discovered that an average boater's reaction time doubled after approximately 3 to 4 hours' involvement in a normal boating environment.[3] (That is, after being exposed to effects such as the sun, wind noise, and vibration, the research subjects reacted twice as slowly.)

The unexpected part of the findings dealt with alcohol. It was found that alcohol in *very low dosages*, approximately one beer or less per hour, actually improved or reduced reaction time in a person exposed to stressors. Apparently the subtle, relaxing factors involved in imbibing relatively *small* amounts of ethanol helped counteract the derogatory effects produced by the environment. (NOTE: We are *not* necessarily implying that water rescuers should occasionally have whiskey in their on-scene coffee.) The main message is that along with the danger of focusing on the victim to the exclusion of everything else, rescuer exposure to stressors at the accident scene must also be considered.

This comes down again to having individuals and a safety supervisor or observer aware of the need to rotate (when and if possible) people away from the scene for short breaks. Individuals also must be briefed about stressors. In some organizations individuals might be reluctant to take short breaks since they might think to do so would indicate that they could not "take it." Such impressions should be clarified as soon as possible.

The rest breaks should be in quiet, covered, and warmed (or cooled, depending on the circumstances) areas removed as far as practicable from the excitement of the rescue site. Additionally, water rescuers or any outdoor workers should not be expected to be at as high a peak or level at the end of their duty cycle as at the beginning. Involvement with the cold, principly in rainy, snowy, or spray-oriented environments in which individuals could be expected to lose heat while *they paid little attention to the cold and environment themselves* should be underscored. Similarly, outdoor workers, especially around the water, should be provided with head (and eye — sunglasses) coverings. Both the sun's rays on the rescuer's head and the subtle, frequently undetected and unnoticed effect of cerebral heat loss can reduce his or her rescue potential.

USING COLD

COLD is an acronym developed by the U.S. Army's Research Institute of Environmental Medicine at Natick, Massachusetts. The acronym represents a number of steps to take to remain warm in a cold climate.[2]

Since there is a good possibility the water-side rescuer will spend much time in cooler, on-scene surroundings, it would be wise to investigate how to protect yourself from all forms of cold. This protection is from the effects of the cold both out of the water and in the water. A basic point is that if you are exposed to prolonged shore-side cold conditions, should you accidently tumble in, the impact of immersion would be increased manyfold. Table 8-3 introduces COLD. Understanding COLD aids your maintaining a high level of internal warmth and

Table 8-3 COLD

C	Clean	Clean clothes allow more insulating, dead-air pockets between threads.
O	Overheat	Remove clothing layers as exertion grows; decrease perspiration buildup.
L	Loose, layered, light	Trap as much dead air in separate clothing cells as possible, with minimum garment weight.
D	Dry	Wet clothing absorbs and wastes body heat.

From U.S. Army Research Institute for Environmental Medicine. McKeown W: New ways to fight the chill that kills, Popular Mechanics, pp 164-166, Dec 1981.

accompanying mental alertness, thereby helping to ensure you do not find yourself suddenly in the water.

- *C stands for Cleanliness of Clothing.* The basic external method used for keeping outdoor humans warm is wearing clothing. The clothing, in turn, does its job by trapping body-warmed air in spaces between fibers. These fibers of wool, nylon, rayon, silk, or cotton are the primary constituents in the layered materials you wear. The more air these spaces or cells can accommodate, the less heat the wearer will lose (also, the better they float). If dirt, grease, or grime is allowed to accumulate in and block these spaces, the clothing loses its insulating value and efficiency.
- *O stands for Overheating.* It is a reminder to, if at all possible, open or remove layers of clothing while exercising. This reduces the possibility of perspiration accumulating inside the clothes. If moisture is in the clothing, a large amount of heat energy must be expended to dry it. This needless waste of energy reserves is a frequent element in the onset of hypothermia. Because the head and neck give off a large amount of heat, removing head covering may reduce overheating. The hands also radiate large quantities of heat. Therefore, removing gloves when strenuously exercising, if possible, might also be advisable.

Some materials are far less likely to absorb and retain moisture. Cotton is a very poor insulator when wet or moist because it absorbs water *into* its fibers. Wool, on the other hand, normally does not retain water.

Certain types of clothing are specifically designed to "wick" away water. Air currents passing over wet wool fibers draw water vapor away from the material. Silk and most man-made fibers are also water resistant. Hollow fill materials such as polypropylene are excellent insulators, especially when used as undergarments. Since the individual fibers are hollow, they provide even more dead air space for insulation. One possible drawback for fire fighters, however, is that polypropylene has a relatively low flash point.

- *L stands for Loose, Layered, and Light.* Since insulation is based on the accumulation of dry, dead air spaces, the more layers of clothing on a person, the more dead (not moving or exposed) air cells there will be. Loose clothing serves two aims. First, by not being constrictive, it allows better blood circulation while not drawing down energy reserves. This energy deficit would occur if the clothing either restricted or made movement more difficult. Second, improved circulation allows the body to shift its warmed or cooled blood into different areas better. The lighter the clothing, the more readily it can be removed or donned. Also, if it is lighter, it can be carried easily.

    Insulation does not necessarily infer great weight. Several lighter coverings are usually more effective than one heavier garment.

    As with trying out PFDs, deciding which garment(s) work best in expected situations is up to the user.

- *D stands for Dry.* As explained previously, moisture or dampness in clothing wastes energy reserves. For this reason, outer clothing layers should be waterproof so exterior water cannot enter. Conversely, clothing should have some provision for "breathing," thereby allowing internal moisture to evaporate and be carried away. A poncho or waterproof outer garment that also allows the expelling of inner moisture, is an example of this clothing. Most modern outdoor winter clothing incorporates this concept as an essential design principle.

LEARNING NOT TO THINK

Initially, the above title seems to be a conflicting statement. Most of this chapter has been geared to ensure that a water rescuer pays close attention to what is happening so he or she does not jeopardize himself or herself or a potential victim. In this context, *not thinking* does not make sense—or does it? The explanation follows.

What is intended is that rescuers must be so practiced in certain aspects of protecting themselves (and their clients—prospective victims) that they instinctively, properly respond to certain situations *without* becoming involved in long analysis and time-consuming thought.

The best way to ensure this semiautomatic processing is in place when needed is to participate in a number of specific drill routines. For the best outcome, these drills take place in the water and are planned on an individual and group basis.

In other words, learning water safety and rescue techniques solely on the job—when they are most needed—is *not* the best method for ensuring individual longevity. But unfortunately, it happens. One reason for putting off this learning is that an individual may think that such an occasion has little likelihood of ever happening to or involving him or her or that water is not that dangerous and that getting someone to safety is simple (at least in a swimming pool). Through the first chapters in this part of the text, elementary, in-water self-survival drills have been presented. If you have tried them, especially the segments dealing with getting out of the water while wearing turnout gear, you should agree that learning water safety and rescue procedures is not easy.

The following exercises will add to the skills you have learned. They are intended more for individual survival than as team events. (Team drills are outlined in Chapter 9.) For best outcomes, try these routines in a safe, supervised, and usually shallow (initially) swimming pool environment; then move to a similar outdoor setting.

Moving water provides the best training situation for several of these exercises. If possible, again emphasizing safety, attempt to incorporate a moving (at first, not too strongly moving) water element in your training.

Moving Water Drills

In the first part of these drills, it is assumed the participants are in a swimming pool. The pool beginning is suggested because this setting provides better group control and safety with new learners and because in some areas moving water may not be available until it is *not* wanted. Try these procedures in a benign pool environment; then practice in the river.

Three procedures are presented:
- Fast water (simulated) tow and throw
- Current circle
- Breaking seas HELP and huddle

The underlying point of the first exercise is to simulate the feeling of being carried downstream in moving water and then to react properly.

Skill Drill 16. The basic mechanism of the drill is that individuals take turns being pulled across a swimming pool by a length of line *loosely* tied around their waist. All participants wear PFDs. The person on the end of the line must attempt a feet first back float as participants standing on the opposite side of the pool pull on the line (Fig. 8-1).

> The speed of the pulling must be gauged and controlled so that the person in the water can move onto his or her back in the proper downstream orientation.

When the person being pulled has traversed a sufficient length of the pool, several others attempt to throw heaving lines, throw bags, or throw bottles across the towed target (Fig. 8-2). The central idea then becomes one of the shore-side rescuers making accurate and usually repeated throws until the person in the water finally receives a line.

When the person receives the line, he or she rolls over several times, wrapping the line around his or her body. The reasoning behind this maneuver is that if you are thrown a line in moving water, especially cold water, you should not attempt to hang on by grip strength alone (Fig. 8-3). Depending on flow rate, water temperature, time of immersion, and size of the person, he or she may not be able to maintain a simple grip

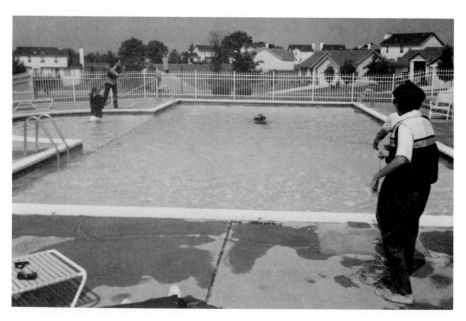

Fig. 8-1 Pool towing drill—feet up and facing "downstream."

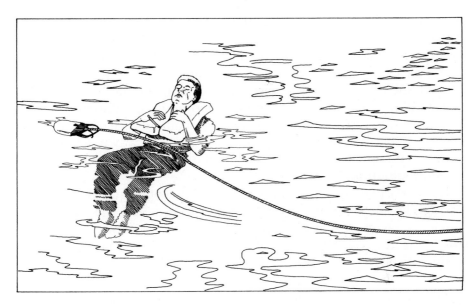

Fig. 8-2 Line thrown across the "victim." In moving current the line must be thrown accurately or the victim will not be able to reach it.

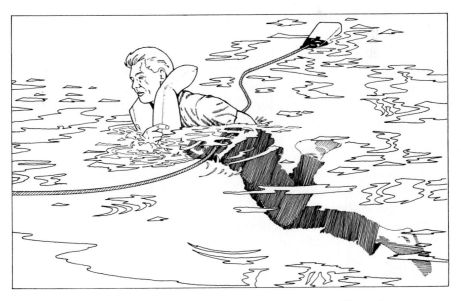

Fig. 8-3 Wrapping up in the line to ensure you will not let go.

on the line. Hence, it is much easier to hold on if additional friction is provided.

There may be controversy about this technique. Some argue that wrapping in the line makes getting out and away from it much more difficult should that be necessary. In addition, should the line become snarled in midstream, with strain developing on the downstream end, the person may be forced underwater. Although this is true, maintaining a sure grip on the line is also paramount. The best way to work this out is to try both approaches in practice and then adopt the one that makes the most situational sense.

Another aspect of this drill is that the line throwers quickly realize that tossing a line across a moving target requires practice. The line throwers should be encouraged *not to replace the line in the throw bags or bottles* should the first toss miss. Rather, they should coil the line, place a small amount of water in the bag or bottle—to weight the thrown end—and heave it again as soon as possible.

The line throwers should also be instructed in using their body as a line **belay.** (*Belay* means to snub or secure.) Just as it is easier for a victim to hold a line wrapped about his or her body, a somewhat similar rule applies to the thrower. Although it has been pointed out that a rescuer must not attach a line to himself or herself lest the victim pull the rescuer in the water, in swift water situations a rescuer, after heaving a line, can quickly place it *around* his or her back (but *not* the whole body). Note that the line does *not* completely encircle the rescuer. Rather, the **bitter,** or shorter, dead end is held in the rescuer's *upstream* hand; the line leads around behind his or her back; and it then is grasped by the downstream hand (Fig. 8-4). In this body belay the "standing" part, or section under strained area leading into the water and to the victim, is on the *downstream* side of the rescuer. This position ensures that the rescuer can work the line without fear of being nudged into the stream.[1]

Current Circle

The concept in this exercise is similar to the tow and throw drill.

Skill Drill 17. Groups of people holding hands and moving in circles can generate a strong current in the shallow end of a swimming pool. Two circles are formed. For best results, they should be formed in the corner of the pool. (Water sometimes rides out of the pool, so bystanders should be warned.) The circles should have at least 10 people each. One group moves in a clockwise direction and the other counterclockwise (Fig. 8-5).

In hip-deep or slightly higher water, a strong current can be generated

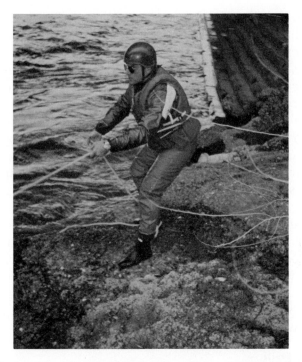

Fig. 8-4 Body belay. Note that (taut) line to victim is always kept on the rescuer's *downstream* side.

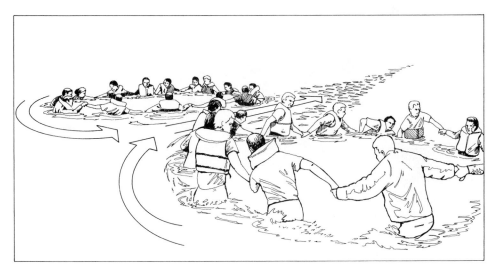

Fig. 8-5 Current circle drill. Groups move in opposite directions, forcing current to flow out into pool.

where the two rapidly moving groups are closest. The rotation should be initiated so that water is drawn from the pool corner out into deeper water. Everyone wears a PFD.

When the circles are rotating as rapidly as the participants can move, an instructor yells, "Break!" When they hear this command, the participants rapidly lie on their backs, attempting to keep their feet "downstream" and in front of them or at least toward the direction they are being carried (Fig. 8-6). If an individual moves appropriately, he or she normally can maneuver to bump into objects and other people with their feet rather than head first. A variation is to have all the participants shut their eyes as if they had fallen into a moving stream at night. They must then become oriented to the flow by feel alone.

Another variant, depending on pool size and group numbers, is to have several individuals attempt to stand in the outrush of the increasingly powerful flow generated by the rotating circles. If respect for moving water was not present previously in these standing individuals, it shortly will be. As they try to maintain their footing while simultaneously dodging the bodies flung at them by the current, they immediately will grasp moving water's force.

Breaking Seas Drill

The purpose of this exercise is to demonstrate that additional forces work against HELP and huddle if they are carried out in a seaway or in rough waters.

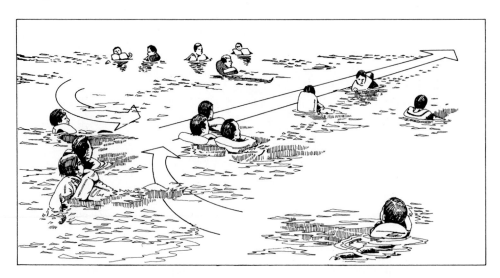

Fig. 8-6 Breaking and "downstream" floating in the current circle drill.

Skill Drill 18. The possibility of this situation ever happening may be remote, but the underlying motivation is to develop a respect for the forces involved with moving water.

Participants wearing PFDs are gathered into the corner of the swimming pool. A canoe, with two persons standing in the water holding its bow and stern, is positioned between the group and the open pool, with one side facing the populated corner. The participants assume HELP positions, and the two people holding the canoe vigorously and alternately pull down on their ends of the canoe. Waves are created that strike the group doing HELP. Most participants will automatically be turned into the waves. If they do not hold their noses, they will very rapidly receive uncomfortably strong doses of water up their nasal passages (Fig. 8-7).

A similar situation can be created for groups doing huddle in the deep end of the pool. If they do not hold each other closely, with their arms underwater and around each other's waist, they will experience much individual bobbing and water cascading down on them.

Moving Water

The ideal training location for initial moving water drills is a narrow stream approximately 25 feet wide and 3 feet deep. The water should be moving at a slow to moderate rate. Training should be scheduled when the water is warmer. Participants should be outfitted in shirts, trousers

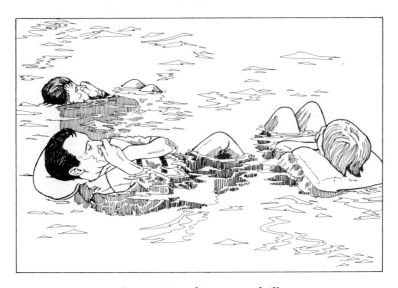

Fig. 8-7 Breaking seas drill.

(or coveralls), and shoes, and everyone should be wearing a PFD. Wearing white water or ice hockey helmets is also a good idea. A safety observer, with no other interfering duties or responsibilities, should be appointed.

This drill would be carried out best as part of the team exercises outlined in Chapter 10. However, this initial set of drills could be used as the first section of a longer outdoor, moving water program.

The tow and throw drill can be used in this setting, with moving water rather than a pulled line providing the motive power.

Before beginning, a search of the bottom should be made to ensure that no snags (e.g., subsurface, bottom-anchored, upstream-pointing tree limbs) and similar dangerous obstacles or hazards are in the stream.

A simple way to check is to stretch a lightly weighted line between banks, then walk it *downstream* along the bottom (Fig. 8-8).

As participants float downstream, lines would be thrown to them. In the actual outdoor setting, several people could be situated at the lower

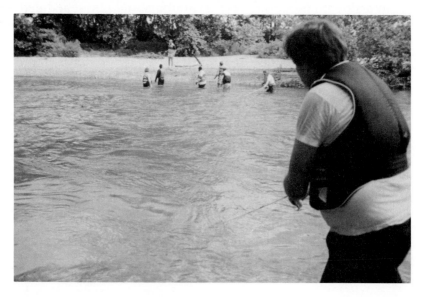

Fig. 8-8 Dragging the stream bottom in a downstream direction, looking for unnoticed obstacles.

part of the stream to ensure a participant is not carried too far. Persons heaving the rescue lines would be cautioned to keep the standing part of the line on their downstream side.

Skill Drill 19. Another appropriate drill is a cross-stream ferry. PFD-equipped participants first attempt to cross the stream singularly. There are two ways to accomplish this in a current. The first is to put your back upstream, then lean on a downstream-positioned pole, canoe paddle, or similar object and shuffle sideways across the current (Fig. 8-9).

The second method is similar, only performed facing upstream. In this method you can see what is coming down the current at you, but the leverage on your staff is less. Try both to find which works best.

Next, attempt the same movement in groups of two or three. In this maneuver the group members form a loose, arms-on-others'-shoulders, heads-down huddle, with their feet farther from the center of the huddle than their shoulders. Leaning in toward each other (and the center of the huddle), they all shuffle sideways across the current. It works best if the largest participant has his or her back to the current. Experiment.

NOTE: Some authorities, pointing out what can happen to a person stepping into an underwater hole, draw the line on this type of ferry at *knee* depth, especially in super-swift, cold, unexamined waters.

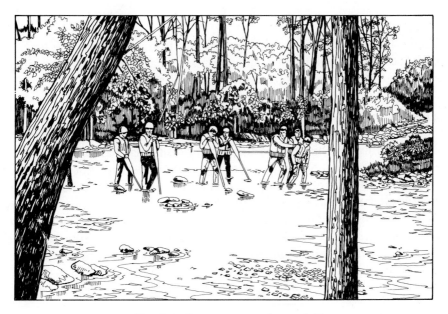

Fig. 8-9 Cross-stream ferry drill.

Shallow Water Search

This procedure demonstrates how difficult finding a small object or body may become, even in shallow water.

Skill Drill 20. The basic concept is to sweep a shallow inshore or beach side area thoroughly, principally in an attempt to locate a child on the bottom. To learn this activity best, practice it initially in a shallow swimming pool setting. A line of rescuers forms in shallow water, with taller individuals placed toward the deeper end of the line. Depending on how far down into the water a rescuer can see, the searchers use different line spacings. The most efficient spacing for poor in-water visibility is gained by searchers locking elbows. In settings with better bottom visibility, they may separate slightly by holding hands.

In swimming pool drills a clear plastic (not glass—it might break) bottle is filled with water and placed on the pool bottom. The line of rescuers then slowly moves across the pool, sweeping the pool bottom with their feet for the nearly invisible bottle. This procedure then could be used in a real search, with the line formed perpendicular to a beach. Depending on the situation, a similar approach could be used in deeper water, with a line of surface-diving rescuers attempting to locate the target.

● ● ●

This concludes the individual-emphasis information in the text. The remainder of the book focuses on group and team functions, building on the principles established for individual safety.

CHAPTER SUMMARY

This chapter emphasized a number of points that can be hazardous to a rescuer. Of greatest importance is remembering not to fix your attention totally on the victim, instead endeavor to follow the one-hand-for-yourself rule. Situational and climate-based safety considerations also were discussed. In particular, points about protecting yourself from cold, both in and out of the water, were covered. Stressors were introduced and explained, along with how to protect yourself from them. Last, a number of simple, in-water routines that primarily assist your adapting to moving water were described.

PRETEST ANSWERS

1. e
2. True
3. b
4. False

REFERENCES

1. Madison A: Swept away, Chatham, NY, 1990, Alan Madison Productions (videotape).
2. McKeown W: New ways to fight the chill that kills, Popular Mechanics, pp 164-166, Dec 1981.
3. Miller J et al: The visual behavior of recreational boat operators, Rep CG-D-31-77, Springfield, Va, 1977, National Technical Information Service.
4. Pozos R and Born D: Hypothermia: Causes, effects, prevention, Piscataway, NJ, 1982, New Century Publishers, p 150.

PART · THREE

Team Rescue Tactics

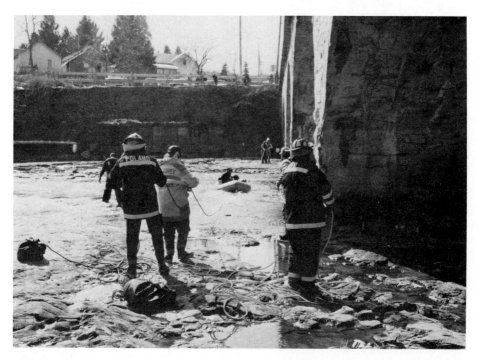

Practicing team water rescue tactics — a boat ferry used to remove victims from moving water.

OVERVIEW

The previous parts of the text have explained the causative factors underlying water accidents and how an *individual* should respond to protect himself or herself from them. This final part of the book examines the basics of *organizational* responses to aquatic mishaps. In particular, it reviews:

- Team preparations for water rescue
- Basic team rescue tactics

- Essential equipment for outfitting a group of water rescuers
- Managing and transporting aquatic trauma victims
- How not to become a victim — *after* the rescue attempt

DISCUSSION

The text has repeatedly indicated that a great deal of work still must be done to update the public's and the professional rescuers' aquatic knowledge. This requirement for modernization also laps into the organizational scene. Many municipal, state, and federal agencies responsible for rescue have yet to expand their aquatic capability or, in some cases, even to realize they need it. That is the bad news. The converse, upbeat side is that proven terrestrial, team-oriented response procedures are both in place and accepted by all emergency resource providers. The primary task is how most quickly and efficiently to marry proper water rescue information and procedures within existing organizational protocols. Efficiency in this case relates to not "reinventing the wheel" nor being reminded, through litigation, that more emphasis on water safety and rescue is necessary in your department's always overloaded training and equipment acquisition agendas.

The usual answer to such dilemmas is to go back to the basics. In this case the basics involve (1) finding out what your organization's aquatic response needs *actually* are or are projected for the future; then (2) discovering and/or reviewing what resources are available from either community, professional, or in-house sources. A relatively large amount of usable information is available. The trick, as always, is knowing where to look for it. The text tries to make this easier by listing a number of resources in Appendix I.

Another key consideration is equipment. If at all possible before concluding a purchase, investigate and compare sample gear, experimenting with it in your typical environment. A number of equipment manufacturers are listed in Appendix I.

The text presents simple team rescue procedures. Once understood, these procedures can form the basis for expanded adaptations suited to fit your particular situations. As a final effort to aid your avoiding aquatic accident pitfalls, several *un*successful, actual water rescue events are analyzed.

9

Preparation for Water Rescue

OVERVIEW

This chapter begins the examination of aquatic rescue from a team or organizational perspective. It identifies areas of potential risk, general personnel and equipment needs, and appropriate training procedures. The chapter also discusses the need to separate rescue from (body) recovery.

OBJECTIVES

After studying this chapter, the reader should understand the developmental relationship of these topics:
1. Why planning precludes peril
2. The necessity for reviewing records — predicting areas and sources of aquatic mishaps
3. Using research in amassing equipment and resources
4. Researching property entry and access routes
5. Clarifying communications and command relationships
6. Specifying training needs and exercise parameters
7. Developing preventive community education projects

PRETEST

1. The hardest job a water rescuer may have is initiating change. (True or false?)
2. Effective water accident prevention programs are (a) based on reviews of past accidents; (b) aided by seeking outside resources and assistance; (c) using educational and informational cam-

---

paigns to promote public awareness of hazards; or (d) all of the above.
3. Conventional fire fighting equipment often can be used in a backup roll for water rescue: (a) plan to use it when required; (b) practice with it if possible; or (c) drill with it to the point of marking its best location for use at potential accident sites. Choose the most sensible option.
4. Initially training in a swimming pool rather than in lake and stream environments allows better supervision and safety. (True or false?)
Pretest answers are at the end of the chapter.

SEPARATING RESCUE FROM RECOVERY

A number of organizations in North America specialize (often along with similar activities in other related emergency service fields) in water rescue. A large portion of these well-intended, caring agencies are in actuality not prepared for water rescue at all. Rather, what they truly concentrate on is after-accident body recovery. They are normally quite proficient since many of them have been providing the service for a long time. They also should be given a great deal of appreciation because their job is usually thankless and emotionally draining.

However, they sometimes inhibit rather than aid assistance. What is the primary reason? They are conditioned to respond in a slower-paced mode since they know the victim after whom they will be sent is beyond help; thus their approach is opposed to the inferences presented in this text. However, with proper dispatch, equipment, and training, aggressive water rescuers *can* and do make a difference, even if intervention takes place many minutes after the victim has disappeared beneath the surface.

The underlying philosophy of this text is to develop an understanding of the basics. Positively approaching obsolete concepts may be the hardest part of a water rescuer's job. Explaining the real causes of aquatic accidents requires knowledge of basic issues. In preparing for team rescue, the same rule holds. The model presented here is just as applicable when you are on scene deciding the best ways to attempt urgent rescue as when initially outfitting your water rescue team with equipment.

Try to comprehensively identify situations with which you presently are involved or may have to confront in your local area of responsibility; then act or plan and organize accordingly.

Long-term planning not only means researching accident records to identify the greatest hazard potentials for which you must prepare; it also means getting your information straight so you can change old and outmoded opinions. One builds on the other. The more you look back, the better you may be able to see ahead.

Three *P*s: Planning Precludes Peril

Courage has been defined as the feeling you have *before* you really understand what you have gotten into. If this outlook is taken literally, true courage does not begin to manifest itself until you must get out of whatever predicament you have created or with which you are involved. Water rescue, or any other similar form of deliverance, best proceeds when participants are more inclined to preincident action, acting with cold calculation and in-depth organization. Another way to present this point is to reflect again on Mr. Murphy's infamous law (Table 9-1).

Perhaps water more than any other potential accident medium allows Murphy's law the fullest play. As noted in the foregoing chapters, water represents many potential, constantly changing avenues for getting into difficulty.

> To defeat "Murphy" positively, assist victims and overcome unbelievers. The three Ps—*p*lanning *p*recludes *p*eril—*must* be used.

An essential bedrock of rescue planning is the philosopher George Santyana's observation, "Those who ignore history are bound to repeat it." Thus the message is do not repeat others' mistakes, especially when historical records are readily available to you. Check into department

Table 9-1 Murphy's Law (With Variations)

Murphy's Primary Law	If Something Can Go Wrong, It Will!
Variation	
No. 1	That which is least expected occurs when it is least desired.
No. 2	That which can never happen does.
No. 3	That which is most put off will find its way to you.
No. 4	What you plan for least, happens most.
No. 5	Murphy never quits.

files for past rescue reports dealing with water incidents. Consult local hospital files on drowning, if available, and other similar sources such as those of the police and fire departments, emergency medical services (EMS), or civil defense units. If your community library or newspaper has an information retrieval system, look for stories dealing with drownings, flooding, and/or aquatic rescues. State or regional organizations such as fire schools or Bureau of EMS Offices may also keep similar records, or they may be able to indicate where this material is available.

Next examine your area of responsibility's natural, manmade, and environmental hazard characteristics. How many different types of water hazards are located near you?

For instance, are there deep or shallow lakes, ponds, or gravel pits; areas of pooled (generally slow-moving or still water) or fast-moving (wide or narrow) streams; numerous swimming pools—mainly in backyards; weather variations that produce ice (short or long freezing periods) and flooding potential; or low head dams (see Chapter 10) or similar attractive nuisances? Is there a great deal of hunting and fishing or white water canoeing? Are there organized sportsmens' clubs? Do large numbers of people go powerboating in either waterskiing, cruising, or personal watercraft modes? Is waterside recreation spread out, or is it confined to a few highly used areas, with people using these same areas seasonally or moving to different locations? Does your area have large water runoff or diversion systems? How easily could someone be swept into them?

INFORMATION EXAMINATION AND PREVENTIVE USE

After gathering the two general groups of information discussed previously (i.e., accident history plus details on present water usage), examine them for three important types of patterns: (1) personal characteristics of victims; (2) commonality of location; and (3) environmental considerations.

> *Personal characteristics of victims.* Do you detect any trends that single out a specific group of people in your particular area as more or most water accident prone?

As an example, a number of smaller communities have discovered the night or weekend of high school graduation is one of their most potent drowning periods. Once this potential is recognized, a few steps similar to the following might be considered: (1) teen-oriented, antidrowning and antidrinking campaigns in the local media shortly before gradua- tion week, which could include a school poster or billboard approach (some state governments provide funding for this type of intervention); (2) increased patrolling in conjunction with that of law enforcement personnel in areas of higher water accident probability; and (3) an EMS and hospital emergency room staff in-service program on near drown- ing (a simple videotape or slide show presentation might suffice; see Appendix I).

Commonality of location. Does your research indicate that any single area or predominate type of locale produces a significant percentage of water accidents?

Is there anything that can be done to reduce accident potential? For instance, simple improvements in the use of signs might reduce the lack of hazard appreciation that causes some accidents (Table 9-2). Can access to the site be restricted? Conversely, how well prepared are you or your organization to deal with aquatic accidents occurring in a specific, high-potential location? As an example, in the case of white water enthusiasts, do you have equipment and training for extrication from semiremote canyon areas? For work in any rural environment, are you aware of the best access routes for personnel and equipment? Have these routes been investigated, and has information on their locations been distributed to potential rescuers? An illustration of using this information in a preventive program follows.

Table 9-2 Sign Usage Basics

Type	Information
Attention	Immediately acquires and holds users' attention; stands out by color, style, placement
Warning	Tells explicitly of danger or hazard
Outcomes	Clearly indicates possible results of interaction with hazard or danger
Avoidance	Explains how to avoid hazard
Repetition	Repeats information as frequently as possible in as many dif- ferent ways as possible
Graphics	Uses pictures to warn illiterates or nonnative, non-English- speaking people

Your research indicates that several duck hunters have died in a local waterfowl hunting area. If there are sportsmen's clubs in your community, have them invite a speaker on water safety for hunters. Each state has a boating law administrator. These officials are usually in the state law enforcement or natural resources department. (A list of state boating law administrators may be obtained from National Marine Manufacturers Association, 2550 M St. NW, Suite 425, Washington, D.C. 20037. In Canada the Canadian Red Cross Society usually has this information.) They are given federal funds to distribute boating and general water safety information. Have an officer from one of these departments make a presentation, or have him or her provide handout materials.

Several states also have extensive audiovisual libraries that lend water safety films and videotapes. To go a step further, if community interest is sufficient, a participative pool demonstration for sportsmen, featuring PFDs, small boat swamping and survival, heavy clothing flotation, plus HELP and huddle is in order.

Environmental considerations. Is there a great deal of seasonal outdoor recreational activity in your area?

How much of it involves water sports? Does ice form and thaw with any predictability? Are there centralized ice locations near gathering places for school children or toddlers? Is flooding or high rainwater runoff a potential hazard? Do you have flood relief (evacuation) plans and equipment? (See Appendix V for flood preparation and planning pointers.) Is there a National Oceanographic and Atmospheric Admin- istration (NOAA) weather and storm advisory service available to your agency or community? Even if there has never been a large-scale flooding incident in your area, are there trailer parks or dwellings built near the bottom of deep-sided creek and ravine locations? Are there any large earthen dams or retaining walls near housing areas?[1] Does early spring bring out a number of high-water canoeists? Does your road network have any low water crossings that might trap vehicles in rising water? Similarly, for more urban or built-up areas, do you know of low-lying underpasses that can receive much water and quickly fill and then empty? Are normally dry, flood-relief channels common in your locale? Can they be, or are they, used for recreational purposes? Are campgrounds or parks located in or near flood plains or creek beds?

What possibility is there of storm waters carrying persons, usually smaller children, into drains and sewers? Do you know how to gain access into these drainage systems?

As an example of this type of information in a preventive program, prepare and distribute a videotape or slide program for showing in local primary schools if storm drains and similar systems do present a potential for danger in the community.

> The goal is to present the information in a way that discourages the more adventurous children who watch the show from performing dangerous behaviors.

As with the other preventive programs, community cable television channels or printed media often may be used for public service messages to bring this information to the public.

ACQUIRING RESOURCES

By generating the foregoing information, you are developing an informational matrix for your area. This matrix helps to indicate locations, seasons, and particular groups of people most likely to become involved in aquatic accidents.

As an example, if your community can be described as an affluent "bedroom" for larger commercial or industrial centers and you are situated in a temperate zone with warmer summers, it presents a large potential for backyard pool near drownings. Your research should indicate this potential. If it does, attention must be given to both the preventive and reactive accident reduction phases to deal with the problem (Table 9-3).

In the case of pools, preventive intervention uses community informational presentations, possibly through dealers of pools or pool equipment. Research and recommendations dealing with building codes and pool fencing are helpful. Home pool safety audits can be offered by departmental personnel, or your department can train neighborhood volunteers to perform courtesy pool audits and distribute information packets. (Such packets are available at low cost from several sources. See Appendix I.)

Reactive intervention includes development of specially trained and equipped teams (should the problem be large enough) who would be on

Table 9-3 Prediction Matrix*

Who	Where	When	How	Why
Preadolescent Age 1-5 yr	Near home, with family, in pool, or bath	Playing, bathing	Unintended fall; curiosity	Unsupervised near hazard
Adolescent Age 6-12 yr	In pond, river; near home	Primarily warm season	Play	Curiosity, uninformed
Teenagers Age 13-20 yr	In larger body of water	Mainly out of school	Fishing, hunting, swimming, diving	Drugs, a dare, uninformed
Adult Age 21-60 yr	In lakes, ponds, rivers	Recreation in season	Fishing, hunting, paddling	Drugs, inability, uninformed
Elderly Age 60+ yr	In smaller waters	Recreation; bathing	Fall; seizure	Physical inability

NOTE: *Drugs* in the "Why" column mainly refer to alcohol. *Uninformed* means to lack information on hazards and proper responses to them such as wearing PFDs.
*Review these items and/or expand on them for your area. For example, do you have any items in the larger bodies of water category, and what is your ability to deal with or to work with them?

call to deal with pool near-drowning situations. (The Phoenix Fire Department has such a team. For more information on their operation call [602] 262-6910 or 262-6370.) Hospital staff members also would be specifically identified and prepared to treat such victims.

The underlying message is to prepare initially for types of cases that have a high historical probability. Then work toward preparation for other types of incidents in decreasing priority based on the potential for their occurrence. Also, do not forget "Murphy." One of his laws says that, "Just because something hasn't happened, doesn't mean it won't." Equipment procurement should be aimed at this goal.

There is a second consideration: what gear is available that could be used in more than one environment or type of water case? An easily recognizable example is your basic item—a PFD. It is ubiquitous and should be found anywhere water rescuers are gathered. On the other hand, what type or style of PFD would work best in your situation? Go back to basic research; attempt to gather a lot of information on different PFDs; then determine which would provide the best cost-benefit. This text presents numerous examples of PFDs, along with detailed information on exactly what they are supposed to do and where to acquire

Table 9-4 Basic Water Rescue Equipment

General Category	Specific Equipment	Comments

Lights and lighting equipment	Flash lights
	  Floatable
	  Waterproof
	Flood lights
	  Easy transport
	Helmet-mounted strobe
		Comments on lights are in Chapter 10.

Lines (ropes)	Carabiner and prusiks Heaving lines Heavy hauling lines Pulleys Throw bags or bottles Vertical lift gear	Line requirements are dependent on training level of team members. Comments on lines are in Chapters 10 and 11.

Line-throwing gear	Bolos (weighted)
	Bow and arrow
	Fly fishing rod
	Guns and projectiles
	  Compressed air
	  Cartridges
	Mortars
		Comments on line throwing gear are in Chapter 11.

Medical equipment	Advanced and basic life support equipment
	Backboards
	Cervical collars
	Medical kits
	Stretchers
	  Floatable
	  Stokes
		Advanced and basic life support equipment is allotted per team members' training and EMS level.
		In-water cervical spine injury management is in Chapter 12.

Personal protective gear	Dry suits
	Helmets
	PFDs
	Wet suits
	  Fins
	  Mask
	  Snorkel
		Short swim fins can be used with (dry) rescue suits.
		Diving-related equipment is allotted per team members' training level.

Reaching rescue gear	Fire hose inflation equipment Reach poles	Chapters 10 and 11 discuss inflated fire hose use.
Signaling equipment	Bullhorns Chemical lightsticks Flags Grease pens and boards Radios Whistles	Additional position-marking gear includes tape (reflective); dye and smoke markers, high-visibility panels.

NOTE: Boats are discussed in Chapter 11.

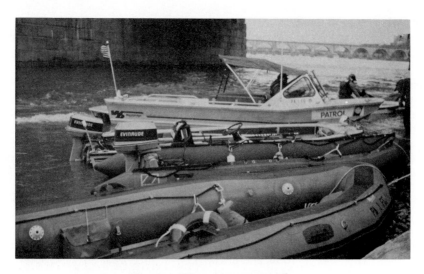

Fig. 9-1 Water rescue craft.

them. In the best possible situation, however, you should experiment with them in your locale before choosing one or more models.

PFDs are comparatively low cost, simple equipment items. In addition, Table 9-4 presents a suggested basic equipment list for review. If, for example, the decision matrix indicates your department needs both open water and ice rescue capability, the answer is to procure a boat. Then you must determine its type, model, size, and capacity (Fig. 9-1). Your rescue craft should have characteristics allowing it to do a number of jobs while safely operating in different environments.

If your department already has a rescue craft, is it really what is needed? For instance, if your probability matrix indicates a high potential for ice rescues in isolated, steep-sided abandoned quarries or gravel pits and if your existing boat is too heavy for manhandling and thus is constrained to a trailer, how do you get it into a steep-sided gravel pit or quarry? You don't! Another avenue must be investigated. Perhaps rescue suits and/or inflatable boats are appropriate alternatives.

PERSONNEL RESOURCES

An effective rescue team is actually a well-balanced group of specialists, sufficiently cross trained to assist each other when needed.

A team should have at least four members, although eight to 10 would be a more ideal number. To be effective, your team members should all be proficient in swimming and (surface) diving, boat operation, and advanced first aid or basic life support (BLS), and they should be trained and qualified in cardiopulmonary resuscitation (CPR). Team members should be required to show their water proficiency by demonstrating their floating, swimming, and surface diving capability. If possible, at least one team member should be an emergency medical technician and be qualified in advanced life support (ALS) (Table 9-5).

Additional qualifications for all members include driving ability, especially in boat trailer hauling and maneuvering; familiarity with radio communications and procedures; and awareness of, or experience with, departmental incident command structure (ICS) practices. Having at least one team member schooled in rope rescue techniques helps.

Note that little has been mentioned about underwater search, rescue, and recovery capabilities. Since this is a basic text and self-contained underwater breathing apparatus (SCUBA) techniques are at a more advanced level, they are not discussed in detail here. However, several sources for information about rescue training in this field are listed in Appendix I. Combining the approaches presented herein with proper underwater tactics would add greatly to the potential of a water rescue team.

Personnel resources include individuals who are not members of the team but who do have particular skills, insights, or local knowledge that might provide assistance. Experienced hunters and fishermen are sources of such assistance, especially if a search phase precedes actual rescue operations. Similarly, informational input or assistance from local (white water) canoeing clubs, hydroelectric companies (operating dams in your area), bridge tenders, marina operators, and other waterside recreational or business resources can be very helpful. An important element included in any resource listing would be the personnel and equipment support available from neighboring communities or emergency service agencies. Special attention should be given to military units, either regular, reserve, or National Guard.

An important resource that might be overlooked is the secondary use of departmental equipment in water rescue. For example, fire department snorkel trucks can be used to reach across ice or moving water to assist victims. One of the basic elements in successful rescue organizations is *always* having a backup approach should your primary or secondary method or means of attack fail. Innovative use of equipment such as the snorkel truck may provide you with such backup. However,

Table 9-5 Rescue Team Assignments

Title	Duties	Equipment
Team leader	Overall supervision Questions witnesses	Radios, bullhorn, charts, notes*
Far-side supervisor	Manages far shore	Specialized equipment; hose inflator and one dry suit
Near-side supervisor	Manages near shore Determines flow rate	Lines, throw bags, one dry suit
Equipment supervisor or downstream supervisor	Provides and operates small craft†	Boats and vehicles, fuel, spare tires, PFDs

NOTE: A fifth important position is safety observer. Each team member provides his or her own PFD. Medically trained member provides medical kit, backboard, cervical collars, and similar gear.
*Notes refers to information about a particular site.
†Becomes downstream supervisor when boat not used.

never plan on using equipment as a stopgap unless and until you have actually tried it. In fact, some municipalities and departments actually try various approaches in drill situations, then mark spots where equipment should be positioned at potential water side accident sites.

PROPERTY ENTRANCE AND ACCESS

Never allow yourself to be surprised, if at all possible, by the circumstances of a water emergency. Scout, learn, and understand your water surroundings and areas and attempt mentally to highlight possible sites for aquatic mishaps. Have someone follow streams, rivers, and canals and similar water-carrying facilities. Know the following:
- Locations where you might have to work a rescue
- What types of equipment you might use and how and where you would transport and launch it
- Any peculiarities about getting into the site

For instance, if there is a dam that might be involved in an emergency, how do you get to it? If it has structures, are they secured, and where can the keys be obtained? Who has permission to open or operate it, and how do you contact them?

Notice how easily all this information can be stored in a central dispatch computer file. *But* someone has to round up these details initially.

In this example, special awareness should be given to hydroelectric facilities that are automatically loaded and discharged. If such a dam is located in your area, is any warning signal, either visual, audible, or both, given to advise persons downstream that the dam is discharging? How far downstream can these warning signals be perceived? Are they reinforced by a system of easily seen and understood signs?

In following a waterway, be attentive to natural obstacles that might trap high-water debris, possibly causing water to back up and flow over or flood surrounding property. At dams or similar hazards, what areas are available and open on either bank to allow your movement or equipment approach? Know what the bottom of the stream looks like and what obstacles are present by observations made during low water levels. Film is not expensive, and a file picture of the underwater terrain might prove valuable during rescues. Visit the area after a heavy rain. Notice if local children congregate or play at certain points. Be aware of upstream dams and their operations. A possible approach to someone stranded in the middle of the stream is to shut down an upstream impoundment, dropping the water level, reducing current and flow rate, and easing rescue at your location.

Another rescue hazard to evaluate is the placement and clearance of overhead electrical wires. Can you move your heavier equipment safely under such obstacles? If necessary, who should be contacted to turn off the power?

Notice the composition of riverbank materials. When muddy, are they firm or soft? Would a vehicle sink or slip in them? Are there trees or other objects nearby to allow winch line attachment, or would it be necessary to bury a log (deadman) in the bank or beach to assist as an anchor in hauling gear from the water? If so, do you have shovels in your rescue vehicles?

> An accurate topographical map displaying all waterways in your area is an indispensable planning and rescue tool. Sources of such maps and how to order them are presented in Appendix I.

What is the most expeditious, rapid route from potential accident sites to a medical facility? Can medical helicopters be called into the area, and can helicopters be made available as a possible midriver rescue tool? Has your team ever practiced with a helicopter in a drill situation? How would you go about setting up such an exercise?

CLARIFYING COMMAND AND CONTROL

In the military the notation *C3I* stands for: command, control, and communications — intelligence. Another similar usage is three *Ss:* swift, simple, and secure. A keystone of effective rescue cooperation and interaction is effective communications. If the three Ss apply to and distinguish your communications, the command, control, and intelligence needs of your situation and organization will be greatly enhanced.

Occasionally everyone is so involved in an activity that radio transmissions might be missed. Heavy head covering in ice operations and the overwhelming engine and rotor noise when working with a helicopter also disrupt most forms of communication.

> Communication at a water rescue location may be difficult for a large number of reasons. If you are working near moving water, the background roar may be deafening. If working at night, you might not be either able to hear or see clearly the persons trying to pass information to you.

The answer to these concerns is as basic as other points made in the text:

- Survival is a direct function of amassing and using alternatives. In other words: *always have a backup.*
- Practice under varying conditions so that you have a good idea what will work and what will not.

After checking into alternatives and what to do in various situations, review the three Ss:

- Swift. The changeability of water conditions has been stressed repeatedly. For this reason, your communications should be as prompt and as precise as possible. In addition, communications loops, or the number of relay points involved in transmitting a message, should be kept to a minimum. The command system should reflect this goal, with decision making given, as completely as the situation allows, to the people at the scene. This also means that priorities and checklists should be developed to ensure that equipment intended for a certain type of rescue scene arrives without there being a time-consuming request and secondary transport operation. In the matter of backup, the swift rule also applies in that through practice, when an initial method does not work, a secondary one can be quickly used.
- Simple. Murphy's law has a special provision for communications,

guaranteeing that the more complicated a communications system or network, the more likely it will fail. Remember that electronics gear and water seldom go together. You may have to use radios in downpours. Can you depend on them?

The message remains the same: have in place tried and simple backup procedures. For example, in high noise areas, writing with grease pens on larger plastic clip boards, which are then held up for everyone to see, might transmit a message better than yelling through a bull horn. Use of whistles, lights, and hand signals should be considered and preferably practiced as backups (Table 9-6).

Consider networking with other agencies and departments. Are everyone's radios calibrated to the same frequency? One of the reasons for large-scale drills is to determine factors like this rather than unpleasantly coming across them during an emergency. Flood relief and evacuation operations are, for example, large-scale, water-oriented emergencies.

- Secure. In military usage this term indicates an enemy cannot intercept and interfere with communications. In our usage Murphy and his laws are the enemy. Therefore *secure* and *simple* work together. Simple means keeping a communication arrangement as uncluttered and uncomplicated as possible. Secure means that the system will not break down or if it does break down, repairs or a backup can be quickly applied.

Clarifying command and control also involves practice and gaining

Table 9-6 Communications Types and Uses

Communication Method	Advantages	Disadvantages
Two-way radio	Compact, effective in a variety of situations	Subject to magnetoelectrical interference; needs power
Bullhorn	Compact, simple one-way mode of communication	Difficult to use in high noise level areas; needs power
Board and grease pen	Effective as backup system in readable distances	Has distance and visibility limitations
Hand signals (including flags)	Low tech but useful at short to moderate distances	Requires standard code; may be misinterpreted
Light signals	Effective at night, in low visibility, at high noise levels	Same as hand signals

familiarity with what must be done and by whom. Rescues that fail usually are condemned by lack of on-scene knowledge *and* unfamiliarity of the persons on-scene with each other and with what they are expected to accomplish.

To return to command considerations, is the table of organization and responsibility for your team known and accepted by all members? Are there any doubts about who is in charge and who has the final responsibility for making decisions? Does everyone know what his or her job responsibilities include? Drills and practice sessions are good methods for determining if these chains of command and linkages are in place and functioning *before* someone's life depends on their working properly (Fig. 9-2).

In working with other organizations, a number of relationships must be clarified:

- In which geographical areas might more than one department respond?
- What are your joint notification procedures?
- How do you call for backup from other agencies?
- Who will be in charge?
- What are the personnel skills, equipment capabilities, and medical assistance levels of other organizations?

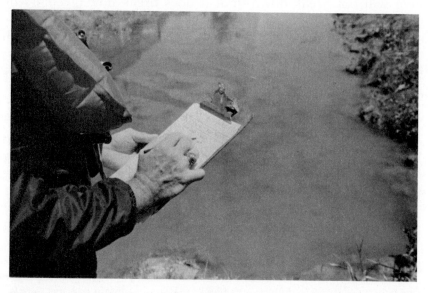

Fig. 9-2 Does your team have a formal organizational chart listing everyone's duties and responsibilities (e.g., the equipment I am supposed to bring to and manage at the scene)?

TRAINING NEEDS AND PARAMETERS

Training needs refer to having people and equipment function as they are supposed to function. Training parameters outline team goals and define evolutions and exercises. Both depend on research to reveal which water emergencies your team most likely can expect.

An example of individual training needs follows. Suppose your area has a number of high-powered speedboat races. Your people, as indicated by historical research and records, should be proficient in stabilizing, extricating, and transporting victims of cervical spine and internal injuries. Similarly, you should have equipment prepared to work in this capacity.

Training parameters indicate you should design drills around significant factors in your zone of responsibility. At this point you might think, "Isn't this just a little too simple? People really ought to understand this." Right and wrong! The first example that began this text cited a water rescue attempt that went awry, costing three rescuers their lives (Fig. 9-3). These people grew up alongside the dam that killed them. Yet they did not recognize or *train* to deal with it as a potential aquatic hazard.

A secondary goal in any type of rescue program is to ensure team members are cross trained sufficiently so they can assist or possibly

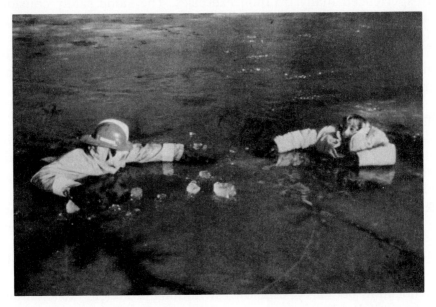

Fig. 9-3 Water rescuer in trouble. What is missing here? (Courtesy Dive Rescue International: Ice rescue [slide/tape presentation].)

substitute for each other. Another goal is to reach the point that team members can adequately explain aquatic accident causes and defenses to the public, underscoring another point to reemphasize: prevention should always precede intervention or reaction. If team members understand the causative factors and preventive actions needed to avoid accidents, they can distribute the message throughout the community. By doing this, they reduce the need for them or anyone else to enter a precarious aquatic situation to perform a rescue.

The goals set in training should be concrete, written, and well known by all team members. They must also directly relate to potential rescue situations in your region. (For simplified examples, see the goals of each skill drill as listed in Appendix IV.)

By following a written outline, progress can be accurately measured, and points that need more work can be identified and repeatedly addressed. This type of compehensive planning is usually followed as a model in other forms of fire, police, and EMS training. It should not be overlooked in dealing with the water.

WATER TRAINING GUIDELINES

Any experienced veteran emergency services provider has attended and experienced many training exercises. The same safety considerations that govern these other types of training should be considered in designing water programs. However, aquatic situations have special facets of which a planner should be aware. These aquatic safety training pointers can be divided into three main branches: individual safety; training site safety; drill, exercise, or evolution safety.

Individual Safety

- *Always* test new members' swimming skills in a safe, initially shallow, supervised pool setting. Individuals sometimes talk about having skills they really do not possess. Make sure that everyone is aware of each other's proficiency *before* depending on each other.
- Be particularly alert for any indications of poor swimming skills such as reluctance to place the face in the water or swimming in a more vertical than horizontal plane.
- Check to ensure that the individual can suddenly, comfortably (diving or falling) enter the water without panicking.
- Do not allow persons of unknown swimming proficiency to enter deep water until they have demonstrated they can handle themselves in the shallows.

Training Site Safety

- All initial training should be done in a pool environment if possible. Training in a pool is much easier because of water clarity and the closeness of instructors to those being trained.
- Be aware of basic water safety rules. Be sure there is strict supervision of poor swimmers; have a swimming buddy accompany them; and provide them with a properly fitted PFD in all deep water exercises.
- Control behavior. Do not allow roughhousing. Large people playing rough games in small boats or on docks can easily result in an unintended injury.
- Do not allow diving in shallow water. Be particularly aware of persons who are falling backward into shallow water.

Evolution Safety

- Appoint a safety observer for all in-water events. This person's *only job is to watch what is going on and be prepared to assist if needed.*
- Be careful when introducing any new element. Talk over and diagram all new drills or changes to old ones. Be sure that all know what is required of them and what *they* are supposed to do. Run through the new drills at slow speeds until all show they know what to do.
- Check to verify that everyone understands the potential hazards involved in each situation being practiced. Make individuals state what the dangers are and how they are avoided.
- Demonstrate a proper and positive safety outlook and attitude through your demeanor. Be and set a good example. *Wear your PFD and make sure all others wear theirs.*

  NOTE: In both training sessions and actual rescue operations, have someone not otherwise involved videotape the proceedings. The tape can be replayed as an aid in reviewing or improving team and individual techniques. In actual cases, it would provide an accurate historical and legal record of exactly what transpired.

CHAPTER SUMMARY

This chapter outlined considerations needed in setting up a water rescue team. It addressed personnel and training particulars. It also emphasized:

- The need for research and planning
- Obtaining resources based on accurate needs evaluation
- How gathering information aids accident prevention
- Understanding and avoiding access and entry problems

- Communications and control considerations
- Water safety training tips

PRETEST ANSWERS

1. True
2. d
3. c
4. True

REFERENCES

1. The awesome power, Washington, DC, 1987, The National Oceanographic and Atmospheric Administration (videotape).

10 Team Rescue Basics

OVERVIEW

This chapter explains the fundamentals of surface-oriented team rescue strategy. It discusses swift water and flooding; ice; low head dam; immersed auto situations; and emergency response afloat.

OBJECTIVES

After studying this chapter, the reader should understand the following topics and increase his or her competence in applying this knowledge:
1. Underlying principles useful in any team rescue event
2. Individual team member duties and equipment responsibilities
3. Tactics and backup strategies appropriate for various common situations
4. Specific hazards, equipment, and extrication details for single-victim and multivictim operations in differing environments and situations
5. Emergency response and fire fighting while afloat

PRETEST

1. Knowing *why* something must be done a certain way aids (a) understanding how to do it best; (b) developing usable, situational alternatives; or (c) both of the above.
2. Launching boats and stationing backups should come before establishing communications with victims. (True or false?)
3. A line leading **downstream** to a victim in a current should be (a) secured; (b) tended at all times; (c) subject to rapid release if

needed; or (d) walked downstream along the bank to reduce strain on the victim. Which of these is least correct?

4. The main consideration in rescuing a child who has fallen through ice is (a) the child's smaller size will allow his or her rapid removal from the water; (b) he or she is more energetic than an adult and thereby is of greater assistance in his or her own rescue; or (c) if the ice did not hold the weight of a smaller child, it probably will not hold yours. Choose the best answer.

Pretest answers are at the end of the chapter.

FUSION AND FOCUS

At this point in the text all the preceding elements are brought together and are focused on a single event or problem. It is unrealistic to believe that all the potential water rescue situations an emergency service provider might possibly encounter can be foreseen and described. Each rescue operation differs from that which precedes or follows it if for no other reason than the people rescued are not the same. Conversely, a primary point is the overall, general similarity that marks the total field of aquatic accidents. A number of basic principles that should apply to each different situation have been presented. The person who under-stands and works with the principles must determine techniques applicable to various situations.

In other words, if you accurately understand the essential *why* behind something that must be done, you are much better prepared to supply appropriately the *how* in doing it.

To review, if you are going to perform your water rescue job in the safest possible way, you must prepare yourself on several different levels, including the following:

- Learn about the potential for aquatic accidents in your area of responsibility by studying three information sources: past accident records; water use (both industrial and recreational) patterns; and potential water dangers characteristic of your region.

- Learn about yourself and other rescuers to the point of understanding what might get you into trouble and how to protect against such an occurrence. This includes the effect of cold and other environmental stressors and the too frequent error of focusing entirely on the victim while neglecting to look after yourself.

- Understand what underlies and causes most water accidents to the point of suggesting how community preventive programs might be developed.

- Know the essentials of protecting yourself in the water, including the use of personal flotation devices (PFDs); heat loss reduction; coping with current; floating with heavy clothing; and getting in and out of water properly.
- Evaluate and practice the basics in one-on-one, reach-throw-row-go procedures, including securely removing the victim from the water. Know that preference of rescue is greatest and safest with self-based (talking the victim into saving themselves); then shore-based; then boat-based; and last, the most dangerous, water-based rescue.

This chapter combines these principles with specific assistance techniques designed for several highly possible aquatic situations. Consider, while working through these scenarios, the following: how these hypothetical situations vary from what you might actually encounter; what parts can or should be considered for modification; and how you best can adapt them.

The following, borrowed from the Ohio Department of Natural Resource's text, *River Rescue,* are general points applicable to most water rescues:

1. Establish communications with victim.
2. Establish command post.
3. Select rescue approach.
4. Launch boats.
5. Station backup. (In swift water situations, exchange 4 and 5.)
6. Position lines.
7. Rescue victim.
8. Administer emergency medical treatment.
9. Salvage victim's equipment.
10. Secure rescue scene.

Note that a three-step process *must* be completed *before* anyone actively begins to interact with the victim. These steps follow:

- Review scene. *Each* team member quickly surveys the situation. Look for potential helps and hazards. A *primary* consideration is to determine if the water level is rising. (If so, it is even more important to keep the rescuers from becoming victims.)
- Review resources. This can be done enroute, but each team member must be aware of his or her own equipment potential. The team leader must know the overall sum of the team's capacity and *endurance.* Consider calling in supporting resources as required.
- Review plan. Quickly integrate the two foregoing points into an action plan. Move only on the team leader's signal.

SWIFT OR FLOOD WATER RESCUES

(To prepare for this section, turn to Appendix V for a number of general suggestions on dealing with potential flooding situations.) Victims involved with moving water will fit into one of two subcategories: either they are in the water and moving with it or they are stationary in it (Fig. 10-1). If stationary, there are two subdivisions: either they are marooned, but mainly above and mostly out of the water, or they are partially immersed, with the water rising around them. Since the marooned person may be considered in a lesser state of jeopardy, persons either being swept downstream or about to be carried away are addressed first.

The following is a list of actions to take to assist those victims in the current (Table 10-1):

■ When arriving at the scene, attempt to communicate with the victims and get flotation to them by throwing PFDs or other flotation objects and devices as soon as possible. Lines should be attached in advance to the thrown objects.

■ Send some rescuers *downstream* in an attempt to catch the victims *should* they be swept away from their initial locations. An excellent

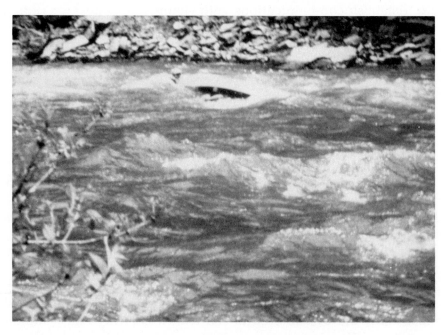

Fig. 10-1 A victim being carried downstream. NOTE: When in moving water with a capsized craft, *always* stay at the *upstream* end.

model is the pickoff in baseball—rescue personnel who have attempted assistance rotate or leapfrog ahead to another position. (Advance scouting of potential swift-water rescue sites is invaluable in this situation to allow you to know how to go from one point to another.) A special situation would occur at night when light sources also must be rotated ahead of the victim.

- Have as many people as possible, including bystanders, point to the victims. Condition all rescue personnel to mark their spot by, for example, making an *X* with their heel in beach sand or mud. (At night, they can mark their position with some type of retroreflective material.) Should the victim go under the water, shoreside spotters could note what was in line with or behind the victim at the moment of disappearance. Comparing several of these lines of position running from the beach *X* to a distant object helps determine the initial underwater search points. (This same marking procedure should be used, when applicable, at any water rescue scene.)
- Always assume worst-case possibilities: the victims are poor or nonswimmers, and they have been seriously affected by cold. With these assumptions in mind, work as quickly as possible. Numerous drownings have occurred when would-be rescuers assumed the opposite—that the victims were not in serious difficulty and it was not necessary to rush the rescue. (One factor in such cases is that the rescuers did not have a plan or know what to do.)
- Check information sources.

Table 10-1 Rescuer Duties: Swift or Flood Waters

Title	Primary Duties
Team leader	Survey scene and resources. Integrate and initiate plan. Oversee operation. Coordinate arriving resources.
Far-side supervisor	Per leader's instructions, prepare to establish position on far bank. Work with equipment supervisor to cross stream, or become lead dry suit swimmer.
Near-side supervisor	Prepare near-side position. Attempt reaching or throwing rescue. Back up dry suit swimmer and line tender.
Equipment supervisor	Per instructions, carry far-side supervisor across stream, aid dry suit rescue team, or rapidly move downstream to secondary rescue site.

Check all possible sources of information to find out *how many other victims may be involved* and what is or may have been happening to them.

- Use witnesses, companions of the victims, and amount of boats or gear (e.g., fishing rods, coolers) present to determine the possible numbers of unaccounted-for persons. Be prepared to search up and down both banks and/or to launch search boats into the stream.

When the Victim Is Stopped

The victim stops because of one of three reasons: (1) he or she is stopped by running into and grasping an obstacle; (2) he or she has grabbed a line; or (3) he or she went underwater. If it appears the victim has gone under the water, carry out last-position marking (as indicated above); alert dive rescue sources; and rapidly move part of the team to the next choke point downstream. This latter group watches for and attempts to snag the body of the unconscious or dead victim if it passes. Someone in the team should be assigned to compute flow rate to determine how far an object can go downstream per time increments. This computation allows downstream parties to position themselves in advance of a body passing their chosen point. Computing flow is always a standard action in any moving water situation (Fig. 10-2). The easiest

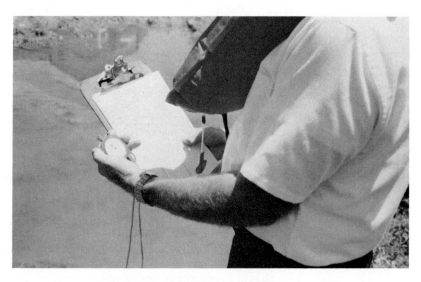

Fig. 10-2 Timing current and flow rate by watching an object move a pre-measured distance as stepped off along the stream's bank.

way to do this is to time a floating object as you walk alongside it on a straight stretch of shoreline. Then multiply the number of feet the object drifts in 1 second times 1.5; the result is number of miles per hour and gives you an approximation of current. If the victim has disappeared by the time rescuers arrive on scene, the rescuers can at least be able to figure how far downstream the victim may have progressed from the time he or she was last seen.

If the Victim Has Grabbed a Line

- Yell at the victim to roll over to wrap the line around his or her hands or body to ensure the victim will hang onto the line. However, if it appears this maneuver might imperil the victim by becoming entangled in obstacles in the stream, tell him or her to hang on and *not* wrap up. This is an on-scene judgment call.
- Current should swing the victim toward the shore on which the line-controlling rescuer is located. As this happens, the rescuer moves downstream. This "dynamic belay" is done to reduce drag on the victim so that he or she will not be swept off the end of the line. In fast water situations do not belay, or secure, a line attached to a person downstream. Rather, as previously explained, use a body belay partially around the rescuer's trunk. A line tied to or fouled on a stationary object can become taut enough to drive an attached person (no matter how much flotation he or she is wearing) to the bottom. It is better to tend a line actively, allowing it to be cast off or repositioned quickly.
- Rescuers with lines snapped to their PFDs should wade to the victim and assist him or her ashore. The rescuers' lines are attached best with a quick disconnect arrangement per the warning immediately above. In other words, if a rescuer's line *does* become snagged, some method

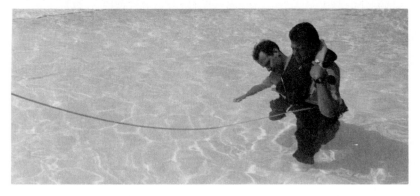

Fig. 10-3 A tethered rescuer assisting a victim from the water.

should be in place to allow its rapid release. (The resources in Appendix I include suppliers of quick-disconnect equipment.)

As a consequence of exposure to flowing cold water, the victim may be hypothermic. If his or her *covered skin is very cold to the touch, do not let the victim move.* Rather, as *gently* as possible, carry the victim (in a horizontal position) to safety; then initiate management and transport protocols as indicated in Chapter 12 (Fig. 10-3).

If the Victim Is Stationary but Partially Immersed

Assuming that the victim will *not* be able to hang on for an extended period of time*:

- Attempt to float a PFD with a line attached to the victim from an upstream location. This float line should be positioned to float past the *far* side of the victim, or closer to the side of the stream *opposite* the person handling the line. This additional scope of line will ensure its arriving at the victim's location. Once the line has floated to a position near the victim, the rescuers can pull it into the victim's reach (Fig. 10-4).

---

*If the victim is pinned against a strainer, the current may be forcing him or her under the water.

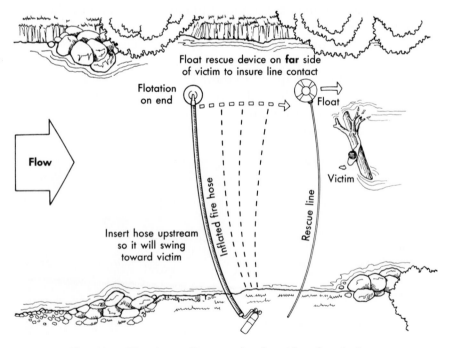

Fig. 10-4 Floating a line on the *far* side of a victim.

- If the victim can don the PFD properly, have him or her do so and then shove off into the stream. Before the victim does this, instruct him or her to float face up as the line attached to the PFD swings him or her toward the shore.
- If the victim cannot manage to don the PFD or appears otherwise unresponsive, the rescue must move from a shore-based to boat- or water-based attempt. The boat-based rescue involves a watercraft with a shore **tether** carrying one or more rescuers aboard. The rescuers paddle the craft to position it. Shore personnel maintain tautness in the line and assist in maneuvering the craft. The line is also kept as high above the water and as parallel to the current as possible. This prevents a **bight,** or loop, of line from catching in the current and sweeping in an unmanageable mass downstream. The team captain positions himself or herself on the shore at a point below the line handlers but above the victim. The captain then uses a bullhorn or agreed-on standardized hand signals to have the line slacked as required by the boat party. A motorized craft may not need a tether because it could foul the screw. See Chapter 11 for information on motorboat operations.

> Should an appropriate watercraft not be available, a rescuer must enter the water. In the best-case scenario, the rescuer has a dry or wet suit and is backed by similarly suited assistants. Short swim fins can be worn over rescue suit boots and are helpful in some current conditions (Fig. 10-5).

The rescuer swims or floats downstream while wearing a second PFD for the victim, but the line attached to him or her is kept as slack as possible per the instructions in the "If the Victim Has Grabbed a Line" section. In this situation the best location for the shoreside end of the line is directly across the stream from the victim, with the rescuer entering the water at an upstream location.

If a rescue suit or wet suit is not available, a rescuer, fully dressed in one or more layers of clothing and wearing a tethered PFD, may attempt the rescue. In these water-based scenarios, the team captain again is in the best position to coordinate the line handlers. (Procedures using river rescue boards—downsized surfboards—have also been developed for this situation.) A rescuer secured at the end of a taut line may be driven underwater. However, in the same situation, a rescuer lying on the

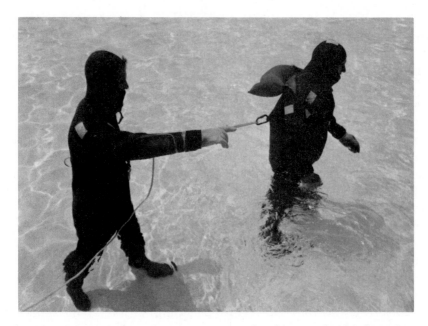

Fig. 10-5 Dry-suited rescuer in water with a line tender backing him.

downstream end of a tethered, upstream belayed backboard may be able to surf across a stream's surface.

If the Victim Is Marooned

The marooned victim is trapped by flowing water but apparently is not in immediate danger of being carried away by it. This time factor may allow your using boat-based rescue systems.

As explained previously, in general, powered boats approaching victims should proceed upstream or into the prevailing wind or current because to do so helps in maneuvering and the opposing forces tend to keep the boat away from, rather than overrunning, the victim.

If, on the other hand, obstructions, floods, high water, or debris situations block downstream approaches, the only recourse is to approach from upstream (Fig. 10-6).

The danger is that the victim may be involved with a strainer. If the rescue craft capsized directly above the strainer, those aboard might be swept into and caught by the same hazard. One solution is to run a rescue craft out into midstream, drop an anchor, and play out the anchor line, using it as a tether as the craft drops downstream. With this maneuver, there is danger in that power and/or control of the craft may be lost before anchoring or after retrieving the anchor after the actual rescue. (Additionally, some bottoms will not allow the anchor to bite, especially

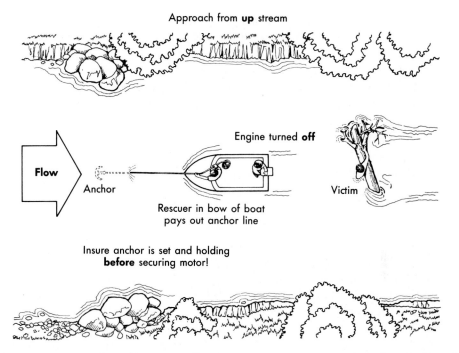

Approach from **up** stream

Flow

Anchor

Engine turned **off**

Victim

Rescuer in bow of boat
pays out anchor line

Insure anchor is set and holding
before securing motor!

Fig. 10-6 Approaching the victim from *up*stream. Rescuer in bow has deployed and is tending anchor line. Engine is turned off.

in a strong current.) The best answer is to use a **ferrying system,** with the rescue craft attached to an upstream line and controlled from the shore.

Ferrying Rescues

Ferrying means to move across a current. In the simplest boat ferrying system, a watercraft is maneuvered up and down and across a stream by shoreside line handlers. There are several methods for rigging a ferry system. The least complex procedure is presented.[1]

To establish a ferry system, a line, usually called a *messenger line,* is passed to team members on the opposite shore. This is probably the most difficult aspect of the entire operation. The primary problem is keeping lines out of the water.

A cross-stream line allowed to belly out in the current is almost impossible to tighten, and the usual solution is to cast off one end of the line and start again. When the rescue team knows the expected area of operations and *has practiced there,* the difficulty of passing the messenger line is greatly reduced. Techniques include using a heaving line (light line with weighted end, or **bolo**) or a throw bag; shooting a line across the area using a line-throwing gun or projectile system (or a bow and arrow); floating a line across at an upstream curve; carrying a line across using a boat; or walking a line across at an upstream bridge or shallow **ford.** A simple fly rod using a large sinker and heavy test line might also work to deliver the messenger line. (Appendix I lists sources for obtaining line-throwing guns and similar gear.) In all these methods pass the line across *as quickly as possible,* taking care *not* to allow a large midstream (downstream) bight to develop in the current. Keep the messenger line out of the water and as taut as practicable (Fig. 10-7).[5]

The messenger line is attached to a heavier line called a *span* or **traverse line.** The messenger line is then used to haul the traverse lines across the stream. If at all possible, polypropylene throw-bag lines should not be used as span lines or in heavy hauling situations. Stronger lines as specified in Table 11-3 are much safer and better suited for this application.

Either a carabiner or a single pulley block is firmly bent (attached so it cannot move) to the middle of the span line. A second line, or **runner,** is **reeved** from the near shore through the block or carabiner to the bow of the rescue craft. The far-shore rescuers then pull the span line, the block, and the rescue craft toward the center of the stream. By hauling on or slacking off the span and runner, the rescue craft is maneuvered to the marooned victim.

Skill Drill 21. Rescuers should consider leading the ends of the span

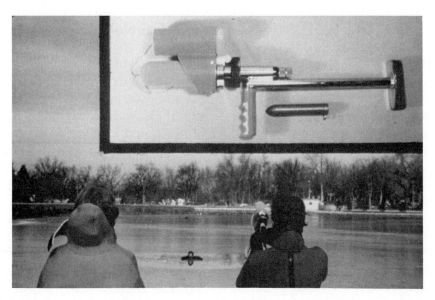

Fig. 10-7 Using a line-throwing gun to assist a victim or to pass a messenger line. (Courtesy Dive Rescue International: Ice rescue [slide/tape presentation].)

and runner partially around trees or similar solid stationary objects to aid their snubbing or possibly belaying the lines should the situation require (Fig. 10-8). Span lines should be twice the width of the stream, and they should be coiled to allow rapid deployment without **fouling.**

In theory, ferrying systems are relatively simple to set up and to operate. *In reality they work best when practiced far in advance of any possible emergency use.*

The system can be expanded by using a stationary span line and movable center block. The block is controlled by near and far shore lines. A simple alternative boat ferry for use on smaller streams is to attach two lines (near side, far side) to the bow of the rescue boat. The boat is launched upstream of the victims and is maneuvered by hauling and slackening the lines. A stationary span line with two movable pulleys or carabiners can be used to power a small craft across a flowing stream. The movable pulleys are attached by short lengths of line to the **bow** and **stern** of a cross-stream–oriented small craft. In this application, called a *dynamic ferry,* water current acting against the side of the boat provides propulsion.

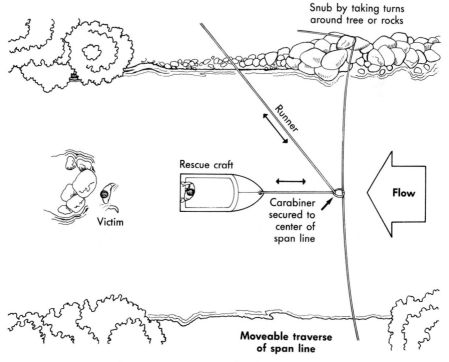

Fig. 10-8 Diagram of a ferrying system.

> The basic ferry system also may be adapted to maneuvering a rescue craft or sled during certain ice rescue situations.

This is possible if the ice-covered area is small enough to allow rescuers to position themselves on its opposite sides or at least opposite each other, with the victim between them. The rescue craft then could be hauled toward the victim.

The foregoing information basically has dealt with swift water as it applies to streams. Flood waters may have some similarities, except the spread of the waters will be too wide to permit shore-side activities. The good news is that the wider the waters, the slower they flow. The bad news is that they increase speed at choke or **convergence** points. Once again, advance scouting and planning are basic tools in responding to floods. Another principle element of flood response is boat-based rescues. They are addressed in Chapter 11.

ICE RESCUE

The basic considerations in *any* ice rescue are as follows:
- Study the ice conditions.
- Watch the victim(s) constantly.
- Throw, slide, or push flotation assistance (in advance of the rescuer) to the victim (Fig. 10-9).
- Do not remove rescuer clothing. (Any decrease in surface weight is far less important than buoyancy and heat retention in the rescuer.) If possible, button, zip, or secure any and all garment openings to trap air better.
- Any rescuer on the ice has flotation and is tethered. A human chain may be considered as tethering *as long as all members are wearing PFDs*.
- Use a rigid reaching device if at all possible. A sturdy tree limb or branch, broom or mop handle, hockey stick, two-by-four timber, board, wooden bench, or ladder may be used to reach the active victim and to spread and support the rescuer's weight.
- When moving across ice, maintain a low center of gravity and distribute body weight as much as possible.

Ice rescues are generally divided into two groups: those involving an active victim or those with an inactive victim. With the active victim, the

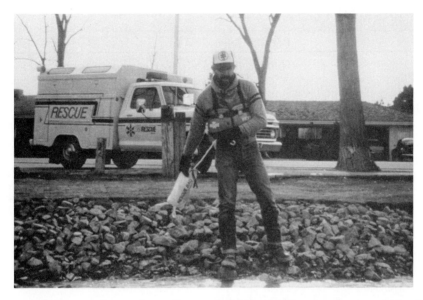

Fig. 10-9 Throw, push, or shove flotation devices or lines to an ice victim both to help the victim float *and to mark his or her position.* (Courtesy Dive Rescue International.)

use of reaching or throwing rescues is highly possible. (Skill Drill 24 in Chapter 11 presents various reaching methods using inflated fire hose. These methods are applicable to ice rescue.)

Anything thrown or passed to the victim should provide for the victim's quickly and easily grasping or using it.[3] (Take into account the victim's increasing inability to feel or to manipulate limbs and fingers.)

Lines or fire hoses should have loops or cross-bars on their ends (Fig. 10-10). The loops allow the victim to encircle himself or herself and then be pulled to safety. A short cross-bar, which could be straddled as an extrication aid by an active victim, also adds throwing weight and accuracy to the end of a line (Table 10-2).

Inactive, cold-debilitated victims call for "go" type rescues. Many unprepared rescuers have died in poorly planned and executed ice rescues. *Do not go unless and until you feel your chances for rescue are at least as great as those of losing the victim.*

Table 10-2 Rescuer Duties: Ice Rescue

Title	Primary Duties
Team leader	Same as in Table 10-1, paying particular attention to ice conditions and potential for hypothermia in victim *and* rescue team members.
Far-side supervisor	Attempt shore or *safe* ice-based throwing rescue.
	Lay out fire hose; attach PFD or other device to far end; tend left-hand steering line; or become lead dry suit swimmer.
	Man boat as required.
Near-side supervisor	Attempt shore-based or *safe* ice-based throwing rescue.
	Assist in laying out and inflating hose; tend right-hand steering line; or become backup dry suit swimmer or line tender.
	Man boat as required.
Equipment supervisor	Rig hose inflation apparatus; push hose on ice as directed; or assist dry suit swimmers.
	Inflate or provide boat as required.
	Tend boat line.

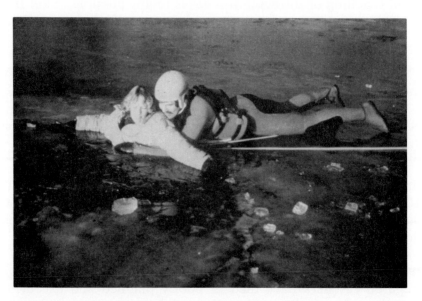

Fig. 10-10 Ice rescuer wearing a dry suit securing an active victim to the rescue line. (Courtesy Dive Rescue International.)

The following are points to consider in ice rescues:
- The victim cannot help himself or herself.
- The victim out of the water is a dead weight.
- If you break through the ice, your ability to help yourself, let alone the victim, rapidly decreases.
- Ice victims may be children who are much smaller and lighter than adult rescuers. If the ice did not support a smaller child, it will *not* support you.
- Your chances of an immediate, unaided rescue are poor to slight unless you do something to better the initial odds. Therefore do not rush rapidly into a go rescue mode without seeking some form of assistance. If nothing else, at least yell for help.
- If confronted with an inactive victim, look for something that will both extend your reach and allow you to hook or grab him or her. (A fire fighter's **pike pole** is a good example of such an instrument.)
- Do not allow yourself to be caught completely unprepared in this situation. In potential ice rescue weather *always have at least a PFD and length of line immediately available in your departmental vehicle* (Fig. 10-11).
- Attempt to loop a line securely (preferably the same one attached to you) around the victim. This step prevents the victim's slipping away

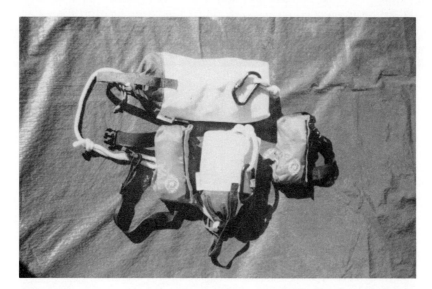

Fig. 10-11 Basic ice rescue equipment carried in a vehicle: PFDs for rescuer and back-up or assistant; tether for rescuer; throw bottle or bag to toss to victim.

from you and aids shoreside efforts to pull both of you back to safety. Put an extra PFD on the victim if you can.

Specific Ice Rescue Team Pointers

The foregoing points primarily have dealt with an individual rescuer's encountering an ice situation. Team tactics build on these pointers. Principle team considerations include responding with dry-suited (preferred) or wet-suited personnel plus backup equipment with which you have practiced. This equipment could include small craft, with inflatable boats preferred; line-throwing devices; inflated (steerable) fire hoses or ramps; and extension apparatus such as snorkel units or an articulated (high-rise) ladder and similar aerial gear (Fig. 10-12). The underlying concept is to realize that you and your organization might be involved in ice rescue and to plan and practice for that possibility. In using any type of backup equipment also look toward access and entry routes and possible problems. Knowing where and how you can use larger pieces of gear around ice may also prevent your having to rescue them (Table 10-3).

> Dry rescue suits (see Chapter 11) are the preferred initial piece of equipment for ice rescue. (NOTE: They are *not* the same as dry diving suits. These preferred suits are for surface rescue only.) They can be rapidly and easily donned, allowing you to wear clothing beneath them for increased rescuer warmth.

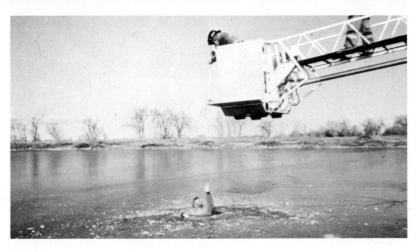

Fig. 10-12 Team ice rescue using a snorkel truck. (Courtesy Dive Rescue International.)

Some suits are manufactured with a **harness** built in; others require the addition of a suitable harness or tethering system. A number of ice rescue approaches can be developed with them. Personnel possessing this equipment should practice, again initially under safe, shallow, supervised conditions, to generate their own departmental guidelines. Even though most of these suits are extremely adaptable, each version has some drawbacks that should be known and appreciated by the user.

Small craft appropriate for ice rescue should be light, extremely buoyant, and easily adaptable to being pushed, shoved, or otherwise moved on an icy or partially frozen surface (Fig. 10-13). Although

Table 10-3 Ice Thickness and Strength

Thickness (inches)	Weight Capacity
< 2	**Stay off!**
2	One man on foot
3	Maximum of two men
4	Ice fishing station
5	Snowmobiles or all-terrain vehicles
8-12	Passenger cars, light trucks
24	Commercial trucks, heavy equipment

Modified from Ice Awareness, Emergency, p 25, March 1984. WARNING: Ice thickness can vary widely in the same general surface area. New ice is stronger than old. Snow may obscure weak ice. Current will undercut ice. Birds and animals flocking or nesting on ice can weaken it.

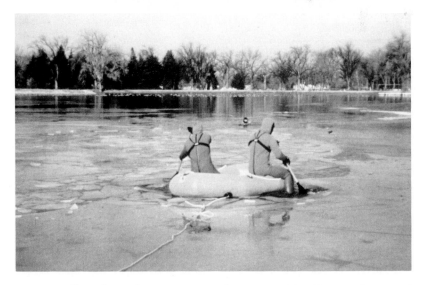

Fig. 10-13 Small craft used in ice rescue. (Courtesy Dive Rescue International.)

smaller aluminum boats, usually provided with extra flotation, have been featured in this role, there are other alternatives.

Inflatable craft generally weigh far less per carrying capacity than any other type of boat. They can be easily carried or, if need be, rapidly assembled or inflated on scene. Their main drawback is price. A number of individuals have modified larger surfboards with runners for ice rescue. Several inventors have also developed similar craft and offer them for sale.

LOW HEAD DAMS

By definition, a low head dam is a uniform barrier across a body of moving water (Fig. 10-14). The dam is level or horizontal, with water falling equally along its entire face.

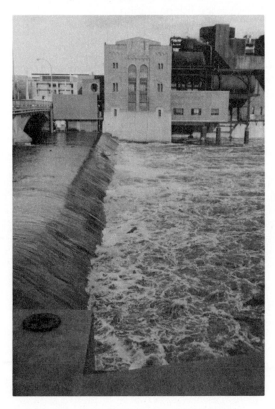

Fig. 10-14 Classic low head dam. A drowning machine.

If the barrier somehow is broken, the extremely hazardous vertical suction that distinguishes this type of danger generally will not form. (However, dangerous *horizontal* eddy currents may still be present.)

Most barriers of this nature have been placed in streams and rivers for one of two major purposes: (1) to slow potential flood waters as they move downstream or (2) to back up water for irrigation and hydroelectric or other similar industrial purposes.

Most of these barriers are artificial. However, they may be created when flash flood waters rush across a highway and drop into a roadside ditch or if a tree or similar object falls across and completely blocks a waterway. The difference in water height between the upper and lower sides of the continuous dam creates countercurrents at the base of the barrier (hydraulics).

As moving water flows over the barrier and falls vertically, part of the flow splits and rotates back toward the barrier. This return rotation generates a *vertical* whirlpool that traps objects at the dam's base (Fig. 10-15).

The area immediately downstream from the dam's face where the descending water splits is called the *boil*, or *boil line*. Depending on the rate of flow, depth of water, and height differences between the two levels of water, the boil line can extend many feet in front of the downstream face of the dam.[6]

Because the water circulating in the hydraulics is extremely **aerated,** most otherwise buoyant objects have difficulty floating. This factor, combined with the hydraulics' downward suction, repeatedly draws floating objects beneath the surface at the dam's lower face, along the

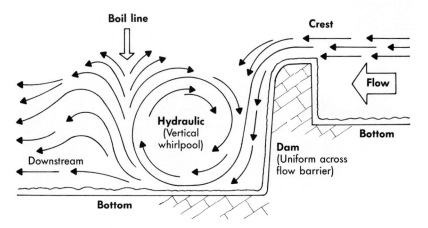

Fig. 10-15 How the hydraulic is formed—a vertical whirlpool.

bottom to the boil, up to the surface, and back toward the face again. The aeration also causes **cavitation** in most boat propellers. This means that small craft drawn into and trapped between the dam and boil line cannot power their way out.

Additionally, because the hydraulics' force is a variable, the boil line itself migrates. In some instances this migration has unexpectedly resulted in downstream safety lines and buoys and unsuspecting boaters being pulled into the hydraulics.

The principal hazard with low head dams is that *most of the time they do not look particularly dangerous.* When water flow decreases, many of these dams can be walked across easily. Children frequently play on or near them, and fishermen climb over their sides. Even when water is running higher, some people are inclined to treat them as a water thrill device, attempting to "surf" down or across them in all types of craft from canoes to air mattresses. Another danger is their upstream lack of presence. When boaters do not know that a low head dam lies downstream, they quite frequently tumble over it. This problem results from the dam's unbroken cross-stream surface.

Because of this seamless upstream optical illusion, the dam is usually undetectable by someone floating down from above. Additionally, sound produced by the falling water is projected *downstream* by the dam's vertical face (Fig. 10-16).

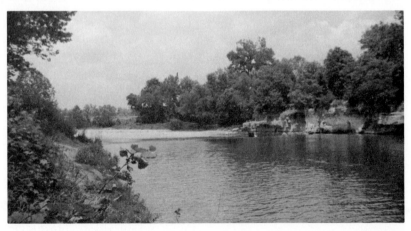

Fig. 10-16 Low head dam as seen from upstream. Note the optical illusion. The top of the dam *cannot* be perceived until the unaware boater is almost on it.

Most of these dams also trap and recirculate large amounts of debris and flotsam at their base. Thus individuals unfortunate enough to fall in may find themselves caught between crashing tree trunks.

The first rule for dealing with these killers is one of prevention. If a low head dam exists within your area, be sure it is well marked, especially with *repeated* upstream warnings. The side walls should be fenced to prevent shore access. Buoy lines and barriers should be placed both above the dam and downstream of the boil. In a number of localities if conditions permit, the dams either have been removed or holes have been created in their faces, thereby destroying the hydraulics. Another remedy is to pile large rocks or **riprap** at the foot of the dam to break the recirculating water pattern.

Rescue from a low head dam is dangerous and chancy. *Never place a rescuer between the dam and boil line* (Fig. 10-17). Always use some form of *practiced* reaching or throwing procedure.

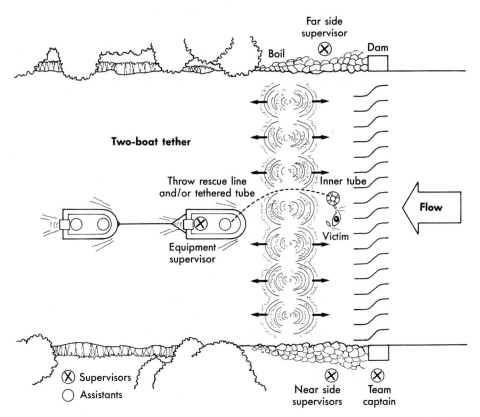

Fig. 10-17 The ideal team rescuer positions for dealing with low head dams.

An inflated fire hose will float against the dam. It can also be rigged with hooks to snare an unconscious victim's clothing. In situations in which too much debris blocks the inflated hose, other techniques can be used (Table 10-4). In some settings with narrower waterways, prepositioned span lines can be used to pull a rescue buoy, equipped with hooks if needed, across the dam's face. If the waterway is too wide to allow either prepositioned lines or some application of a thrown or shot line, a line must be carried across the stream.

Towing a line across the water *well above* a dam may be easier than attempting the same maneuver below it, for generally deeper, slower moving water above the dam presents fewer obstacles to the line.

On the other hand, should the towing craft lose power, it might be swept over the dam. If the team manning the on-shore end of the messenger line were to haul it in rapidly, the disabled towing craft could be pulled from trouble. In any instance all due precautions should be taken to prevent fouling lines in *any* boat's propeller anywhere near a dam. A general rule of thumb is to position the line-crossing point twice as far above the dam as the river is wide. In addition, sufficient line equal to twice the stream's width should be on hand. Managing long lines at high speeds promotes friction burns on the line haulers' hands. Therefore anyone involved in this aspect of the rescue must wear gloves suitable for working with line.

Once a line is established across the stream, it could be allowed to float downstream, over the dam, and into the hydraulic; or it could be pulled upstream across the boil. In either instance a *floating* line must be used. A flotation or rescue device then could be taken to the victim (Fig. 10-18).

Table 10-4 Rescuer Duties: Low Head Dam

Title	Primary Duties
Team leader	Same as Table 10-1, paying particular attention to victim situation and endurance plus location of boil line and access areas.
Far-side supervisor	Attempt shore-based or throwing rescue.
	Take messenger or span line to far side.
	Assist boat operator in boat-based rescue.
Near-side supervisor	Attempt to talk victim into self-rescue.
	Provide shore-based, throwing rescue as needed.
	Tend span line as required.
	Tend boat line from shore in boat-based rescue.
Equipment supervisor	Inflate, launch, and operate boat.
	Direct both boats in two-boat tether operation.

See Skill Drill 22 in Appendix IV to review rescue procedures at low head dams.

> The victim then should be moved *directly across the stream* to the nearest shore. Pulling a victim or a small craft downstream and over a boil line generally is not recommended. The water's force could flip a boat or pull the victim off the rescue line.

Boat-based rescues involving two craft can also be used. One boat is used as a downstream anchor. It is tethered to an upstream craft, with this upstream boat approaching but remaining clearly *below* the boil line. A rescue device such as a type IV ring buoy or an inner tube with a line attached is thrown from the upstream boat across the boil. (See Skill Drill 23.) The downstream boat can then pull both the upstream craft and the victim away from the dam. Fire fighting equipment such as aerial ladders and snorkel trucks have also been used.

Using helicopters is an additional alternative, but their use also has drawbacks. The downdraft under a hovering helicopter may approach 100 miles per hour. Thus, with cold victims or rescuers, wind chill may be a serious problem. Because of helicopters' high noise levels, communications must be extremely dependable, preferably including at

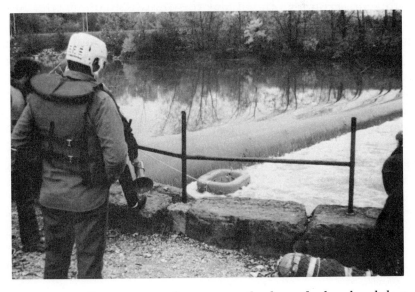

Fig. 10-18 Pulling a rescue float across the face of a low head dam.

least two radio channels (a primary and a backup). The unpredictable effects of a helicopter's surface downwash can shove or even capsize small boats. Do not count on helicopters as your primary source of providing rescues unless you have practiced with them.

Several rescue publications have carried diagrams indicating how self-contained underwater breathing apparatus (SCUBA)-equipped rescuers can defeat hydraulics. Such techniques may work in lower intensity flows, but they generally should not be trusted. Even well-trained divers can become confused in the hydraulics' zero visibility turbulence. Additionally, the possibility of snags and debris holding anyone underwater cannot be discounted.

IMMERSED AUTO

Cars and trucks enter the water for several reasons. A fairly common occurrence during northern winters is for vehicles driven on ice to sink through it. Drivers may lose control while driving alongside a lake, stream, or river and crash into the water. Small children, left alone in a car parked by the water, can either release the brakes or engage the gears, resulting in immersion of the auto. Occasionally, heavily traveled bridges fail, causing a number of vehicles to tumble into the water. In addition, flash floods claim many lives when rising waters engulf stalled cars, trucks, and buses or when flooded streams unexpectedly rush through campgrounds. In all the foregoing situations, the primary response is prevention.

Although experienced persons on frozen lakes should know that at least 7½ to 8 inches of ice are needed to support a small car, many unseen and unexpected hazards may be present (see Table 10-3). For instance, pressure ridges can fracture and weaken ice and then be lightly covered with snow. Large schools of milling fish can send warmer bottom water toward the surface. Currents beneath the ice can introduce warmer waters. Pipes running from houses located alongside lakes may contain warmed water, thereby melting ice located above their ends.

If someone is caught in an ice-entrapped vehicle, the first response should be to *get out immediately on the surface.* Do not plan to ride the car down. Too many hazards such as turning upside down in deep silt are extremely probable.

Because most vehicles will float for 30 to 60 seconds on the surface, bailing out as quickly as possible topside should be the rule.[2]

A similar rule exists for rising flood waters. Essentially, if others have stalled, so will you. Do not attempt to cross a flooded area unless you *know* that the depth of the water is insufficient to stall your vehicle. Most smaller autos will float in 2 feet of water. Once the car has two wheels off the road surface, it and anyone inside are subject to the water's whims. Even as a car gradually fills and settles, it still can be subject to the not-too-gentle aspects of current, especially when carried into deeper areas.[4]

As a rescuer, you have two main concerns with immersed vehicles: getting everyone out as quickly as possible and being sure you have accounted for everyone. Auto-immersion cases can be divided into four categories: those in fast water; those in still water; deep submersions; and shallow submersions. Two other subcategories include (1) intact cars and (2) wrecked or inverted cars. Extrication possibilities run from the very complex (a wrecked or inverted car in deep and flowing water) to the relatively simple (an undamaged vehicle in a shallow, still situation). In this spectrum of potentials, your order of priorities should flow as follows:

- Find and mark the vehicle. Detailed shoreside searches may be needed to determine exactly where the car entered. (Maintaining a list of underwater hulks near roadways might sound silly, but noting where junkers are located when the water is low can help on cold, rainy night searches.) Once you find the (right) car, mark it in some way, either with a PFD with a fairly long length of line tied to it or by shoreside lines of position. In the former case, should the car shift into deeper water, you will still be able to tell where it went. Be sure a wrecker has been called or that you have operating, shoreside winch capability. Also be sure that divers have been alerted if they have not already dispatched to the scene.
- Depending on the situation, decide if you want to attempt to enter the car in the water or wait until it can be hauled into a shallower setting. An important consideration is how long you or your crew can remain functioning in the water. In addition, is the water rising? Will the vehicle be carried further into the stream? If you decide to enter the car, first try a door on the *downstream* side. If the door does not work, a simple center punch hammered against the lower front corner of side windows will usually break them. If you are using a punch or a similar device, be sure all the tools have lanyards on them to prevent their being dropped and carried away by the water. If the vehicle is

stable and the rear window is exposed, breaking the window may be your quickest route. However, be sure you are not deflating an air pocket, which may provide oxygen to occupants and/or flotation for the vehicle.

- If you enter the car in *moderate* current, you are probably less likely to get into trouble if you enter from the downstream side. In *strong* current, entering from downstream is unwise because the car might roll over and trap the rescuer. In this case breaking an upstream window may have to suffice since the current will keep upstream doors closed. Do *not* open all doors in a current, for doing so allows the water to race through the vehicle and pull smaller occupants out. It also sets up a strainer that could imperil you and your team. Opening an upstream door could also result in debris or silt entering, making search and extrication more difficult.

- *All* personnel working on, in, or around the vehicle must wear PFDs. If current is involved, everyone must have a safety line properly attached to him or her.

- Attempt to read the license plate, even as you go about extricating occupants. Find out who owns the car; then have someone quickly contact them. This step greatly assists in determining how many people might have been in the car and whether or not one or more may

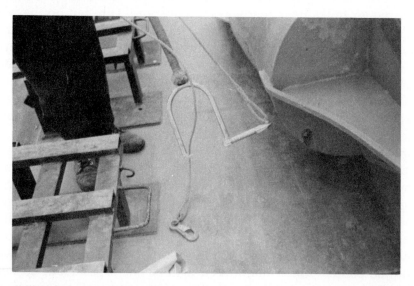

Fig. 10-19 A "Snatch" hook (initially designed for placing a tag line through the lifting eye on a buoy). Used in passing a line around or through semisubmerged objects.

have been carried away or thrown out somewhere on the bank. (NOTE: This same procedure can be of assistance in boat cases in which tracing the boat's hull registration numbers can assist in determining who is missing.) If anyone is available on the scene who might know how many occupants were in the car, immediately have the witness questioned.

In addition to the foregoing, especially if there is a large probability of your department's responding to auto immersions, consider obtaining or rigging the following: a "snatch" hook device and an air hose "roof penetrator" insert. The first device allows the attachment of a line around an object such as a car bumper, even when it is under water (Fig. 10-19). This would facilitate hooking a winch line onto a submerged auto. The second device is designed to penetrate the roof of a vehicle, allowing the insertion of high-pressure air, possibly driving the interior water level down while making the auto more buoyant.

SPECIAL CIRCUMSTANCES
Multivictim Incidents

A special vehicle-immersion situation involves buses or passenger-carrying aircraft in the water. The two prime considerations are expeditiously extricating as many victims as possible and accounting for everyone.

Carrying large inflatable devices on every type of rescue vehicle might be impractical. A usable alternative is to have all hose-equipped fire trucks provided with air inflators. Inflated fire hoses can support large numbers of people being pulled to safety. Incident command system protocols should be followed in multivictim water accidents, and a primary effort should be directed toward determining as soon as possible exactly how many victims are involved.

Many large metropolitan airports are built alongside or project out into river flood plains, bays, or other large bodies of water. For this reason, the potential for responding to commercial aircraft downed in the water is not remote. Consideration and planning given to this possibility may pay great future dividends.

Shallow Water Line Searches

A rule of thumb useful in those cases in which no clear indication of the victim's last location can be developed follows: *10 feet from safety and 50 feet from the beach*, depending on bottom conditions and water flow. In other words, most aquatic victims die 10 feet from safety and within

50 feet of a beach. This usually means that a line of searchers perpendicular to the shore can join hands or link arms and sweep an area 50 feet out from the beach. Usually, the closer the spacing, the more quickly the object is found, even if repeated passes must be made through the area.

If the water is too deep for wading, the offshore end of the line is comprised of surface divers, at least until self-contained breathing apparatus (SCBA)-equipped personnel arrive. As many people as possible should be wearing PFDs, particularly those on the deeper end or if the bottom is unknown or irregular. This same technique can be used in clouded, underwater-vision–impaired swimming pool situations. It is better to walk the pool bottom with a line of rescuers than to swing safety poles.

As a practical indication of just how difficult searching for an underwater object can be, review the shallow water line search exercise in Chapter 8 (i.e., Skill Drill 20), which involves searching for a nearly invisible clear plastic bottle on the pool bottom. This experience teaches everyone to be very careful and methodical in conducting *any* type of in-water search.

ON-WATER FIRE FIGHTING AND EMERGENCY RESPONSE SAFETY

Fire fighting and emergency response over or on the water have three special considerations in addition to normal, terrestrial procedures: (1) flammable fluid-water interactions and dynamics; (2) personnel disorientation; and (3) sudden, unexpected immersion potential.

Flammable Fluids

> Fires have the potential for developing, spreading, and enveloping fire fighting parties much more rapidly on water than on land.

The basic reason is that most flammable fluids are lighter than water. They are rapidly distributed or spread by wind, tide, and current. Thus fire fighters should attempt to contain flammable fluids if at all possible *before ignition*. Even after ignition, attempts should be made to establish boundaries to prevent further spread of surface fires because of potential wind shifts or tidal changes.

Depending on circumstances, one possible alternative, especially in an area with a small circumference, is the use of an inflated fire hose containment boom.

Of particular importance is the fire fighters' knowledge of wind and current potentials in the fire area. Just as terrestrial fires should be fought with the wind at the fire fighters' backs, a similar stance should be taken relative to current and tide. If all the dynamic forces are aligned in the same heading, there is a greatly expanded potential for spreading the fire. But there is little question of the attack direction. Conversely, when wind and current (or tide) are running *against* each other, a number of measurements and decisions must be made to determine which is the greater or lesser hazard.

Additionally, there must be a definite awareness of potential changes in prevailing dynamic patterns (e.g., the wind's suddenly changing direction or growing in intensity). Thus in water situations fire fighting personnel must be extremely mobile (able to move or get away from harm rapidly) and in *constant* communications (including having available in-depth backup) with command personnel.

Personnel Disorientation

Any fire scene involving dense smoke and flames has the potential, through reduced visibility, to cause disorientation to involved personnel.

> Of particular importance in the water area is the fact that wind and current may intervene by moving floating structures or fire fighting platforms. This movement can readily confuse and disorient emergency responders.

Rescue personnel entering a low visibility area afloat *must be tethered with a fire-resistant steel cable.* Because of the dynamic potential of sudden changes in the fire scene, a simple set of pull signals must be understood by everyone involved on both ends of the cables. Shipboard fire fighting procedures now include communication wires centered in the tethers to allow the fire fighter and line handler, who both are wearing lightweight headsets, to communicate with each other. However, since this system might be interrupted, the pull signals still should be practiced. Naval or Coast Guard Reserve centers should be able to provide information on this equipment.

Sudden Immersion

As previously indicated, fire fighters and other emergency providers, especially at nighttime accident and fire scenes, might suddenly find themselves in the water. For this reason, any emergency response organization potentially responsible for responding to an on-water (or over-water) call *must* provide its people with sufficient flotation equipment (*and* suitable training in its use).

This need is reenforced by the fire dynamics and disorientation potential indicated in the foregoing paragraphs. As with other aspects of water-related emergency response, practice and understanding of what can and might happen are essential. Again, the idea is to set up on-water training practices if and where the need is identified.

Although responding to and controlling many types of terrestrial accidents is difficult, the possibilities for chaos on the water are near limitless. For example, picture a scene in the passenger-filled compartment of a river gambling boat such as those now operating on midwestern rivers. Should fire break out or the vessel be rammed and start to settle, how would *you* go about removing a thousand passengers from a sinking vessel — in midriver, at midnight, over near-freezing water — that might be on fire? To this scenario, add the possibilities that all light and power aboard may have failed and that your compartment is not only continuously tilting to one side but is also rapidly filling with cold water. Although neither a pretty nor an inviting picture, this *is* the possible scene of the water emergency response.

If such a potential exists in your area of responsibility, do *not* become involved with reinventing the wheel. Instead, attempt to contact your nearest Navy or Coast Guard Reserve Training Center. It should have specialists well schooled in systematically approaching this type of event. In fact, if your neighboring naval reserve training facility is large enough, it may have a shipboard damage simulator, wherein you might have an opportunity to experience and to practice basic responses to the foregoing situations safely.

CHAPTER SUMMARY

This chapter has presented *basic* team-oriented considerations for use in a number of common water rescue situations. In particular, procedures were covered concerning:
- Swift water rescues.
- Ice rescues.
- Rescues from low head dams.
- Team member responsibilities.
- Elementary equipment requirements.

- Backup equipment and procedural suggestions.
- On-water, large-scale emergency response.

REFERENCES

1. Bechdel L and Ray S: River rescue, Boston, 1989, Appalachian Mountain Club Books, pp 100-105.
2. Fawcett W: Water: The timeless compound, Wayzetta, Minn, 1980, Fawcett Communications (film).
3. Ice rescue, Fort Collins, Colo, 1981, Dive Rescue International (slide/tape).
4. Madison A: Swept away, Chatham, NY, 1990, Alan Madison Productions (videotape).
5. River rescue, Columbus, Ohio, 1980, Ohio Department of Natural Resources, pp 11-13.
6. The drowning machine, State College, Pa, 1981, Film Space (videotape).

11

~~~~~~ **Equipment**

OVERVIEW

Water rescue equipment and suggestions for its use, specifications, and training involvement constitute the focus of this chapter. Situation-specific tactics are discussed for certain types of gear. Hazards and hindrances also are examined. Different types of water craft and their rescue potentials are compared.

OBJECTIVES

After studying this chapter, the reader should comprehend various kinds of equipment used in water rescue. Particular points include:
1. Ship abandonment and dry (rescue) suits
2. Tactics and safety considerations for use of dry suits
3. Inflated hose options
4. Basic waterside rope and rigging considerations
5. Identification of rescue boat requirements
6. Rescue boat tactics and safety specifics
7. Design of drills and procedures combining equipment use
8. Equipping fire, police, and emergency medical services (EMS) vehicles for water rescue

PRETEST

1. One drawback of the **neoprene** "dry" water rescue suit is that a fully clothed wearer may suffer an internal temperature drop after wearing it in the water for an hour. (True or false?)
2. Proper procedure for use of a rescue suit includes (a) having a

tether snapped to the suit; (b) having the line tender also in a dry suit; (c) back paddling for best speed; or (d) allowing the victim to grab the suited rescuer's head. (Which of the above is not true?)
3. In a rescue craft, which of the following is most important? (a) speed; (b) maneuverability; (c) survivability; or (d) loading capacity.
4. The primary operating requirements for a rescue boat operator are (a) knowing the weather; (b) knowing what is going on around and in the boat; (c) keeping a good lookout; or (d) carrying proper signaling equipment. (Which two are most important?)
Pretest answers are at the end of the chapter.

DEVELOPMENT OF THE NEOPRENE WATER RESCUE SUIT

The text has stressed that many techniques basic to swimming pool water rescue training simply do not work in the usual rescue environment. One solution for bridging this need for providing professional rescue personnel with all-around water safety equipment has been development of the dry rescue suit.

During the late 1960s and early 1970s a number of ship sinkings, especially on the Great Lakes, caused the Coast Guard to look into going beyond personal flotation devices (PFDs) for in-water protection. Many survivors perished while wearing PFDs because of the effects of cold. Research projects were established to develop some form of garment that would both float a potential victim and protect him or her from the cold.[1] The basis for these developments was the neoprene self-contained underwater breathing apparatus (SCUBA) diver's dry suit. The dry diver's suit grew out of the classic neoprene "wet" suit. The wet suit, by trapping a layer of warmed water between the diver's skin and the suit's inner surface, provides protection from heat loss. The dry diving suit completely isolates the diver's body from the water, allowing the diver to wear dry thermal undergarments. Although this was a cold-protection step forward, dry diving suits are expensive because they must, for best all-around effects, be closely cut to conform to the diver's body. This also means that they are difficult to don quickly.

By working with these essential elements, ship abandonment suit designers generated a loose-fitting, easily worn garment that would float the wearer while isolating him or her from cold water. The only part of the wearer directly touched by water is the face. It must be covered by both gloved hands when initially entering the water, especially if the water is extremely cold (Fig. 11-1). Although earlier attempts at such suits were made by military designers, their greatest dilemma was designing an effective, simple watertight zipper. Research into space suits solved this problem. A number of Canadian and American manufacturers produce these neoprene immersion suits primarily for the shipping and offshore oil industries. Donning time is usually specified as a minute or less, with heat loss in an otherwise naked adult in ice water allowed at no more than 1° F per hour. In a fully clothed (multilayered) person the heat loss is far less than 1° F per hour. Some persons have been adrift at sea for several days without serious internal temperature difficulty.

There are three types of federally approved immersion (ship abandonment) suits: child universal; adult universal; and adult oversize. The child universal suit fits children weighing up to 110 pounds. The adult universal design fits people up to 6 feet 3 inches tall, weighing up to 330 pounds. Adult oversize suits accommodate wearers up to 6 feet, 9 inches tall, weighing up to 375 pounds. Being made of neoprene allows the suit

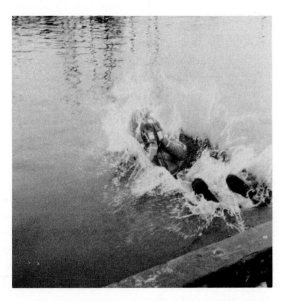

Fig. 11-1 The only place for water to enter in the dry suit is the face. Attempt to cover the face when entering the water. Torso reflex can also be a very large problem.

to stretch. Additionally, the "Gumby" style feet allow rapid donning over almost all kinds of boots and footwear. Flotation provided by the neoprene in the suit is 55 pounds. An inflation pillow behind the head adds another 15 pounds of buoyancy.

If a wearer enters the water on his or her back and does not stand upright when immersed, two other people can usually float on top of the suit. Although trapped air is not needed to float the original occupant, buoyancy provided by air trapped in the oversized feet and legs helps to support the extra riders.

The neoprene *water rescue* suit is a modified ship abandonment design. It is *not* approved by the Coast Guard because it has fitted boots attached to the suit, which require a wearer to remove his or her shoes or boots. It also does not have the hypothermia-protective head pillow. Hence the rescue suit's flotation is less than that of the ship abandonment style. Conversely, with its boots and reenforced knees and elbows, it can be comfortably worn both in the water and on shore (Fig. 11-2). Both types of suits come with retroreflective materials on their upper surfaces and whistles on the zipper pulls (Fig. 11-3). The rescue suit and most ship abandonment suits normally have an attached belt or harness strong enough to allow deployment from a helicopter or lowering and lifting from other overhead positions.

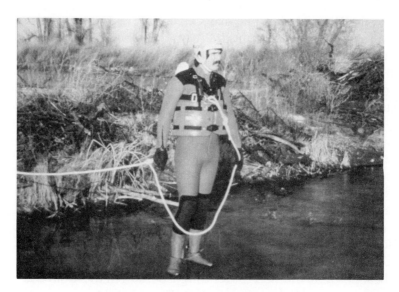

Fig. 11-2 Rescue suit boots and reenforced knees and elbows are designed for rugged streamside environments. This rescuer has added an additional layer of flotation. (Courtesy Dive Rescue International: Ice rescue [slide/tape presentation].)

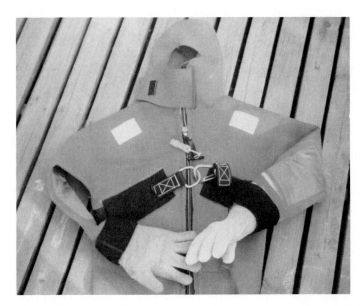

Fig. 11-3 The whistle, retroreflective tape, and harness are all part of the rescue suit package.

USING RESCUE SUITS

Although the rescue suits are extremely user friendly, absorbing almost all kinds of punishment, there are points to consider in their use. If the suits are not used frequently, zippers tend to jam. A paraffin-based lubricant is usually provided by the manufacturer to remedy this problem. The suits are *not* designed as hazardous material protective. They can take a lot of rough use without tearing, and small holes can be repaired easily with plastic cement. However, if repeatedly used for training in highly chlorinated swimming pools, the glue attaching the suit panels may be affected. Always thoroughly rinse the suits, inside and out, after a pool session. The suits must also be completely dried on the inside before being stored. The insides of glove fingers are particularly prone to mildew and rot if not cared for. Finally, although the suits are extremely buoyant, they *can* be submerged under certain conditions, one of which—downstream in fast-moving current on the end of a taut belayed tether—is very dangerous.

The best possible method for tending a person in these suits is with the line across, *not parallel to*, the current (Fig. 11-4). As another safety tip, the line tender should wear a suit so that if required, he or she can be ready to assist the primary rescuer (Fig. 11-5). Use of quick-release

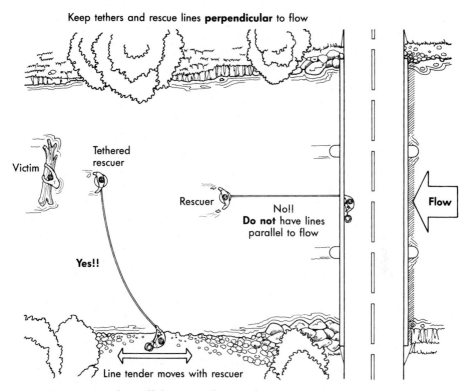

Keep tethers and rescue lines **perpendicular** to flow

Victim

Tethered rescuer

Rescuer

Yes!!

No!!
Do not have lines
parallel to flow

Flow

Line tender moves with rescuer

Fig. 11-4 Be sure that all lines with people on the ends of them are worked *perpendicular* to the flow.

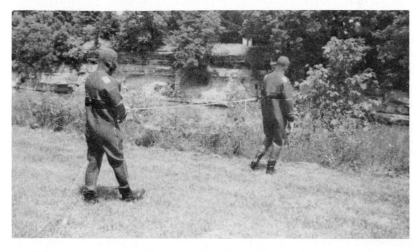

Fig. 11-5 Two people should be suited and ready. The line tender is wearing a suit to provide for quick assistance should the primary rescuer require help.

devices, mentioned in Chapter 10, might also be considered.

As with all other forms of rescue equipment, repeated practice with the suits and proper maintenance ensure best results.

Although when not immersed the suits appear bulky and unmanageable, a *practiced* person can become agile while wearing them in the water. One of the first lessons most users learn is that, because of the relatively large area of the gloves, they form effective paddles for back stroking. Also, because of the outsized feet, kicking is normally ineffective. Note that remaining on the back produces the best speed in the suits. When initially practicing with the suits, techniques that encourage victims to grab the wearer's feet, then possibly ease themselves up on the rescuers thighs (while the shore-tethered rescuer talks to and calms the victim) seem to work best.

Skill Drill 23. In this drill the rescuer is securely tethered to a line handler, and the rescuer passes a loop of line around the victim before they are both pulled to safety. What a suit user most definitely does *not* want to happen is to blunder head first into a victim. If this occurs, with the victim pushing down on the rescuer's head, trapped air in the suit's feet may make escape and stabilization extremely difficult.

Again, in almost all instances the suit should be tethered. Tactics should be developed in which the line tender can warn the rescuer, who is usually swimming on his or her back, to turn around *before* the rescuer is within the reach of the victim.

As mentioned previously in the text, the neoprene suits are not the only waterproof garments available for water rescuers. Comfortable, lightweight, loose-fitting nylon dry suits are also on the market. These suits are generally less expensive, more easily worn when out of the water, and less confining than the bulkier neoprene models. However, they do not provide as much flotation or in-water warmth. Rapidly donned wet suits, featuring accordion zippered closures, are another option rescue team members might consider. Each of these suits has definite pluses and drawbacks. The best idea is to try them whenever possible; then match the proper garment to your needs. The resources listed in Appendix I can provide a starting point for learning more about this equipment.

INFLATED HOSE USE

An inflated fire hose is one of the simplest, yet most universally applicable water rescue devices imaginable if the people using it are well practiced and inventive (Fig. 11-6).

As indicated in the accompanying illustrations, rigging the hose is

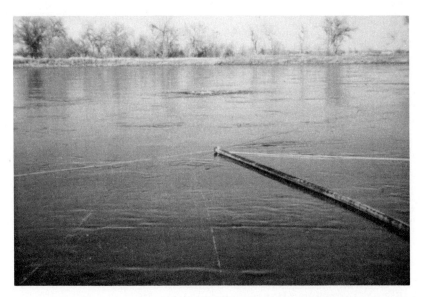

Fig. 11-6 Ice rescue is made much easier with an inflated fire hose. (Courtesy Dive Rescue International: Ice rescue [slide/tape presentation].)

extremely simple. Making this inflation device and developing procedures for its use are relatively elementary. The three elements of the system—hose, hose caps with adapters, and self-contained breathing apparatus (SCBA) tanks with appropriate fittings—are easily transportable and normally can be quickly delivered at most rescue scenes (Fig. 11-7).

The usual hose is a 2½ inch fire hose capable of sustaining 100 to 120 pounds per square inch (psi) pressure. Depending on pressure, one fully charged SCBA tank should be able to inflate at least four sections of 2½ inch hose. All hose connections should be as tight as possible, and checked with spanners.

Skill Drill 24.

> The offshore end of the hose should be supported with a PFD because the weight of the fittings may cause it to submerge.

If possible, the hose sections should be laid out and connected in a straight line before inflation. Repeated practice with the hose under different conditions such as still water, ice, and fast current is a must (Table 11-1).

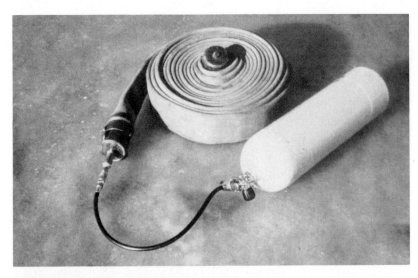

Fig. 11-7 Separate elements needed to inflate the hose. (Courtesy Dive Rescue International: Ice rescue [slide/tape presentation].)

Table 11-1 Hose Inflation Components

Component	Use
50 feet long fire hose	Inflate to 120 lb pressure.
2½ inch male and female caps	Cap hose.
	One cap is drilled, with truck tire stem inserted and seated.
Pressure-reducing valve	Reduce pressure from SCBA bottle down to 120 psi.
Tire and hose inflator	Attach from pressure-reducing valve on SCBA bottle.
	Inflate hose in manner similar to that for tire.
Alternate method:	Connect SCBA bottle to shutoff valve on male cap.
½ inch flexible hose with quick-connect fitting	Inflate hose to 120 psi.
Shutoff valve and pressure relief valve on male cap	Secure bottle and hose valves.

Although the inflated hose is fairly rigid, poking it toward a victim requires some skill and practice. Even when steering lines are attached to the offshore end, the hose may have a tendency to curve or bend. Two methods may improve this situation. The first is to twist continually or rotate the hose as it enters the water. Care must be exercised not to foul the steering lines when this is done. The other alternative is to double the hose because two sections laid alongside each other provide a much more rigid, easily aimed device. The problem generated by this approach is that twice as much hose and compressed air is needed.

Practicing with the hose in different conditions of current is the best way to learn how to steer it during a fast water rescue. Pushing it into the current at an angle while tending the upstream line is one method for reaching a target. Laying it in the water parallel to the bank, then allowing it to pivot with the upstream end falling downstream and farther out into the current may also work.

As with the low head dam situation, and when a number of victims are encountered, simply pulling the hose across a waterway could be an acceptable alternative, but current will attempt to move it downstream.

In using this technique for ice rescue, a smaller diameter hose might be more manageable. The problem is not as much one of total hose flotation as it is of overcoming sliding friction with the ice surface. The best practice procedure would be to try both sizes of hose — 1 ½ inch plus 2 ½ inch — to see which works best for you. Since the hose caps are so easily modified, having caps for both sizes of hose should present no great problem. Another ice-specific modification is to rig the offshore cap or end of the hose to receive a piece of 3-inch polyvinyl chloride (PVC) plastic tubing 2 feet long. When the PVC is capped at both ends and attached crossway to the end of the hose, it both provides a seat on which the victim can climb and aids overall flotation.

INFLATION AND IMAGINATION

Because use of inflated hose is continually developing, other applications have been suggested and have undergone experimentation. Since these applications are tentative and highly dependent on the situation, they should be practiced to determine if they can be used by you before their acceptance as basic response ploys.

The first alternative is using inflated hose as a "quicky" flotation barrier in an oil or chemical spill. Lengths of hose can be inserted into the water to encircle smaller patches of contaminants, forming an initial containment boom.

This procedure would work only for smaller areas in still water, with the hose connections securely fastened to prevent eventual air leakage and sinking of the hose.

If enough hose and compressed air are available, multiple loops can be laid alongside each other to increase the barrier effect. Using hose in this manner would result in an extensive job of cleaning the hose exterior and returning it to service.

A high-capacity raft capable of carrying several people or their weight equivalent in equipment can be rigged quickly by doubling or faking several lengths of hose and loosely securing them to each other before inflation. This tactic would be a last-gap step if flotation were needed and no suitable watercraft were in the area. A similar application would involve loosely jamming hose under or encircling an object with the hose to lift it off the bottom of a stream or lake. Depending on the size and number of hoses used, after inflation of the hose, a considerable lifting force could be developed, if not to bring an object to the surface, at least to get it off the bottom so it could be towed or pulled into shallower water.

Dealing with a passive victim or recovering a (floating) body in ice or at low head dams might be easier with inflated hose. Hooks similar to those used in body dragging operations can be attached to the hose end. Hopefully, the hooks would snag the victim's clothing without injuring the person. As previously mentioned, a length of 2½ inch hose can support a large number of people either hanging onto or straddling it. Tests indicate that eight to 10 people can be supported per 50 feet of hose length. This is a very useful application if large numbers of people are adrift in a relatively small water area, depending on how much time is involved in rigging the hose, the numbers of rescuers, and the condition of the victims. Last, an inflated hose placed at an angle completely across a flooded, fast moving waterway may help corral victims floating downstream. Victims should be directed to throw their upper body (per strainer) across the hose. The force of the moving water will shove them toward shore and waiting rescuers. The hose is angled because when the hose is perpendicular to fast flow, victims have a difficult time maintaining their grip.

INFLATABLE BOATS

Inflation provides high buoyancy with reduced structural size or weight. For instance, a double-ended johnboat 10 to 12 feet long has a *maximum* capacity of approximately 400 to 600 pounds, but all too commonly it is found as a standard water rescue device (Fig. 11-8).

A 10- or 12-foot inflatable boat of the same length and width will have at least *twice* this loading factor.

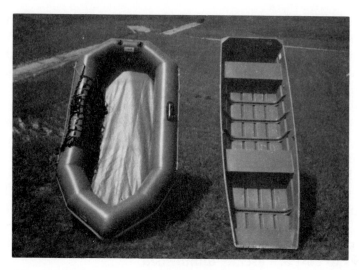

Fig. 11-8 Although both of these boats are approximately the same length, the inflatable is rated at three times the carrying capacity of the johnboat.

Placing two or three adult rescuers in the above-mentioned rigid (usually aluminum) craft begs the question of where to place the sodden victim who, when initially brought aboard, may weigh a quarter of a ton. Too frequently the johnboat is overloaded and sinks or is capsized. Inflatable craft are normally four times as expensive as the same-sized aluminum-hulled boat. Is this initial difference in expense worth it? Definitely yes! As an example, almost every smaller rescue craft now used by the U.S. and Canadian Coast Guards is inflatable. Why? Survivability and then ease of use are the answers.

Inflatable boats are essentially catamarans. Thus their buoyancy is multiple hulled or redundantly chambered and is distributed outboard. This design feature protects them against suddenly capsizing or flipping and makes them hard to sink (puncturing an air chamber in the average inflatable craft normally requires a force such as a gunshot). Repairing damage in most cases requires little time and a tire patch plus glue. Even when fiercely swept or pounded against rocks, trees, or strainers, inflatables hold up very well.

In real life situations inflatable boats can be easily carried or lowered just about anywhere by a few crew members. Actually, two people can carry most 12-foot inflatable boats, with one more person carrying a small outboard engine and gas can.

Because of weight and displacement factors, inflatables normally can develop relatively high speeds with smaller power plants. Also, their extremely simple inflation packages mean they can be toted uninflated almost anywhere and quickly pumped up, using either small air bottles, SCBA tanks, or foot pumps.

On the other hand, inflatables do have some drawbacks. Their rubber surfaces can degrade when continually exposed to abrasion and sunlight. Their rounded sides, although making victim retrieval easier, can become a formidable boarding obstacle to an unpracticed person if no one else is aboard. Should the boat deflate, getting air back into it requires simple equipment that may not be immediately available.

The final consideration in obtaining or upgrading to an inflatable boat depends on the user. However, rescue work demands survivability, which is inherent in inflatables. When all factors are reviewed, objections to cost are greatly diminished.

RESCUE BOAT CHARACTERISTICS

Various types of watercraft have been used successfully in rescues. They include but are not limited to canoes, rowboats, kayaks, and surfboards. Although a large amount of information is available on these nonpowered craft, our primary interest focuses on powered types. However, many of the following points are equally useful on any form of vessel, including unconventional water vehicles such as airboats, personal watercraft (jet skis), and hovercraft.

Survivability is *the* overwhelming need in a rescue craft. It—and you—may be placed in interesting and exacting situations. In fact, how well does your rescue craft float? Has it ever been swamped in safe, shallow water to ensure its floating full of water and people? Have you added extra, out-of-the-way flotation such as foam blocks or sealed, plastic jugs under the seats, decking, or gunwales?

In addition to survivability, an ideal rescue craft should possess the following capabilities:

- Stability. The design of the craft should allow working along side or over the side without undue heeling or tipping. The normal weight factor is the equivalent of a crew of two attempting to lift or roll a third person aboard over the side. It should not be top heavy because of large aerials or elevated light fixtures.
- Maneuverability. The craft should be able to move sharply or crisply in confined areas. If powered by an inboard engine, the rudder should have a wide range of motion and should be positioned for maximum

deflection of thrust from the screw. If an outboard motor is used, it should be able to swing through a large, maximized arc. If steering is in the stern with an engine **tiller** or control handle, nothing should be in the way of moving this handle from one side of the craft to the other. In this situation the gearshift lever should also be readily available and smooth in its operation.

- Speed. Good response time achieved with a fast-moving boat is a desired point. On the other hand, especially in dealing with outboard motors, speed can be gained by installing a larger, heavier engine. This may, in turn, reduce the boat's carrying capacity and maneuverability. A wise move in powering any craft is to check the Coast Guard capacity plate to determine maximum powering capacities. If the boat is to move at high speeds, provision should be made to shield the crew and possible on-board patients from (cold) wind and spray.

- Power train. With both inboard and outboard engines, screws or propellers should be matched with the engine for the normally intended use. For instance, if the boat is expected to do a large amount of towing, maneuvering, or pushing with the bow, a speed propeller would be inefficient. A rescue craft can be expected to operate in many types of water conditions and depths. For this reason, consideration should be given to checking into slip clutches versus shear pins. If an inexpensive shear pin breaks, the cost factor for replacement is minimal, but should the powerless boat be carried into danger, the value of the slip clutch arrangement far outweighs its cost.

  Use of ducted, shrouded, or jet-type lower units should be considered. Although protecting the screw does reduce power while taking away some top speed, *not* having lines or debris foul the propeller and kill the engine is a proper consideration. These determinations are made according to how and where the boat will be used. If at all possible, testing with different types of powering before the purchase is a good idea.

- Freeboard. Freeboard has a lot of impact on survivability, but it also affects ease of retrieval of persons overboard. As Chapter 7 indicates, the stern provides the most stability for bringing people aboard. However, on some craft the engine gets in the way, and it is necessary to work over the side. If so, the higher the side, the harder is the lift. Some trade-off is usually needed, with most rescue craft having lower sides **aft.**

- Rescue equipment and accessories. Depending on the size of the craft, some allowance should be made for a light source in addition to the navigation lights. In its simplest form, should the craft have a 12-volt battery, a spotlight can be plugged into a cigarette lighter arrangement. The craft should have a lot of retroreflective material topside so that it can be easily spotted at night or in reduced visibility. It should have a dependable sound signaling system in addition to and independent of a radio system. This system could include a battery-powered bullhorn or compressed gas-powered, hand-held horn. The boat should have *several* forms of alternative power such as oars and paddles. The craft should have enough space to carry extra PFDs, throw bags, lines, ring buoys, and possibly two different types of anchors. These anchors would be a small stockless type for use in sand or mud and a **grapnel** (with corks on the prongs if used in an inflatable craft) type for use on stone or rocky bottoms. Depending on the size and possible use of the craft, the operator could be provided with a kill switch if an outboard engine is used.

- Boarding aids. The boat, regardless of its size, when responding to an accident, should have a manrope, or grab rope, continually draped along its gunwale. These loops of line allow victims in the water to hang on while preparations are made to bring them aboard. The manrope's best position on the side of the hull should allow someone in the water to reach it *without* its snagging on brush alongside a steep river bank. This line should be of moderate diameter because line that is too thin can cut a person's hands. Some form of boarding net or

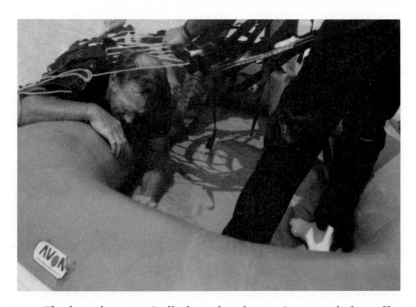

Fig. 11-9 The boarding net (roll-aboard technique) is simple but effective.

ladder should be included. The net, which can be made of small diameter rope, nylon strapping, or plastic snow fence and construction barrier netting is secured to and is normally carried under the gunwale (Fig. 11-9). Although someone could climb aboard using the net, its primary use is to roll an incapacitated person over the side and into the boat. (This is further discussed in the section on rescue lines.) A major consideration with smaller, unpowered rescue craft or vessels without outboard stern drives is how to get back on board if no one is available to help you.

A knotted "climbing-in" line (possibly a modified stern line or painter) may be needed in addition to the manrope. This is definitely a point to include in rescue boat training.

RESCUE LINES

All proficient water rescue personnel should have some basic knowledge of lines and knotting techniques. Basic line knowledge includes general information, as presented below, on which types of lines are used in certain situations. Knots (e.g., square, bowline, half hitch, clove hitch, and figure eights) are indispensable (Fig. 11-10, Table 11-2). You should be able to bend (tie) them in the dark and, even better, behind your back. They are simple to learn and, once learned, are difficult to forget. These five knots are illustrated on p. 248. Appendix I lists references for other knots, bends, and hitches.

The proper (salty) terminology for small-sized cordage is *line* rather than *rope*. In fact, in older sailing ship days very few "ropes" were found on vessels. There were, however, halyards, lanyards, sheets, braces, cables, outhauls, and downhauls. In the rescue business little differentiation is made between lines and ropes except to indicate that lines usually have a smaller diameter than ropes. Lines and ropes used by water rescuers have similar characteristics: they float, are resilient, and resist rot and mildew. Most of them consist of manmade fibers. Table 11-3 lists some of the more specific qualities of different line types.

A very prominent point involves breaking strengths. Lighter, more flexible (having a looser weave or braid) lines are designed for throwing and towing individuals through water. These lines also have a large expansion factor to reduce the jerk or shock to the person on the end if he or she is brought to a sudden stop. These types are *not* intended for

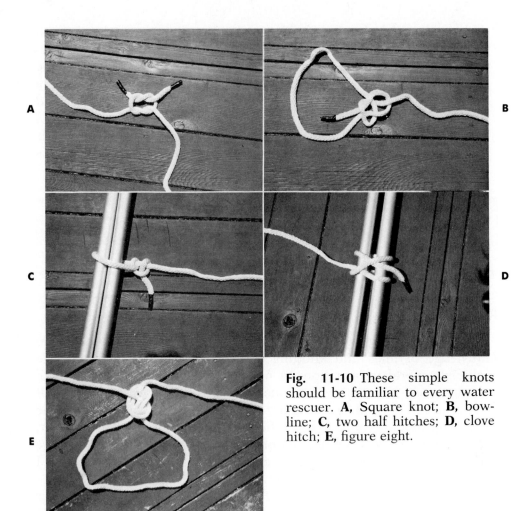

Fig. 11-10 These simple knots should be familiar to every water rescuer. **A**, Square knot; **B**, bowline; **C**, two half hitches; **D**, clove hitch; **E**, figure eight.

Table 11-2 Basic Water Rescue Knots

Type of Knot	Use
Square	Joins lines of same size; will not slip; easily untied
Bowline	Makes nonslipping bight or loop on end of line
Half hitch	Backs up primary knot with shorter end of line; securely ties or tightens around object
Clove hitch	Normally bends line around stationary objects
Figure eight	Makes loop(s) on line

heavy lifting, pulling, or dragging duty. This distinction must be understood. Numerous accidents and injuries have occurred when lighter lines were substituted for the heavier hauling variety (Fig. 11-11).

Other general line safety tips follow:

- Do not stand in the bight (loop) of any line that is or *may be* placed under a strain. This also means that if you are hauling on a line, stay away from the inside of any moving parts and as far back as practicable from bends, pulleys, and carabiners under stress. It is usually a good procedure *not* to turn your back on moving or working (under a strain) lines (Fig. 11-12).
- Always wear gloves while working with moving lines, or serious cuts or abrasions may result. Similarly, always use as large a diameter line as possible when passing it around victims and/or when lifting them. Never allow lines to pass over bare skin if at all possible. Rather, especially in practice sessions, be sure that the "victim" is generously insulated and padded from line cuts and friction burns.
- Trust *no* knots or bends unless you have tied them or are well aware of the proficiency of the person who did. If you suspect the propriety of a knot, double check it *before* someone's life depends on it. Since knots can fail, use heavy duty snaps, rescue and safety harnesses, and carabiners as much as possible.

Rescue lines are used for throwing and towing aids and, as previously described, in rigging ferrying and other systems. Another use is in rolling or lifting victims into boats. The lifting technique illustrated in the accompanying illustrations shows a two-to-one mechanical advantage lifting rig called a **parbuckle** (Fig. 11-13). This is a method developed by sailors to role cargo up the sides of and aboard ships before

Table 11-3 Rope Types, Strength, Uses

Type	Use	Strength
Natural fiber: manila	General purpose Stiff, nonelastic	Low to moderate (depends on size)*
Nylon (polyamide)	Elastic and pliable	Moderate (twice that of manila)
Dacron (high-intensity polyester)	Nonelastic, stiff Does not float	Very strong
Polypropylene	Light, pliable Floats, stretches	Low (½ inch diameter breaks at approximately 1800 lb)

*One-half inch manila rope has approximately 1500 lbs. breaking strength.

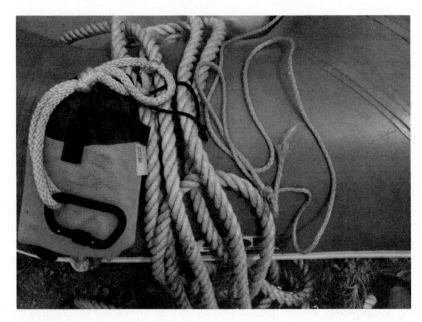

Fig. 11-11 Line varies in strength. Be sure you are using line heavy enough for the job at hand.

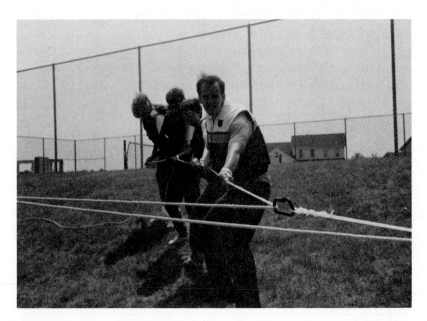

Fig. 11-12 Stay clear of any lines that are moving or under strain such as this "Z" drag.

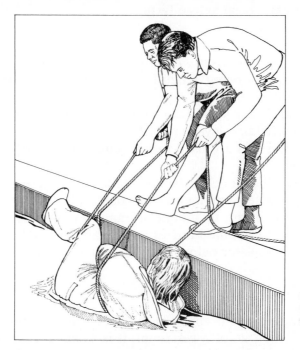

Fig. 11-13 In parbuckling, the line leads around the strong backs, or stationary members, *under* the victim's *midback* and knees, and back to the rescuers. Rescuers work inside the line, raising the victim slowly, being careful not to allow the line to ride up on the victim's neck.

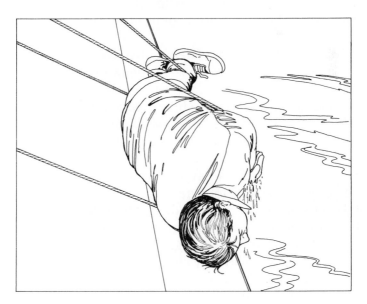

Fig. 11-14 Parbuckle technique may be used for a large vertical lift up a flat surface.

the introduction of powered winching equipment (Fig. 11-14). It is a very effective way to bring a helpless (but *non*cervical spine injured person) aboard a small craft, especially from the standpoints of boat stability and muscle use. When done properly (after lots of practice), the boat should remain fairly level, even though there is a large over-the-side weight factor. The legs are used rather than depending solely on back and arm power.

Skill Drill 25. When a net or expanded plastic mesh (e.g., that used as a snow fence or a safety barrier around construction sites) is substituted for the line, this rescue technique is made even easier. (NOTE AGAIN: Victims with cervical-spine injuries are always splinted and placed on a backboard in the water before they are lifted. See Chapter 12.)

RESCUE BOAT TACTICS

The most pressing requirement of someone who is conning (steering), operating, or in charge of a rescue craft is to *know what is going on*. Chapter 8 warned of the danger of a rescuer's totally fixating on the victim. This is an even more compelling hazard when you are responsible for a small craft bearing one or more other individuals potentially at the mercies of weather, moving water, and "Murphy's law." Therefore just as outlined with other rescue methodologies, quickly review the following before committing your craft and yourself (Table 11-4):

- What are the water conditions? How swift and deep is the current, and where is it coming from? What is in the water, and what must be looked out for and avoided (e.g., timbers, rocks, lines, strainers, snags, deadheads [sodden logs floating slightly beneath the surface], pilings, bridge **abutments,** bottom anchored or floating debris)? What are the wave factors — size and direction (particularly if on a lake or large body of water)?
- What is happening with the weather? Where is the wind coming from and at what force? What is the wind chill and potential icing factors? How well protected is the crew? Is there a lee (shelter) from the wind? Into what can the craft possibly be blown or carried? What is the weather going to do — improve, degrade, stay the same? What are the lighting conditions and will they change — which way? What artificial lighting is available?
- How much power does the craft have for maneuvering? How quickly will it go backward and respond under the present conditions? Is all the rescue equipment aboard and correctly positioned? What are the

Table 11-4 Boat Dangers

General Type	Subsets	Considerations
Lookout	Barriers, structures, and distractions Other duties and responsibilities	Failure of or improper lookout causes most boating accidents.
Weather	Visibility Wind and wave force and direction Temperature changes?	Can boat or crew respond to markedly different weather conditions?
Water	Obstructions (visible) Wave height and force Flow rate	How well can boat handle current or waves?
Craft capability	Size: width, length, draft, power, maneuverability, endurance Crew	Can craft do job and survive? How many people can be brought aboard?

qualification levels of the crew? What are the victim's situation and condition? What is the general plan for approaching and assisting the victim? What is the backup plan, and *where are the escape routes?*

The primary cause of most boating accidents is failure to maintain a proper lookout. The same deficiency can be thought of as degrading boat rescues.

As an emergency craft operator, can you clearly see everything that is happening, and can you envision what might happen in the immediate future?

The foregoing considerations cover almost any rescue boat situation. The following examples, however, are much more specific in dealing with river running or flood operations. The tactics you must develop for actual situations fall somewhere within this continuum. Relying on this knowledge plus understanding, after practice, how your particular craft (and crewmates) respond will allow you to deal your best with real situations. To aid this interaction, examine a few basic boat and shore (co)operation drills.

COMBINED EQUIPMENT PROCEDURES

The following sections deal with elementary boat-based rescues incorporating all the information discussed up to this point. Space is not taken in the text to explain how to operate a boat properly. Appendix I lists several sources for this information.

Single Boat, Single Victim

Skill Drill 26. The purpose of this drill is to practice, using a two-person crew, basic boat-based approach and extrication maneuvers. The drill has two variants: the first is a calm water approach, and the second involves wind and current. The two crew members act as operator and lookout, respectively, exchanging places after a few practice pickups. Emphasized points follow:

- Work as a team to locate and approach the victim.
- Follow proper safety precautions in placing the engine in neutral and/or stopping it altogether as needed. With some outboards, the screw will continue to windmill, even when the gear shift is in neutral.
- Practice — as a team and as individuals — one-on-one, two-on-one, and parbuckle and net pickups. (As explained in Chapter 7, two-on-one pickup features a short piece of line passed under the victim's armpits and around his or her back, with one rescuer on each end of the line jointly bouncing and lifting the victim.)

After everyone, including the "victim," has had an opportunity to operate the craft, seek a position that provides some wind and/or current potential. In this procedure it may be necessary to include some provision for maintaining the position of the boat when two-on-one pickups are practiced. If practice is not held in a clear area, the craft may be carried ashore or may drift into an obstacle. Simply anchoring the craft while attempting to "land" the victim may work.

Taking the victim, while held alongside, to a less exposed area is another alternative, but it is not recommended because of (1) the potential for danger with the engine running in close proximity to the victim and (2) the greatly increased heat loss of persons overboard in moving water.

Single Boat, Multiple Victims

In this exercise the same procedures as above are followed except two or more victims are brought aboard. The essential idea is to understand how difficult it may be to work one person while tracking a second. Since some propeller-related maneuvering danger may be involved, it is recommended that the second victim be a weighted, approximately human-shaped dummy. A set of coveralls stuffed with rags and wearing a PFD works well as a dummy. One important aspect of the drill is tossing flotation to the second victim while the first is picked up.

Do not drag the first victim; instead, have him or her safely aboard before going to the second victim. A variation on this drill, particularly if you believe there may be a large number of victims in the water, is to practice towing and maneuvering an inflated fire hose. The hose would be pushed toward a group of PFD-wearing victims, and all would then be *slowly* taken to the shore. However, *at all times* observe where the moving propeller is relative to *anyone* in the water.

Two-Boat Tether

The object of this drill is to practice jointly maneuvering two tethered craft as in the boat-based low head dam rescue scenario presented in Chapter 10. The tether is secured by a buoyed bridle to the stern of the forward craft. In the downstream craft the tether is held by a crew member in the bow (Fig. 11-15). Approaches are made on a dummy in flat, then moving water situations, with everyone having a chance to operate both craft. Both boats must remained aligned with each other and the wind or current, whichever is greater, to run this drill successfully.

Depending on the water area used, a line can be stretched across a stream or river to imitate the boil line of a low head dam. Or if water depth and other conditions allow, the boats can approach a beach where a throw bag is tossed from the forward boat.

These drills can also be run at night (under safe, supervised circumstances).

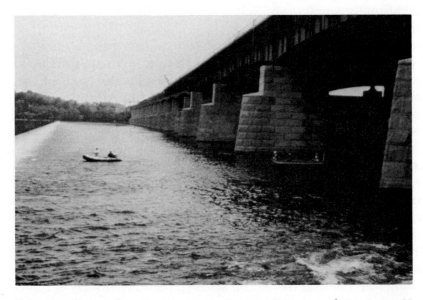

Fig. 11-15 Two-boat tether in operation. (Courtesy N. Joseph Ketterer, Harrisburg River Rescue.)

Surf Rescue

Rescues performed in breaking surf are dangerous and should be attempted *only* by trained, experienced personnel. However, since a number of fire and police rescue units are located by the sea or at large lakes, the following basic surf operations guidelines are given. Inflatable boats are recommended as the rescue craft.

- Study surf conditions, noting where the largest waves break and the pattern between large and smaller swells. Note that higher waves accumulate over shallower bottoms or shoals. Attempt to launch into the calmest waters.
- If you must launch into surf, *always* keep the boat's bow facing into the seas. A **broaching** or capsizing small craft can crush crew members caught between it and the bottom.
- If using a powered craft, place some type of guard around the screw. A shrouded propeller will suffer less damage if it strikes the bottom, does not foul lines easily, and provides better protection to the crew and victims than an unguarded one.
- Securely stow all gear so that it is reachable but will not be lost if the boat flips.
- Crew members should be wearing helmets and Type I PFDs or dry suits with Type II, III, or V PFDs.
- Attempt shore-based rescues or talking victims into self-rescue before committing a small craft. Self-rescue may include swimming *across* rather than against current, rip, or undertow.
- Larger line-throwing apparatus can be modified to fire a small grapnel or folding **fluke** sand anchor. Attached to it is a small pulley with a double strand of messenger line. A small inflatable boat or raft can then be hauled out to the victim. Line throwing guns are available to fire a self-inflating float. Note that these projectiles should be fired *beyond* but *not at* a victim.
- If launching into surf, the anchoring system noted above can be used to keep a small craft's bow into the seas while being pulled beyond the breaker line.
- When attempting rescues from seaward toward shore, deploy an anchor beyond the breaker line, allowing the craft to be carried stern first toward the victim.
- Personal water craft with a floatable stretcher towed immediately astern are highly usable in surf rescues. A crew member rides the stretcher and assists the victim aboard, then lies on top of the victim on the trip to safety. This technique requires practice, situational expertise, and flawless timing.

EQUIPPING FOR WATER RESCUE

Two general types of equipment lists have been given, with the first covering equipment needed for any form of team water rescue and the other pertaining to boat-based assistance. Suppose you arrive on scene from your vehicle but initially have no afloat capability. What could you carry in the vehicle that would be of assistance until watercraft arrived?

> In *any vehicle* that might respond to a water call, be sure you have at least one PFD and a 100-foot length of polypropylene line.

For storage sake, the PFD could be inflatable, and the line could easily be stowed in a throw bag or bottle. (A throw bottle is usually a plastic gallon milk jug containing 70 to 100 feet of polypropylene line. The lighter end of the line is secured to the bottom of the jug similar to a throw bag.) At night, having a spotlight, either fixed or portable, is helpful.

In *larger vehicles*, again depending on their size and storage capacity compared to the potential need, keep the following:

- Several PFDs, enough for the crew plus at least two extras (inflatables take up less space)
- More and heavier line (at least 200 feet of 1-inch nylon) plus several throw bags
- Appropriate first aid kit
- Provision for towing boat trailers

On the *largest vehicles*, carry all of the foregoing plus the following:

- At least two dry (water rescue) suits, harness, and tethers
- Hose inflation equipment (NOTE: Fire department pumpers should carry the basic attachments for hose inflation using compressed air from SCBA bottles.)
- Carried inflatable craft or provision for towing a watercraft

Since much of this equipment is seasonal or event specific, stowage may be aided if some parts of this equipment were kept in likely response areas and broken out during times of anticipated need. For instance, dry suits, hose inflation gear, extra line, and extra PFDs might be kept in a trailer-mounted boat that would be made ready on a seasonal or weather-warning basis. The trailer could be taken as quickly as possible to an incident site. Note that not all the equipment would be in a a centralized location. Some of it would be brought to the scene by responding vehicles.

Additionally, key water rescue team members should be assigned to the location where the stowed gear is kept or vice versa so they would be available to take it to the water response scene.

Any individuals using this gear or carrying it in their vehicles should always be trained and practiced in the basics of its application.

CHAPTER SUMMARY

This chapter has expanded aquatic assistance knowledge by presenting specifics on water rescue equipment and team usage. In particular, you should be familiar with:
- Water rescue suits.
- Elementary rope rescue information.
- Inflated fire hose tactics.
- Safety and operational needs for water rescue craft.
- Simple boat operation and rescue exercises.
- Suggestions for outfitting units with water rescue apparatus.

PRETEST ANSWERS

1. False
2. d
3. c
4. b, c

REFERENCE

1. Experimental evaluations of selected immersion hypothermia protection equipment, Rep No CG-D-79-79, Springfield, Va, 1979, National Technical Information Services.

12 Medical Management and Transport of Aquatic Trauma Victims

OVERVIEW

Locating and rescuing the aquatic accident victim do not complete the process. The traumatized or potentially injured person must be properly extricated, stabilized, and transported to a medical facility. Of particular importance is understanding which assessment techniques to use at *all* treatment levels for aquatically induced hidden trauma.

OBJECTIVES

After studying this chapter, the reader should understand the proper methods for dealing with aquatic trauma. In addition to indicating methods for removing victims from the water with the least likelihood of aggravating an injury, the following also are emphasized:
1. Understanding potential factors affecting an aquatic injury victim
2. Extrication procedures
3. Review of water-oriented field and clinical transport and treatment basics
4. Primary factors involved with near drowning
5. Expanded definition of physical (neurological) reactions to cold
6. Suggestions for dealing with hypothermic patients
7. Rewarming procedures

PRETEST

1. In responding to an accident involving an entrapped or pinned white water paddler, your response priorities would include protecting from cold; aiding breathing; and preventing further injury. What is the correct order for providing the foregoing?
2. Under certain conditions, the same technique can be used in both shallow and deep water rotation of a cervical spine injury victim onto his or her back. (True or false?)
3. The inward circulation of cooled blood in a hypothermic victim (a) may continue for up to an hour after rescue and removal from a cold environment; (b) can be fatal; (c) is called *afterdrop;* or (d) can be prevented by having the victim sit up and exercise. (Which of these is incorrect?)
4. The less a drowning victim struggled before submerging, the greater is the chance that a small residue of oxygen is trapped in his or her lungs. (True or false?)
5. **Barotrauma** may occur in water depths as shallow as (a) 4 feet; (b) 15 feet; or (c) 30 feet. (Pick the correct answer.)
   Pretest answers are at the end of the chapter.

FIVE CATEGORIES OF AQUATIC INJURY

Accidents involving water activities tend to produce major injuries in five principle groupings:
- Cervical spine or fractured or displaced vertebrae
- Multiple lacerations caused by boat propeller strikes
- Near drowning I, revived at scene
- Near drowning II, *not* revived at scene
- Barotrauma, or underwater, pressure-related injuries

Although persons can be injured in many ways around the water, ranging from scalds at a kitchen sink to stepping on a fish hook, the five listed categories represent the most frequently encountered *primary* aquatic trauma concerns. The following are initial considerations pertaining to each of these groupings.

Cervical Spine

A cervical spine injury usually is incurred as a result of diving into shallow water, although other situations also can cause this injury (e.g., high-speed boat collisions, falling head first off a height). A fractured skull might also be involved; however, skull fractures usually result from collisions rather than water-related falls or diving. Apparently water tends to protect the head by providing a partial cushioning effect.

Conversely, when a diver's head hits an unprepared bottom layer of sand or silt, although somewhat cushioned, the head is generally held in place. This inability to move laterally tends to concentrate downward momentum or force, and the rest of the body massively presses on the upper part of the spinal column, frequently resulting in damage (usually compression fractures) to the fourth, fifth, or sixth cervical (C-4, C-5, C-6) vertebrae.[6]

If the bottom is smooth and slick such as in a slippery swimming pool, the diver's head may slide a short distance after impact. The result of this cranial displacement is either **hyperflexion** or **hyperextension,** with the head bent violently forward or backward as it supports the body's plunging weight. This may also result in fracturing or displacement or disruption of the vertebrae.

> In many of these instances, the victim is paralyzed on impact, unable to do anything either to gain attention or, more importantly, to roll over on his or her back and float face up. If the victim is allowed to remain face down, he or she will drown. On the other hand, if the victim is not rolled over correctly and supported properly, the initial damage to the spine may be worsened.

Multiple Lacerations

This kind of aquatic injury has a high potential in areas where speeding watercraft are close to swimmers, generally in one of two locations: (1) swimming areas, marked or otherwise, near boat traffic lanes (e.g., near a busy dock or boat ramp); and (2) waterskiing zones. A secondary place is in anchorages or offshore mooring areas that might be used as shortcuts between harbors and high-interest locales such as fishing grounds. These accidents are usually the result of inattention on the part of the boat operator or swimmer. They are quite serious from the standpoint of blood loss and possible amputation. The victim must be removed from the water, stabilized, and transported as expeditiously as possible.

Special preparations should be made to provide high-flow **intravenous (IV)** intervention procedures and equipment for use by emergency response providers responding to calls in these high-risk areas.

Near Drowning I

In this occurrence the victim may be seen to have difficulty and/or to have been submerged, yet he or she spontaneously begins breathing at the site of the incident and is alert and responsive within a few minutes after being taken from the water. With this type patient, the main concern after restoration of breathing, is hidden lung damage resulting in secondary drowning.

In *any* case of this nature the victim should be seen as quickly as possible in a clinical setting, with his or her being held for observation for *at least 12 hours.*

Near Drowning II

This is the classic, long-term case in which the victim who has suffered a hypothermic cold water accident appears dead. This appearance may be present when the victim is removed from the water and when presented at the emergency room or clinical facility. This may be the most difficult of the five situations with which to deal in that the hypothermic victim, even after a relatively short underwater duration, may have no apparent signs of life (Fig. 12-1). The overwhelming requirement placed on the emergency responder in this instance is to deal with the patient completely and comprehensively while *not* wasting time at the scene. In other words, stabilize and transfer the patient as *quickly and as efficiently as possible.*

In the clinical setting this means that basic resuscitation and core temperature stabilization efforts must be *jointly* sustained until the victim begins to gain body temperature and vital signs have been given an opportunity to manifest. These sustained efforts may also include transfer to a medical facility where definitive rewarming can be accomplished.

Barotrauma

The National Underwater Accident Data Center (NUADC) at the University of Rhode Island reports an average of 130 scuba or underwater diving fatalities yearly.[9] Approximately half these deaths are

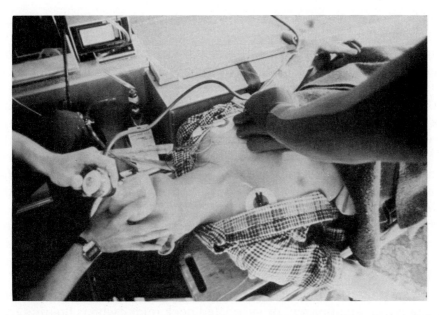

Fig. 12-1 When transporting the hypothermic aquatic accident victim, lightly cover the patient's trunk, but leave arms and legs at room temperature (approximately 70° F). (Courtesy Dive Rescue International: Cold water near drowning: emergency care.)

primarily listed as drownings. Other leading causes are barotrauma or **embolism** (gas in the bloodstream), head injuries, cardiovascular syndrome (mainly cardiac arrest in overstressed or exhausted older divers), and aspiration of stomach contents. As a very rough rule of thumb, consider there are 10 serious aquatic injuries for every fatality. According to the NUADC statistics, approximately one fourth of all scuba deaths involve barotrauma (literally, pressure-related injury). Therefore expect a minimum of 350 such cases per year. Note that there is potential for more than one of these types of injuries to affect the same person.

The next sections examine what must be done when you arrive on scene and are confronted with one or more of these cases.

IN-WATER PROCEDURES: STABILIZATION

The most difficult overall water extrications involve the occupant of a canoe or kayak pinned in a crumpled craft under a torrent of crashing water.[3] Three main dangers are present in this situation. First, if the victim cannot keep his or her head above the moving water, he or she will quickly drown. Second, the trapped person may suffer increasing physical trauma as he or she is buffeted by the water. Third, the chill factor of any body of moving water affecting a person in this condition, regardless of the time of year, is awesome. The only favorable aspect of this scenario is its relative rareness.

Usually when persons are involved with this situation, they are part of a group of practiced white water paddlers, some of whom normally have experience in dealing with similar events. Nevertheless, the prioritized actions taken to assist the pinned kayaker still apply in less tortuous waters. In other words, aid breathing; reduce the potential for increased injury; and protect the victim from cold (remove from the water).

Specialized rescue equipment and procedures needed in white water accidents are presented in Appendix I. If you believe there is potential for such occurrences in your area, acquire these references and attend a white water training session.

The next most difficult water extrication task involves handling someone with an apparent or suspected neck injury who is floating face down in *deep* water. Comparatively speaking, rolling a neck injury victim in shallow water while splinting or stabilizing his or her spine is simple. In shallow water you can stand on the bottom and gain leverage from your legs. This is not the case in deeper water. The following are two deep water procedures.

Deep Water Roll

If you respond to an accident scene with a nonmoving person face down in the water, *always* assume spine injury unless clearly informed otherwise. This injury can result from a boat collision, and there is a good chance that no one will be able to indicate the victim's status.

This rotation involves the rescuer's placing his or her arms against the victim's upper back and chest, then dipping under the victim. Because of this maneuver, a PFD may interfere with a smaller rescuer attempting to work with a much larger victim. Hence two variations to the initial approach and splinting are suggested. Practice with both methods to determine which works best for you.

First variation (smaller rescuer working with larger victim):
- Approach the victim, remove your PFD, and slide it up your arm on the side closest to the victim.
- Grasp the victim's nearest wrist and *gently* slide the PFD as high as possible up his or her arm (Fig. 12-2, *A*).
- Push the victim's arm down alongside his or her body. The PFD now is sandwiched between the victim's arm and torso.

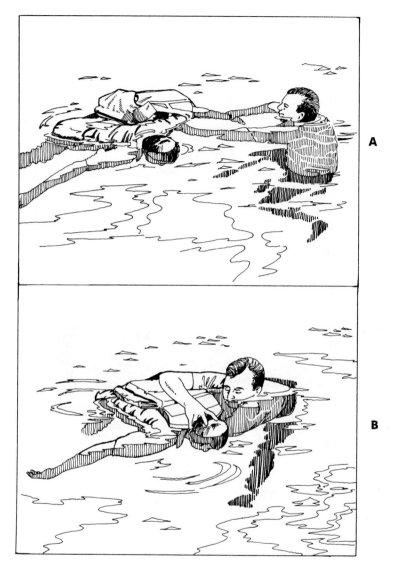

Fig. 12-2 A, Gently sliding a PFD from rescuer's arm to that of the victim. **B,** Splinting the deep water neck injury victim.

- Splint the victim with your arms by placing one elbow in the middle of his or her back, with your hand on the rear of his or her head. Place your other elbow in the middle of his or her chest, with your hand cradling his or her chin (Fig. 12-3, *A*).
- Take a deep breath, firmly hold the splint, then swim *under* the victim, using your legs to kick as the victim rotates onto his or her back. *Do*

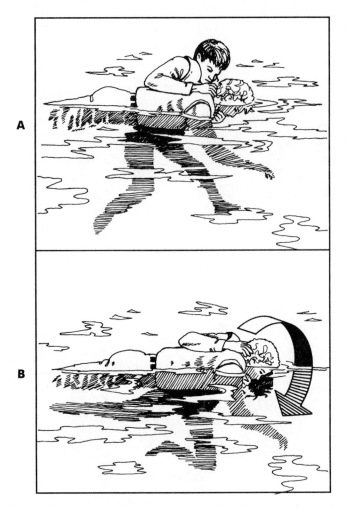

Fig. 12-3 A and **B**, Rolling the victim over by ducking beneath the victim.

not twist the victim over by solely turning his or her chin. Instead, lever
the victim onto his or her back using your *elbows* (Fig. 12-3, *B* and *C*).
- You should now have the victim splinted and floating on his or her
  back, with both of you supported by the PFD (Fig. 12-3, *D*).[5]
  Second variation (larger rescuer working with same sized or smaller
victim):
- *Keep your PFD on,* and skip the first two steps.
- Go directly to ensuring victim's arm is alongside his or her body. Then
  do splinting and rotating.

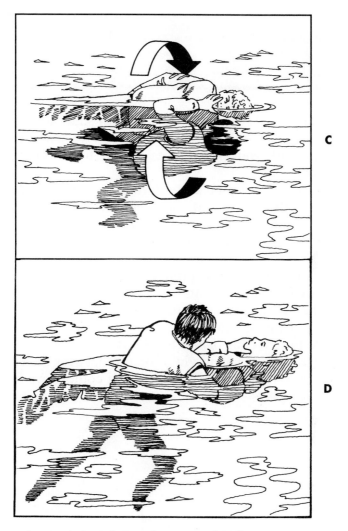

Fig. 12-3, cont'd **C** and **D**, Completed maneuver.

Your next decision is whether to remain stationary, awaiting assistance, or to attempt to swim the victim slowly into shallow water. (This splinting, rotating, and swimming are not easily done unless you are a good swimmer and have seriously practiced.)

Shallow Water Roll (Dry Suit Modification)

The second alternative is the rotating procedure normally used in shallow water.

As a result of the extreme buoyancy provided by a dry rescue or ship abandonment (immersion) suit, a rescuer can *stand* vertically in deep water and rotate the victim.

Here is the process (it can also be used in shallow water):

- Stand alongside the victim (in shallows, hip- to low-chest-deep water works best) with your side perpendicular to the victim, facing the victim's near arm.
- Reach across the victim's back with your closest hand, grasp his or her arm between the elbow and shoulder, and *gently* pin his or her far upper arm against the far ear (Fig. 12-4).
- Pin the victim's near upper arm against the near ear.
- Push down on the victim's near arm while pulling up with your other hand. Keep his or her arms pinned to his or her head as you do this.
- The victim will roll over with their upper back cradled in your arm. Squeeze the victim against your chest to maintain the splint as you remove your nearest hand. (As a test in practice, the "victim" should not be able to move his or her head.[13])
- With your free hand, you might, if required, cover the victim's mouth to do mouth-to-nose resuscitation, or you could wave for assistance.

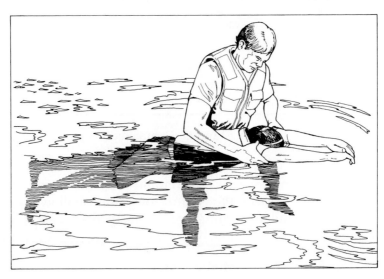

Fig. 12-4 Stand alongside victim, facing his near arm, and reach across his back, pinning the victim's upper arms to his ears.

(Your arms will be positioned so that you cannot do mouth-to-mouth resuscitation.)

In deep water you must decide whether you wish to kick slowly toward land (if wearing the dry suit) or remain where you are.

In both instances, you must place the victim on a backboard and place a cervical collar on him or her before extrication from the water.

IN-WATER PROCEDURES: EXTRICATION

Placing a backboard under a victim in the water should not be attempted without practice. Since most backboards are quite buoyant, gently submerging one under the victim is not easy. Also, because a full board usually is required when removing someone from the water, *total immobilization* of the victim is necessary; thus using a shorter board with less buoyancy is not the answer. The best procedure is to have at least three rescuers in the water to maintain spinal alignment as the victim is gently leaned to one side while other rescuers slowly slide the board sideways beneath the victim. Again, practice this maneuver before you ever need it (Fig. 12-5).

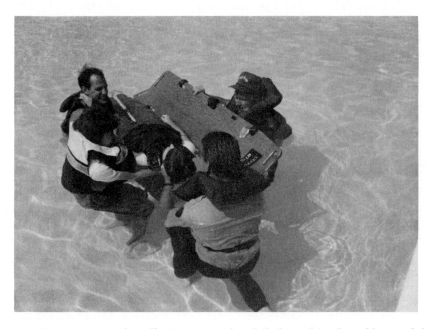

Fig. 12-5 Rescuers gently roll victim to side while board is placed beneath him. Using a backboard in deep water requires detailed practice.

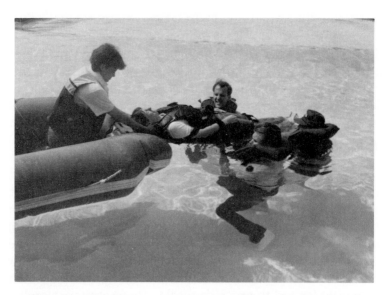

Fig. 12-6 Passing a patient on a backboard into a boat.

If he or she is in deep water, the victim must be taken up and onto a boat. If available, a four-point, horizontal lift works best (i.e., the backboard or, even better, a Stokes litter containing both the board and the victim is supported evenly on all four corners by lifting straps). If a lifting strap or sling system cannot be rigged, the next alternative is to slide the backboard, attempting to keep the victim level, over the lowest point of the boat's side. The stern is usually the best location for this maneuver (Fig. 12-6). The backboard should be placed perpendicular not parallel to the gunwale.

Practice before actual application is definitely needed. Should all other alternatives be exhausted, a *securely* boarded victim can be gently net-rolled or parbuckled into a boat or up a vertical face.

In-Water Resuscitation

Part of the extrication process may involve in-water resuscitation. Testing of various methods for chest compression while afloat has not proved successful. Under certain conditions, mouth-to-mouth resuscitation (rescue breathing) can be used, but the rescuer should understand both his or her limitations and the potential for further injury to the victim. (Mouth-to-snorkel resuscitation is a modification that might work in high seas. The mouthpiece of the snorkel is held securely in the victim's mouth, and the rescuer blows into the snorkel tube.)

The following are basic in-water resuscitation guidelines:

- Do not impede taking the victim to safety by attempting prolonged mouth-to-mouth efforts.
- Two quick breaths may be tried when the victim is brought to the surface. Make sure the airway is open by proper (standard CPR) positioning of the head and neck.
- Do not attempt any further in-water rescue breathing *unless the victim's head (mouth and nose) can be continually maintained above water.*
- If providing further mouth-to-mouth resuscitation, do so *only* with some form of flotation device supporting the victim's neck and head.

Follow these precautions because if the victim's face repeatedly goes under water as rescue breathing is applied, water may be forced deeper into breathing passages or the victim might reflexively gasp while underwater, thereby ingesting more fluid.

A related problem is the mistaken belief that allowing a person's face to remain in the water will extend the protective effects of the diving reflex. If dive reflex occurs, it is only present at the beginning of the drowning incident. The best response is to get the victim's breathing passages out of the water as soon as possible.

Water Extrication in General

These general principles govern extrication from water:

- Treat the patient as gently as possible. Try not to bump, rub, manipulate, or exercise the victim or his or her limbs.
- Keep the victim horizontal. Do not allow the person who has been immersed for more than a few minutes to sit up suddenly or stand erect. Extended exposure to water temperature and pressure may adversely affect the vascular system. In most people these effects eventually are normalized after removal from the water as the body nears average temperature levels. The time taken to complete this normalization process is directly proportional to the time spent in the water.

- Keep the victim warm. A person exposed to immersion or to prolonged terrestrial cold may suffer from **afterdrop**,[8] or reduction of inner body temperature, even when he or she has been placed in a warm, dry location.

> This inward circulation of cooled, exterior blood as a result of shell or outer warming may last for up to an hour after rescue or extrication and can prove fatal.

- Be alert for increased bleeding in the lacerated victim after removal from the water.
- *Do not attempt to rewarm the victim in the field.* Rewarming of a hypothermic victim is a highly detailed, clinical procedure. Do apply *monitored, insulated* hot packs to primary heat loss areas — head and neck, groin, armpits — in the unconscious hypothermic victim. This is *not* a rewarming technique.

   In cases of severe hypothermia (victim unconscious or approaching unconscious state as a result of cold — body temperature at or below 30° C or 86° F) — warm *only* from the core out. Avoid *all* external heat application techniques.[17]

FACTORS INVOLVED WITH SURVIVAL OF NEAR DROWNING

Persons underwater in a hypothermic condition for up to (and sometimes more than) 1 hour may be alive, yet they may have no observable vital signs. The following *general* guidelines are applicable as an indication of potential survival conditions:

- The colder the water, the better. The less warmth there is in the body, the less oxygen needed to maintain metabolism. The body requires 50% less oxygen for each 20° F reduction in internal temperature. Therefore at approximately 60° F (15.5° C), oxygen needs for cellular maintenance are one fourth that at normal temperature levels.[4]

> Note that this requirement is simply for cell maintenance, not overall physical activity. The amount of lung tissue required for maintaining the comatose body is far less than the total lung capacity.

Similarly, estimates of lung occlusion (filling) during the initial portion of the drowning progression indicate that approximately 1 quart of water enters the lungs for every 100 pounds of body weight.[10] The average adult's lungs may hold up to 5 quarts of water. Therefore the lungs may not be completely filled with water, and the small amount of lung-entrapped air, coupled with lower oxygen needs induced by cold, may provide part of the underwater survival envelope. Additionally, hypothermic victims who become unconscious before totally submerging may have minimal water accumulation in their lungs as a result of cold-arrested respiratory function.

Moving water is also cooler than standing water. Therefore do *not* predicate survival chances simply on ambient air and water temperatures and time of year alone.

Note that depth of water usually correlates with coldness. Temperature drops as you descend. For instance, during the summertime in a 4-foot deep, above-ground pool, there might be as much as a 10° or 15° difference between surface and bottom temperature (providing the pool's pump and filter system are off and not mixing layers of water).

- The smaller the person, the better. Smaller objects lose heat faster than larger objects. Tests on drowned dogs have indicated that a 30- to 40-pound animal may lose up to 1° F per minute of total submersion.[15] In children these heat loss rates could produce an 80° F (26.6° C) body temperature after 20 minutes submersion in 80° F water. (Children have comparatively larger skulls than adults, with a major portion of heat loss occurring in the neck and above.) This profile may also extend underwater survival potential.
- The younger the person, the better. Children apparently tolerate hypoxia better than adults. Some of the reasons are children have fewer preexisting physical problems than adults; children have not debilitated their lung tissue through smoking; children are not taking abusive drugs; and rescuers are more inclined to resuscitate children aggressively. Even after resuscitation, a child's brain is still growing, and this progression may allow compensation for near-drowning–induced cerebral damage. Also, because of larger surface area–body mass ratios, children cool much more quickly in hypothermic water accidents.

- The cleaner the water, the better. Contaminants or biological growths ingested into the lungs frequently cause massive infections secondary to pulmonary injuries after the initial immersion incident.
- The shorter the time underwater, the better.
- The less the victim struggles in the water, the better. If the victim submerges with a minimum of struggling, more oxygen remains in his or her bloodstream and lungs for cellular maintenance.

The point must also be made that a number of older individuals have been resuscitated after up to 40 minutes submersion, with some of these cases occurring in southern waters during summer months. (On June 30, 1983, in Miami, Florida, a 59-year-old man found floating and believed dead astonished rescuers by suddenly sitting up. Note date and place. According to the police records, the victim had been seen floating *face down* for 2 hours![7])

Additional Factors Influencing Long-Term Submersion

Three general processes apparently are involved in protecting submerged individuals:

- The physiology of drowning. As discussed in Part I of this text, drowning humans instinctively perform acts that increase the oxygen loading available to their lungs. They automatically create as large and as clear an airway as possible and move their arms in a manner that expands their lungs. Notwithstanding the fact that they are struggling and are therefore burning oxygen, the struggling is performed in a manner that maximizes oxygen uptake.

  Also, depending on the position of the face relative to the water's surface, torso reflex, or sudden, automatic inhalation when entering a cooled environment, when occurring *above* the water, may be seen as another method provided by nature to maximize lung oxygen loading.
- Dive reflex. Despite the controversy surrounding the possible presence and effect of this reflex in humans, some triggering agent accomplishes the two primary effects normally attributed to dive reflex: (1) redistribution, or **shunting,** of cooled blood from the exterior to the interior of the body, and (2) rapid reduction of metabolism.[1] The first effect produces an increased level of oxygen within certain parts of the body, primarily the heart, lungs, and brain. The second effect further slows the rate of oxygen consumption. The presence of these factors in many types of diving vertebrates such as whales, penguins, turtles, ducks, and diving iguanas is undisputed and has been proved by the surgical insertion of monitoring devices. To date and for obvious ethical reasons, no similar invasive testing has been accomplished on

panicked, fearful humans. The results indicating lack of its presence have been based on after-the-immediate-incident analysis of blood chemistry and breathing reactions.[11]

On the other hand, most researchers do accept that something similar to dive reflex does occur in the human birthing process when the neonate (newborn) emerges from the womb and is subject to relatively sudden changes in temperature and pressure. It has been noted that increased depth means cooler temperature. Could depth as reflected in changed exterior pressure also affect oxygen consumption in humans?[2]

- Hypothermia. Researchers who reject the potential for dive reflex in humans state that the powerful effects of hypothermia, usually acting on the smaller body of a child, comprise the single underlying cause of survival in long-term submersion. It has previously been indicated that the body automatically goes through processes that both reduce blood flow to the periphery and result in gross physiological shut down. (Table 12-1 indicates autonomic responses to cold.) Outside of the World War II Nazi studies of hypothermia in concentration camp

Table 12-1 Body Reactions and Responses to Cold (Autonomic or Automatic)

Peripheral Vasoconstriction (PVC)	Shivering (From Approximately 87°-98° F [30.5°-36.6° C])	Physiological Shut Down
Body temperature falls approximately ½° F below normal.	If body heat loss not reduced by PVC, involuntary exercise begins.	If heat loss not reduced, shivering stops; remaining heat is *drastically* conserved.
Blood vessels in periphery (directly beneath skin) begin to contract, reducing heat radiated to air.	Ten times as much heat production results from rapidly expanding and contracting muscles as during resting state.	Body and brain begin to shut down; vital signs diminish; cells shift to *maintenance* oxygen levels.
Blood begins to trap in periphery; sets initial stage for "afterdrop."	If heat loss continues, blood becomes acidotic, with build up of toxic exertion byproducts.	*Victim may appear to be dead, with severe potential for harm to internal organs as a result of perfusion by toxic blood.*

Modified from Smith D and Smith S: Waterwise, Imperial, Mo, 1984, Smith Aquatic Safety Services.

inmates, no one has had the opportunity or has been permitted to discover exactly what happens as a healthy but panicked and hypoxic human is subject to severe cooling (patients undergoing open heart surgery have been cooled to as low as 48° F). However, the observed end results of this non-clinical cooling process are as unpredictable in terms of survival as they are profound.

MEDICAL MANAGEMENT AND TRANSPORT OF THE NEAR-DROWNING VICTIM

Your responsibilities toward a potential victim of drowning follow:
- Rescue and remove victim from the water as soon as possible.
- Initiate CPR as soon as practicable, maintaining it until relieved by higher authority.
- Provide 100% high-flow rate oxygen, warmed and given through a nebulizer if available.
- Transport victim to a clinical facility as rapidly as you can.
- Remove victim's wet clothing; insulate and protect him or her from wind chill.

For those seeking more detailed information on this subject, the following are important aspects of the management of near-drowning patients as taken from *Guidelines for Cardiopulmonary Resuscitation and Emergency Cardiac Care*, 1992, American Heart Association.

Near-Drowning

The most important consequence of prolonged underwater submersion without ventilation is hypoxemia. The duration of hypoxia is the critical factor in determining the victim's outcome. Therefore, restoration of **ventilation** and perfusion should be accomplished as rapidly as possible.

Basic Life Support Rescue From the Water

When attempting to rescue a near-drowning victim, the rescuer should get to the victim as quickly as possible, preferably with some conveyance (boat, raft, surfboard, or flotation device). The rescuer must always be aware of personal safety in attempting a rescue and should exercise caution to minimize the danger.

Rescue Breathing

Initial treatment of the near-drowning victim consists of rescue breathing with the mouth-to-mouth technique. Rescue breathing should be started as soon as the victim's airway can be opened and protected and the rescuer's safety can be ensured. This is usually achieved when the victim is in shallow water or out of the water.

Appliances (such as a snorkel for the mouth-to-snorkel technique or buoyancy aids) may permit specially trained rescuers to perform rescue breathing in deep water. However, rescue breathing should not be delayed for lack of such equipment if it can otherwise be provided safely. Untrained rescuers should not attempt to use such adjuncts.

In a diving accident, neck injury should be suspected. The victim's neck should be supported in a neutral position (without flexion or extension), and the victim should be floated supine on a back support before being removed from the water. If the victim must be turned, the head, neck, chest, and body should be aligned, supported, and turned as a unit to the horizontal, supine position. If artificial respiration is required, rescue breathing should be provided with the head maintained in a neutral position; i.e., jaw thrust without head tilt or chin lift without head tilt should be used.

Immediate ventilation and rescue breathing should be initiated if the submersion victim is not breathing. Management of the airway and ventilation of the submersion victim are similar to those of any victim in cardiopulmonary arrest. There is no need to clear the airway of aspirated water. However, rescuers may need to remove debris, **gastric** contents, or other foreign materials using standard techniques for obstructed airway. Usual airway management with adjuncts, such as bag-mask ventilation and intubation, can be accomplished in the near-drowning victim. At most only a modest amount of water is aspirated by the majority of both freshwater and seawater drowning victims, and it is rapidly absorbed from the lungs into the circulation. Furthermore, 10% to 12% of victims do not aspirate at all because of laryngospasm or breath-holding. An attempt to remove water from the breathing passages by any means other than suction is usually unnecessary and apt to be dangerous because it may eject gastric contents and cause aspiration.

A **Heimlich maneuver** delays initiation of ventilation and breathing. Its value is not proven scientifically and is supported only by anecdotal evidence, and its risk-benefit ratio is untested. Therefore, a Heimlich maneuver should be used only if the rescuer suspects that foreign matter is obstructing the airway or if the victim does not respond appropriately to mouth-to-mouth ventilation. Then, if necessary, CPR should be reinstituted after the Heimlich maneuver has been performed. The Heimlich maneuver is performed on the near-drowning victim as described in the treatment of foreign-body airway obstruction (unconscious supine) except that in near-drowning the victim's head should be turned sideways unless cervical trauma is suspected.

Chest Compressions

Chest compressions should not be attempted in the water unless the rescuer has had special training in techniques of in-water CPR, because the brain is not perfused effectively unless the victim is maintained in the horizontal position and the back is supported. It is usually not possible to keep the victim's body horizontal and the head above water in position for rescue breathing.

After removal from the water, the victim must be immediately assessed for adequacy of circulation. The pulse may be difficult to appreciate in a near-drowning victim because of peripheral vasoconstriction and a low cardiac output. If a pulse cannot be felt, chest compressions should be started at once.

Advanced Cardiac Life Support

The near-drowning victim in cardiac arrest should be given advanced cardiac life support (ACLS) including intubation without delay. Every submersion victim, even one who requires only minimal resuscitation and regains consciousness at the scene, should be transferred to a medical facility for follow-up care. It is imperative that monitoring of life support measures be continued enroute and that oxygen be administered if it is available in the transport vehicle, since pulmonary injury may develop up to several hours after submersion. Although survival is unlikely in victims who have undergone prolonged submersion and require prolonged resuscitation, successful resuscitation with full **neurological** recovery has occurred in near-drowning victims with prolonged submersion in extremely cold water. Since it is often difficult for rescuers to obtain an accurate time of submersion, attempts at resuscitation should be initiated by rescuers at the scene unless there is obvious physical evidence of death (such as **putrefaction, dependent lividity,** or rigor mortis). The victim should be transported with continued CPR to an emergency facility where a physician can decide whether to continue resuscitation. Aggressive attempts at resuscitation in the hospital should be continued for the victim of cold water submersion.

Secondary considerations influencing your performing the foregoing are the following:

- In the past, the time limit to achieve positive results from resuscitation efforts has been *1 hour* underwater. However, several considerations temper this limit, and it may be expandable. First, accurate timekeeping *before* the information is inserted into an emergency response system is usually sketchy at best. *Time seems to pass slowly for people involved in emergencies.* Second, in at least two North American cases (a 3-year-old girl revived on June 10, 1986, in Salt Lake City, Utah, after 66 minutes under water and another 3-year-old girl resuscitated in November 1980 in Alaska after apparently being submerged for 63 minutes[14]), complete recovery occurred in victims documented to have been underwater for 60 to 70 minutes. This means that your timekeeping should err on the broader rather than narrower side.
- As information on this and the immediately preceding pages has indicated, too many factors are involved in surviving near drowning

to allow anyone to predict automatically the potential outcome, *regardless of situation or setting.* In other words, no one can tell absolutely at the scene what will happen with the application of clinically based, aggressive resuscitation practices.

- Best resuscitation results apparently follow expeditious transport to a medical facility possessing a heart-lung bypass capability. *Your plan for dealing with near drowning should include a procedure for getting the victim, as soon as possible, to a trauma center.* The heart-lung capability allows effective and exact rewarming, oxygenation, and medicating plus immediate analysis of internal chemistry and lung activity.
- Do not attempt to rewarm the patient in the field. *Do* keep the patient from growing colder by *not* allowing his or her placement directly on a cold surface such as the ground or exposure to wind. After placing the victim in a vehicle, lightly cover his or her trunk. Do not increase the heat in the vehicle. Transport the patient horizontally at normal room temperature (i.e., approximately 70° F). As previously explained, hot packs may be applied to heat loss areas, but this should be done only during a long transport of more than 15 minutes and only if the (monitored and insulated as required) hot packs do not interfere with resuscitation efforts. (This localized application of hot packs is *not* done to rewarm the patient; rather, as cold blood circulates past the areas where large blood vessels are close to the surface, heat is transferred to the blood. The concept is to moderate the temperature of the blood as it moves toward the heart, not to rewarm the patient.)

External rewarming should *never* be done on an unconscious, hypothermic patient; but warm, humidified oxygen can be used in the field to stabilize core temperature.

- Medicate only at the order of higher authority and only after initially indicating the temperature level of the patient to the higher authority; and do so guardedly in patients whose core temperature is at or below 86° F. Depending on temperature levels, circulation may be greatly compromised. If medications are applied per normothermic protocols, they might only have the effect of overdosing the patient when circulation begins to return to normal.

The ability to take an accurate temperature in a moving vehicle is questionable. At least feel covered parts of the body to see if they

remain cold to the touch. If so, include this finding in your initial report.
- When arriving at a medical facility, indicate the following:
  Total time submerged
  Water temperature (if possible at the depth containing the patient)
  Any changes in body temperature
  Type of water such as contaminated, salt, or brackish or discolored by organic growths; provide a water sample if possible
- Since you or members of your family may be potential water accident or near-drowning victims, be sure that someone in the emergency room staff with which you normally work understands the following: (1) the effect of cold, even in the summer, especially on smaller submerged children is *profound;* (2) an individual in such a situation may have the potential for resuscitation while exhibiting *no vital signs whatsoever;* (3) resuscitation efforts should be continued *until* the patient's body has been rewarmed to near-normal body temperature *without* corresponding return or improvement of vital signs; and (4) until rewarming takes place, the effects of submersion and/or cold may do the following:
  Reduce or nullify electroencephalographic or electrocardiographic monitoring results
  Reduce heartbeats to less than one every 2 minutes (with a corresponding reduction in breathing), possibly completely obliterating them

Table 12-2 Apparent Signs of Death in Cold, Living Persons

Sign	State	Reason
Cold	Cold to touch	Heat loss to cold water or air
Color	Unusual skin color or pallor	Peripheral vasoconstriction (see Table 12-1)
Pulse	Lacking (apparently)	Slow; hard to find in cold person
Pupils	Fixed and unresponsive to light	No response if body < 85° F
Rigid	Induced by cold	Effect of toxic, poorly oxygenated blood in muscles
Respiration	Lacking (apparently)	Shallow; four times slower than heart

Modified from Emergency care for cold water near drowning, Fort Collins, Colo, 1981, Dive Rescue International.

Completely obscure brachial blood pressure
Induce physical rigidity (in some cases) similar to rigor mortis
Completely block any pupillary or pain response.

Table 12-2 summarizes apparent signs of death. Because a large percentage of present emergency medical responders may not be completely aware of them, share the hypothermia and near-drowning protocols in Appendix I. Note that the 1992 Emergency Cardiac Cardiac Care Guidelines of the American Heart Association, dealing with hypothermia and near drowning, are of particular importance.

REWARMING PROCEDURES

As repeatedly indicated, field rewarming is not advisable unless it is impossible to transport the patient to a clinical setting. On the other hand, since there may be some misunderstanding regarding the best rewarming techniques, the basics in this process are reviewed. The underlying principle is to remember that cold, acidotic blood contaminated with the harmful by-products of exertion (i.e., metabolic steroids) permeates the cooled body's periphery. When a copious amount of this blood is allowed to circulate rapidly toward the heart and other organs, it can cause complications as serious as cardiac arrest. This *afterdrop* phenomenon will occur in any hypothermic patient as circulation increases. The goal is to slow and not aid its progression.

Most earlier suggestions for treating the hypothermic patient such as wrapping him or her in warmed blankets or immersing the torso in a warm bath were more harmful than helpful because of the overall effect of such procedures actually speeding afterdrop.[12]

Research has indicated that beside heart-lung bypass procedures, rewarming from the inside out is less harmful to the patient. A number of methods of warming the interior such as peritoneal lavage (flushing warmed fluids through the abdominal cavity) or mediastinal irrigation have been tried. The simplest and apparently most efficient all-round method is warm, moist oxygen inhalation. Since the lungs jacket the heart, warming them will in turn warm the heart, thereby protecting it best from afterdrop.

In the past few portable oxygen provision systems outside of a hospital had the capability for warming and nebulizing (moisturizing) oxygen. This situation is improving (see Appendix I).

Dry oxygen has a very low specific heat content. Thus by itself dry gas does little to carry or provide warmth. Conversely, compressed gases expand from their storage tanks at *very low temperatures*. There is a

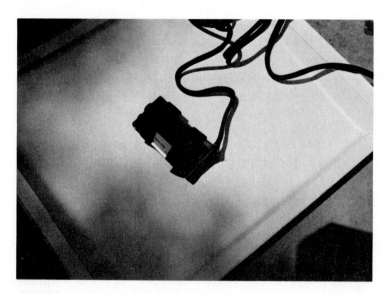

Fig. 12-7 Battery-operated, variable temperature intravenous (IV) fluid warmer. It is simple to use, with the IV tubing placed between the upper and lower warmer halves, which then are held together with Velcro strapping.

possibility, especially in the very small chilled victim, that the low temperature of even the dry gas may interfere with rewarming. Therefore always attempt to do something to warm both inhalants and IV solutions given cold patients. A simple field procedure would be to wrap oxygen and IV tubes in a hot pack or around someone's leg, or possibly coil them in a plastic bag or container filled with warmed fluid. The ideal inhalant and IV temperatures are 108° to 115° and 109° F, respectively. Some methods, possibly placing a clinical thermometer in the warming fluid, should be used to ensure that the fluid is not too warm (Fig. 12-7).

This technique might also prove helpful if shared with emergency room providers because cooler air temperatures, unheated inhalants, plus room-temperature IV applications may be unthinkingly applied. It is strongly recommended that all emergency room staff be made aware of the need to obtain body temperature readings as a basic initial assessment procedure with *any* patient.

TERRESTRIAL HYPOTHERMIA

Mouth-to-mouth resuscitation provides a warmed inhalant to the victim. However, rescue breathing may be harmful to a cold *terrestrial* hypothermia victim, but you *must* provide mouth-to-mouth assistance to the hypoxic, otherwise not breathing *aquatic* victim.

> In *purely terrestrial hypothermia cases* a change in **protocol** may be needed.

Severely cooled terrestrial victims are extremely susceptible to **ventricular fibrillation** (spasmodic beating in which very small quantities of blood are moved through the heart's chambers). This highly dangerous type of arrhythmia (irregular heartbeat) is induced in hypothermic patients by their being dropped or by their being subject to some other form of sudden physical shock. Apparently either chest compressions or rapid inflation of the lungs such as used in CPR can produce fibrillation.[16]

Again, purely in terrestrial hypothermia victims, feel their covered skin and compare its temperature to their uncovered areas to develop an impression of how cold they are. In the case of the very cold, apparently lifeless terrestrial hypothermic victim, *take a careful 45- to 60-second pulse check on each side of the carotid before initiating CPR.* If a pulse, however slight, is detected, do *not* apply chest compressions. Instead, help the victim to rewarm himself or herself by getting him or her off the ground and out of the wind. Take care to handle the victim gently while also trying to insulate his or her head.

After the victim is in a warmer area, have someone buddy breathe with the victim. In this process a person breathes *across* a patient's mouth rather than into it. Use a torso wrap if the victim is very cold. Arms and legs are left at room temperature, and the head and trunk are covered. This is done to reduce the effect of afterdrop.

When dealing with victims of hypothermia, some provision should be made for rewarming if transport is *un*available. This is a last-ditch, stopgap approach, which should be used only if *no other transport option is usable.* Probably the least injurious field method is naked body rewarming. In this technique one or more donors lie in a sleeping bag with the victim, from whom all wet clothing has been removed, positioned between them. This technique may prove dangerous, however, because well-meaning but isolated rescuers may themselves die of hypothermia while attempting to rewarm a corpse.

FINAL IMMERSION HYPOTHERMIA NOTES

If *you* are subject to immersion in cold water, remember these points:
- Even though wind chill may make you uncomfortable initially, you usually are much better *out of the water* than in it.
- In addition to losing heat rapidly to the water, thinking ability and grip strength will be downwardly affected.
- Should you make it to shore in layered, wet clothing, you usually are best advised to keep *all* your clothing on, getting to warmth, shelter, and dry clothing as rapidly as possible. If you are in an exposed position without warm, dry clothing, and materials to make a fire, layered wet clothing tends to act as a "wet" suit, trapping warmer water next to the skin. Removing *any* of these layers in extremely cold air may markedly reduce this insulation factor. Therefore you are in better shape by getting to shelter quickly, rather than taking time and energy to remove wet clothing.

> If you have a *victim* (including one with potential hypothermia) with wet clothing, do everything you can to remove these items expeditiously and replace them with warm, dry garments. Base this action, however, on the total situation. Should you be within 5 minutes of a medical facility, the time taken to remove and replace wet clothing would unnecessarily delay transport.

BASIC BAROTRAUMA PROTOCOLS

The following statements are taken from pages 5 to 7 of the Divers Alert Network (DAN) *Underwater Diving Accident Manual:*

Two life-threatening conditions may occur as a result of a diving accident — air embolism and decompression sickness — grouped together as Decompression Sickness.

Air embolism occurs when bubbles entering the bloodstream from a damaged lung obstruct the blood flow to an area of the brain, usually causing unconsciousness and paralysis.

Any person who has breathed air underwater, regardless of depth, may have an air embolism. This can occur at depths as shallow as *4 feet* with a breath-holding ascent. Even a well trained diver breathing properly during ascent may embolize because of medical problems affecting the lungs, causing air-trapping during ascent. The pressure of this expanding air may be sufficient to rupture lung air sacs, and the escaping air may enter the bloodstream as an air embolism.

Decompression sickness is the syndrome of joint pains (the bends, caisson disease), numbness, paralysis, and other symptoms caused by gas dissolved in tissues forming bubbles upon surfacing after a dive.

Decompression sickness can occur in any individual who violates decompression limits either willingly or unintentionally when surfacing from depths greater than 30 feet.

Fatigue or unusual tiredness and itching are considered mild symptoms and may respond to treatment with oxygen. Joint pain has sometimes been considered a mild symptom. *No symptoms should be ignored as the progression from mild to serious can occur rapidly.*

If a diver experiences mild symptoms on surfacing, place the diver horizontally on left side, head low and give oxygen. Oxygen treatment may relieve the symptoms or prevent them from getting worse. If the symptoms appear relieved after an interval of oxygen treatment, *do not* remove the oxygen immediately as the symptoms may recur. The victim should continue to receive oxygen for at least 30 minutes for mild symptoms, and then the flow chart (per the DAN *Underwater Diving Accident Manual*) should be followed for further instructions.

Any symptom such as pain, weakness, numbness, dizziness, nausea or decreased consciousness can be a symptom of serious decompression illness. When these symptoms occur shortly after a dive, a serious diving injury is the likely cause.

Serious symptoms are a *medical emergency*, which requires urgent medical evaluation and treatment at the nearest hospital, followed by emergency evacuation to an appropriate recompression chamber. Calling the DAN physician *(DAN's 24 hour emergency number: 919-684-8111)* from the emergency room helps establish an early, accurate diagnosis and speeds transfer to a recompression chamber if needed. If a diver shows any serious symptoms within 24 hours after a dive, place the injured diver in a horizontal left-side-down-head-low position and provide oxygen during transport to the nearest medical facility.

If you suspect there is any potential for barotrauma injuries in your area of responsibility, contact DAN at the above number, or write them per their address in Appendix I. The *Underwater Diving Accident Manual* and other DAN materials are relatively inexpensive but are invaluable as aids during an actual emergency. Additionally, through DAN, determine where the nearest recompression chamber is located; then review the procedures needed to transport a patient from your location to the chamber.

CHAPTER SUMMARY

This chapter has focused on the basic principles involved with extricating, stabilizing, treating, and transporting aquatic accident victims. In particular, it has examined:

- Common types of serious aquatic injuries and where they may be expected to happen.
- Extrication procedures for various types of aquatic patients.
- Elementary water injury treatment and transport concepts.
- Factors involved in survival of near-drowning victims.
- Various pointers on dealing with both aquatic and terrestrial hypothermic victims.

PRETEST ANSWERS

1. Aid breathing; prevent further injury; and protect from cold.
2. True
3. d
4. False
5. a

REFERENCES

1. Anderson H: Physiological adaptations in diving vertebrates, New Haven, Conn, 1966, John B Pierce Foundation.
2. Anderson H: Physiological adaptations in diving vertebrates, New Haven, Conn, 1966, John B Pierce Foundation, p 26.
3. Bechdel L and Ray R: River rescue, Boston, Mass, 1985, Appalachian Mountain Club Books, p 9.
4. Cold water near-drowning: Emergency care, Fort Collins, Colo, 1980, Dive Rescue International (slide/tape).
5. Deep water lifeguard training, Washington, DC, 1988, American Red Cross, pp 61-63.
6. Gabrielson M: Diving injuries, a critical insight and recommendations, Indianapolis, Ind, 1984, Council for National Cooperation in Aquatics, pp 27, 44.
7. "He's alive!" cop shouts as 'corpse' sits up, Chicago Tribune, p 2, June 30, 1983.
8. Martin T: Near drowning and cold water immersion, Ann Emerg Med 13:4, 1984, p 266.
9. McAniff J: US underwater diving fatality statistics, 1989, Kingston, RI, 1991, National Underwater Accident Data Center, p 7.
10. Mohammed WF: St Francis Hospital, Waterloo, Iowa, unpublished protocol, 1983.

11. Orlowski J: Drowning, near drowning and ice water submersions, Pediatr Clin North Am 34: 79-90, 1987.
12. Resuscitation from hypothermia, Rep CG-D-26-79, Springfield, Va, 1979, National Technical Information Services, p 47.
13. Shallow water lifeguard training, Washington, DC, 1988, American Red Cross, pp 59-60.
14. Smith D: Accidental hypothermia, Postgrad Med 8:3, 1987, pp 38-47.
15. Tisherman W: Cardiovascular resuscibility of dogs after up to 90 minutes cold water drowning using cardiopulmonary bypass, Ann Emerg Med 13:5, 1984.
16. Webb JQ: Cold to the core, J Emerg Med Serv 14: 33, 1989.
17. Weinberg A and Hamlet M, editors: Cold weather emergencies — Principles of patient management, Branford, Conn, 1990, Medical Publishing Co, p 22.

13 Legal Considerations

OVERVIEW

This final chapter examines several water rescues that went amiss. Along with these scenarios are discussed some of the common reasons water rescues flounder and how to avoid such miscues. The benefits of positive public relations and why knowing and using them may be of special importance to you are examined. Litigation pointers are reviewed: why legal suits occur and what might be done to avoid them.

OBJECTIVES

After studying this chapter, the reader will have (a) come full circle back to the opening scenes that introduced the text and (b) should gain a reenforced understanding of the easily correctable elements that have been known to doom miscarried water rescues. Other issues include:

1. A sample analysis of disastrous and near-disastrous water rescue attempts
2. Why we fail
3. On-scene safety observers
4. Note and record taking
5. Videotaping when and if possible
6. Victim follow-up
7. Proper public relations pointers
8. The overwhelming importance of being up-to-date
9. Knowing your information resources
10. Review of training plan necessities

PRETEST

1. As a rescuer, Good Samaritan laws will protect you from being sued in all cases and events. (True or false?)

2. In cases of failed water rescues the following points stand out: (a) improper or insufficient equipment; (b) lack of training; (c) failure to cooperate or coordinate with other available training or rescue resources; or (d) all of the above. Select the most appropriate answer.
3. Postincident debriefings should become routine for (a) legal; (b) professional; (c) psychological; or (d) recreational purposes. Pick the least important of the above.
4. A simple way to acquire and to extend community support and involvement is to provide safety programs to and through children. (True or false?)
Pretest answers are at the end of the chapter.

TWO TARNISHED TALES

In both of the following incidents, which actually occurred, a number of mistakes were made. The author was involved as an expert witness in the cases' litigation and therefore had access to many of their details. In retrospect, the errors in the actions of the involved rescue personnel appear obvious. "How can such things be allowed to take place?" you may ask. They do; they have; and they may again. The reason— essentially not thinking ahead or not preparing to deal with circumstances that can be foreseen. Complacency may also be a key issue.

In the first occurrence the actions or reactions of salaried members of a fire department in a midsized town in northern mid-America are examined. The fire department in this town is responsible for water rescue on the river within the city limits. The incident begins near 11 PM on an evening in early spring. Two brothers are clocked speeding in their car on a city street. An officer responds and gives chase.

The brothers' vehicle, when approaching a sharp turn by the river, bounces off the road, skids across a lawn, and plows into the water. Both occupants are swept out of the car by the current. A police officer spots one of the brothers hanging onto a low-lying tree limb; a passerby sees the other. Both are grasping branches while their torsos are mostly awash. The fire department rescue team is summoned, arriving jointly with the town's fire chief. The fire fighters see the people in the water *but do nothing immediately to aid them.* One of the victims eventually is swept away from the shore and drowns.

The second victim finally is rescued. He is immediately placed in jail for manslaughter since, it is reasoned, as the driver of the car, he was directly responsible for his brother's death.

After a defense lawyer is hired, the surviving car occupant not only is freed from jail, but the city is successfully sued for negligence by the dead brother's family. What really happened?

- Although the fire department had responsibility for water rescue and the call sent by the police officer specified a river incident, there was *no water rescue gear* in the fire department's vehicles.
- The rescue team driver responded *without the department's boat*, which also contained all the water rescue equipment.

The boat was kept at the second of two stations, which was located twice as far from the river as the first. The driver had to go back for it. When the boat was finally placed in the river, instead of at the accident point, it was launched at a site 10 minutes away.

To clarify the action further, here are excerpts from the author's report prepared in defense of the incarcerated brother[2]:

These particular fire (and police) department personnel were apparently unaware of the potential effects of hypothermia. The human body loses approximately 25 times as much heat to still water as it does to air of the same temperature. If the water is moving past an immersed individual, this heat loss rate can approach 250 times that of still air. For this reason, rescuers must attempt as quickly and as comprehensively as possible to remove accident victims from cold, moving water. A paramount consideration is the rapid loss of muscle control and grip strength which reduce a victim's ability to grasp and/or retain sources of safety or assistance. The longer rescue personnel wait to approach an immersed fast water accident victim, the less the probability of the victim's maintaining his position, and the greater the degree of difficulty in successfully effecting the rescue.

. . . Although the fire department rescue truck was called to the scene, it carried no specific water safety equipment such as personal flotation devices. . . . Failure to provide first, on-scene responders with proper water rescue equipment is analogous to fire fighters' arriving at a fire without a pumper or hose truck. . . . These oversights clearly demonstrate both a lack of training and inadequate understanding of the basic requirements of water rescue. Underscoring the foregoing are the inability to use rescue lines or lengths of rope which were in the rescue truck; and not requesting assistance from neighboring facilities, even though aid was offered which could have provided timely backup, both in rescue and subsequent search aspects of the incident.

Drag and Bag

The second event occurred in late winter in a large city; in this municipality the city police department was mandated as the lead water rescue agency. The state in which this major city is located has one of the nation's primary water rescue training programs. Apparently this police department did not partake of this learning opportunity.

An individual determined to commit suicide by jumping off a bridge over one of the rivers bordering the city. The rescue boat crew was contacted by an officer who had last seen the victim being carried down the river. The primary *rescue* boat, which was located 6 miles downstream, was in the shop for repairs. The backup boat had engine problems and took 25 minutes to reach the scene. When the victim was finally located, his heavy water-logged winter clothing, plus his own weight, prevented the boat crew's bringing him aboard easily. They opted to tow him—*by wrapping a line around his ankles*—11 blocks to an *upstream* boat landing where a paramedic waited. When they reached the landing, approximately 1 hour after the incident began, the rescuers were amazed to hear the paramedic shout, "His heart's beating!"

Nevertheless, the victim died 4 hours later. His family eventually and successfully sued the city; a number of city employees lost their jobs or were reassigned to other duties; and a general interdepartmental shakeup followed. The city now has a well-trained and highly capable water rescue unit. But at what price was it bought?

What went wrong? As with the previous case, here are excerpts from a legal report concerning the incident[1]:

... adequate rescue doctrine should emphasize rapid dispatch and mini-mum transport time to accident scenes. In this case, rather than providing a means of trailering a rescue craft as closely as possible to the scene, and launching as quickly as possible in proximity to the victim, the rescuers traveled approximately 25 minutes upstream, against the current, to arrive at the victim's location. This six mile trip is a prominent error when consideration is given to a number of nearby launch sites, including a marina. Due to this delay and the effect of river current, the victim eventually became lodged under a barge, thereby adding a further unnecessary impediment to the rescue.

... Despite the known, predictably unacceptable performance available from the department's apparently poorly serviced, inadequately maintained rescue craft, no backup was initiated or requested from neighboring commu-nity or federal resources. Hence, the unreasonable choice of water transport to the scene was compounded by the rescue boat's breaking down enroute. . . . Notwithstanding the presence of only two rescuers in the police department boat, the height of the boat's freeboard, and the victim's weight, simple, easily learned practices are available whereby two men can lift or roll a third out of the water and into a boat. Evidently, even though they were responsible for providing this very basic service, police personnel were neither familiar with, trained, or practiced in it. Apparently only a very limited number of water rescue practices were employed by the police department . . . the normal method was to use a craft with a stern mounted, water level, "divers' door" to allow victims to be brought aboard. However, if the highly predictable unavailability of a door equipped craft was known in advance, why weren't other methods of in-water retrieval practiced and used (Table 13-1)?

...ignorance of cold water (37 degrees F at the scene) near-drowning principles and protocols by emergency personnel in this case indicates a culpable level of negligence. Expert and highly knowledgeable community resources were available to train and advise the police department in up-to-date procedures required in treating any near-drowning victim. (One of the nation's initial, leading proponents of CPR regularly taught classes in a hospital within two miles of the incident.)

Table 13-1 Water Extrication Methods

Method	Rescuers	Description
Self (heavy clothing)	Self	*Gently* bounce; lay chest over edge; *drain water;* roll away.
One on one*	One	Hold *both* victim's hands together; bounce or bend victim over edge; move hands down victim; pull in victim.
Two on one*	Two	Rescuer is on each end of line. Pass line *behind* victim's back and under armpits; bounce into boat.†
Parbuckle roll into boat† (can use small cargo net)	Two or four	Extend line from rescuer(s) with strong back(s), with one end *under* victim's midback and one end *under* knees. Victim's arms are *inside* line. Rescuers pull ends of line.†
Cervical spine deep water (can do shallow roll *if* wearing dry suit)	One for roll over; five for backboard	Splint: one elbow is in victim's mid-chest, with hand on chin; one elbow is in victim's midback, with hand on head; swim *under* victim. Await cervical collar or backboard, or swim victim to beach.
Cervical spine shallow water (can do mouth-to-*nose* rescue breathing)	One for roll over; five for backboard	Stand alongside victim. Pin victim's upper arms against ears. *Push down near* arm; *pull up far* arm. Hold victim cradled against your chest. Await cervical collar and backboard.

*NOTE: *Not* for cervical spine–injured victim.
†Prevent rope burn by doubling smaller line and/or increasing clothing around victim.

. . . .The officers involved in the recovery had a limited, inadequate awareness of the potential for revival as they: A, Stated that they attempted (but failed) to keep the victim's head above water; and B, Tried to get him to the paramedics waiting at the marina. If so concerned why did they not:

1. Pass a line under his armpits to elevate his head, rather than securing his ankles?
2. Immediately take him to the nearest shore where waiting paramedical personnel could more rapidly approach and treat the victim?

Similarly, why was the victim towed a considerable distance upstream, against the current? Movement through the water markedly increases heat loss, and heightens the deleterious effects of hypothermia. . . . Likewise, depending on the victim's in-water positioning, water pressure developed by the foregoing motion can force additional fluid and associated contaminants farther into the victim's lungs and stomach, thereby greatly complicating resuscitation and physiological recovery. These last facts relating to towing the victim are sufficient to precipitate his death.

In conclusion, the clear contradiction and unbelievable non-appreciation of so many basic emergency assistance principles is plainly apparent in this disastrous rescue attempt. The lack of even nominal levels of expertise expected of rescuers in a case of this nature greatly compromised the victim's chance for survival.

WHY WE FAIL

Perhaps you think the foregoing is too strongly worded. "Surely someone should have compassion for the misguided rescuers," you may say. Sorry, but when the legal chips are down, whatever you may have done or have not done is fair game, *and* the more you can be placed in the worst of positions by the other side, the better! Therefore the word to the wise is plain: do not allow yourself or your agency ever to be caught in situations such as the preceding ones.

A detailed analysis of "what went wrong" requires a broadened perception. As examples, a few sample considerations are represented in the above and other similar cases. Think over these considerations carefully to see how your or your department's actions compare with them.

Rescue Versus Recovery

The beginning of Chapter 9 discusses the need for separating rescue from (body) recovery. Do you think that both departments in the foregoing cases emphasized recovery too much and were way behind in learning about *modern* water rescue techniques? Where does your agency stand? One outstanding aspect of the best departments is they are always seeking methods to improve their performance. "But we don't have the budget," you may say or be told. Fine. However, there certainly is a super chance of your department having even *less* of a budget if the foregoing types of catastrophes engulf your people.

Disputes Between Agencies

An arresting aspect of the second tragic tale was that a lot of good, timely information was readily available to the water rescue providers, but apparently they did not want to partake of it. Why? Since maintenance of their craft was consuming a great deal of budgeted funds, perhaps they did not have enough money available to send people to classes. Although this reasoning sounds good, it is not, for much of the information that would have helped them was free. In reading other material related to the incident, the reviewer begins to see that a sizable amount of animosity may have existed between the police department water rescue team and fire department EMTs. Although this type of antagonism is sometimes an unfortunate part of a provider's professional scene, water is a great leveler. Anybody can drown; and if you do not want to work together, you might be the one.

Attorneys representing the victims of failed rescues like to hear about disputes. Such disputes give them an opportunity to bring more parties into the case. In other words, more people may be sued. Another problem is the otherwise action-oriented rescue team supervisor who cannot seem to take the time to cross train. He or she will attend classes in his or her own specialties but is reluctant to find out what is going on in other areas such as water safety. A number of situations have arisen in which this person responds to a water scene, takes charge, orders people and boat usage, fails to don a PFD properly himself or herself, falls in the water, and becomes a casualty.

If you find yourself working in such a situation, offer to present a simple in-house, in-service water training session, featuring some of the basic ideas presented in this text. One of your key objectives would be to model a properly fitted PFD.

Back to the Basics

An in-depth review of the majority of recently failed water rescues in which either the victim and/or rescuer died tends to highlight the same factors—*the rescuers were not trained or equipped* (Fig. 13-1). Their intentions may have been of the highest order, but they simply did not

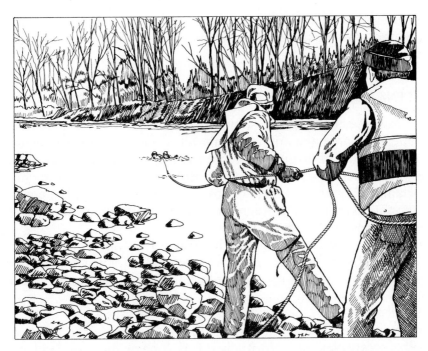

Fig. 13-1 Practice does make perfect. Rescuers use body belays to snub and swing swimmers into shore.

know what to do. Resulting errors include recovered persons underwater for relatively short periods of time that no one attempted to resuscitate. Even with all the information on this subject, many providers remain ignorant about it.

Some instances and circumstances are too difficult to handle, even with very sophisticated equipment and tactics; *but* you stand far less chance of being taken to court over a rescue if you have done your best and can readily explain how your actions were based on proper training and procedures. In fact, as explained later in this chapter, your chances of ever being taken to court are greatly reduced if the majority of the people in your community believe you were acting as capably as possible in a tough situation. In the two ill-fated examples, the plaintiffs sued primarily because the rescuers *clearly* were less than adept.

Being basically prepared for water rescue is undoubtedly the best defense against a legal suit. Basically prepared relates to having simpler gear and equipment and practicing with it. Fielding a dive rescue team or a helicopter response is laudable, but these advanced response modes rarely become involved in legal actions because the individuals who perform them must be well trained and competent. Their probability of making the gross mistakes so easily apparent in the examples is greatly reduced.

ON-SCENE OBSERVERS AND OBSERVATIONS

Just as some emergency response providers need to have their water awareness updated, the public is generally even more undereducated in aquatics. This means to guard against possible legal actions, (1) you must have your rescue procedures organized and practiced, and, just as importantly, (2) you must, if at all possible, take a few simple steps to aid an after-action reviewer's understanding of *exactly* what you were doing when you tried to rescue someone.

To achieve this second goal, there are a number of shortcuts to use: safety observers; automatic videocameras; voice-activated tape recorders; victim follow-up protocols; and debriefing procedures.

Safety Observers

Somewhere in your team responsibilities, someone should be given the job of safety observer. Normally this is done by the team leader *until* enough personnel arrive to allow another person to assume the job. In both exercises and actual operations, the safety observer should not only monitor proper or potentially dangerous aspects of the operation, but he or she should be specifically designated to record, through some noninterfering medium such as a voice-activated recorder, what is being done, when, and if possible, why. This person would have the overall responsibility of giving a chronological commentary of exactly what transpired during the rescue and when it occurred. A double benefit accrues during drill sessions because this observer not only practices his or her own duties but more importantly is in a good position to critique constructively the overall operation.

Automatic Videocameras

The use of pictures is far better than written commentary in describing any event, especially if it is as potentially confusing as an involved water rescue operation. Many police and fire agencies use low-level-light video equipment to record rescue operations as a standard procedure. Smaller, less well-subsidized municipalities might also use this technology. After clearing the largest hurdle, that of obtaining a videocamera, the next step is either to plan and train with someone to use it or as an alternative, to develop an automated use scheme. Depending on your area of operations, if lack of personnel and physical security of the camera present potential problems, rig it for mounting in the cab or on the dash of a rescue vehicle, which usually is the vehicle carrying water rescue gear and would have parked closest to the scene. On arrival at the scene, plug the camera into the dashboard's cigarette lighter, aim the lens at the scene (making sure the self-focusing mechanism is *not* misled by the nearness of window glass, turn it on, and then leave it. Extension microphones are usually inexpensive. One of them could be plugged into the camera and left hanging outside the vehicle's locked window (Fig. 13-2).

Someone might object to this monitoring, saying, "If we make a mistake, it'll be on the record." If your group is far enough along to attempt this recording alternative, the probability of your committing the classic errors described is remote. The chances of videotaping being an aid are far greater than its chances of being a hindrance.

Voice-Activated Tape Recorders

Perhaps videotaping is not a good alternative for your agency, or perhaps you want even more precision in piecing together the flow of an

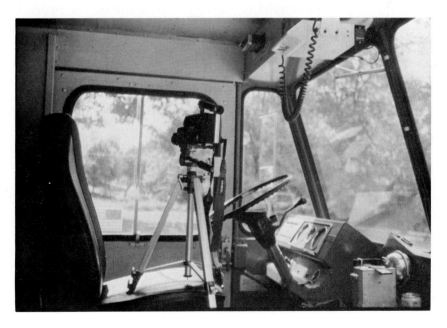

Fig. 13-2 A secure videotaping setup.

event. Small, relatively inexpensive, breast-pocket mounted, voice-activated tape recorders offer a suitable alternative. They can be used with either their built-in microphone, which might be muffled, or a plugged-in miniature microphone clipped to a user's outer lapel. If only the team leader and one or two other key persons have these "hands off" recorders, a comprehensive ability to determine what happens during the course of an exercise or actual operation still is provided. If your group depends on hand-held radios, teaming a small voice-actuated recorder with an on-scene transceiver can be a valuable move. The idea is to provide as much detailed information as simply as possible should you ever have to fall back on it legally.

Victim Follow-Up

Chapter 10 emphasized the need for quickly getting information from an accident victim whenever possible, primarily to determine if anyone is missing and the missing person(s)' last known location. The following may seem like a lot to do, but if at all available, attempt to record, in written notes if nothing more technologically sophisticated is handy, *what the victim thinks happened.* If you ever have to defend your actions in court, this timely information can be invaluable. If the victim makes sufficient statements to indicate his or her own irresponsibility for initiating the event and requiring you to put your life on the proverbial line to save him or her, the potential for litigation will be markedly reduced.

Any notes or recordings taken in this manner must be safeguarded and maintained in a custodial chain of evidence. Do this so no one can imply later that the information was altered. The best way to maintain this chain is simply to have each person handling the material sign for it, stating the time, date, and place it was transmitted to and from him or her.

Like it or not, litigation is becoming an increasingly common aspect of our society. Public service providers must be prepared to deal with it, if for no other reason than the mental and social outlook of many of the individuals who get themselves into situations requiring rescue. When chain-of-evidence procedures for handling case information become routine, as they easily can, the imposition of any related perceived hassle is largely diminished. Sad to say, you often must be prepared to protect yourself as thoroughly *after* the rescue as during it.

Do not think that Good Samaritan laws will protect you totally. If it can be proved that a person is negligent by not knowing about or doing something that is *clearly and reasonably part of his or her job responsibility,* he or she is "fair game" for an aggressive attorney.

THE CASE FOR DEBRIEFINGS

Perhaps your service has gotten into the habit of discussing an event immediately after it has transpired. Conversely, the numbers of cases you deal with may prevent the luxury of such a postincident meeting. Seriously consider establishing such a procedure within your group for several very important reasons—legal, professional, and psychological.

- *Legal reasons.* If you can talk over and record exactly what transpired in an incident as close in time as possible to its happening, the ability to recall important details is much greater than when attempting the same process days or months later.

> Key elements, which may not seem important in themselves and likely will soon be forgotten or mentally misplaced later, can be entered permanently in the record *immediately* after the incident.

Additionally, it is far less likely that a gathering of individuals jointly reliving something that has just happened will be seen as tampering with or bending essential information.

- *Professional reasons.* By reviewing an event while it is still fresh in perspective and close in time, a team might perceive which existing procedures and equipment were less than sufficient. This information may allow and encourage improvement for the next occurrence. Similarly, a short and simple review may provide information about items for inclusion in the next training exercise or syllabus.

  Frequently equipment is procured and protocols are established based on a limited group of outlooks. Since survival is based on considering expanded alternatives, the more input, the greater is the likelihood of discovering superior alternatives. In addition, such discussions provide an opportunity for a more personal "buy-in" on the part of group members. This is an especially important element in maintaining volunteer organizations.

- *Psychological reasons.* The final point of the preceding paragraph leads to the consideration of behavioral factors.

> An opportunity to talk over what went right is just as important as reviewing what may have gone wrong. The first instance builds group morale. Solidarity has a lot to do with good memories of rewarding interactions with others.

On the other hand, if the interaction did not go as well as planned or as hoped, the group can provide an excellent opportunity for unloading debilitating feelings. In Chapter 1 the term *macho* was examined as a cause of accidents. In the present context machismo may also be harmful because it can be (mis)taken as a manly excuse for not sharing emotions, beliefs, or opinions. When the "chips" are really down, the group members must be "out of their collective minds" (and just possibly might be) not to allow themselves an opportunity to dump or vent possibly harmful internal sentiments. If such debriefing opportunities are routine and habitual, the chances improve that inner doubts, insights, or observations will be aired, shared, and potentially minimized or dissipated in the privacy of the group's closed circle.[5]

PUBLIC RELATIONS POINTERS

In the "Why We Fail" section of this chapter, the disturbing effect of intradepartmental friction was addressed. Practical public relations wisdom follows the same course. For a number of obvious reasons, one of the essential conflicts you and your team or agency do *not* need is an *us-against-them* (everybody else) outlook or mental set. Positive and productive public relations is part of the water rescuer's job. *You want the public on your side.* One of the underlying reasons you will not be called out at 3 AM under absolutely atrocious weather conditions is that you have worked with the public in an effective educational mode.[3] Education is hinged on trust. With no trust, there is no belief, and if there is no education, there will be more rescue calls.

Maintain a positive image in the community both to *give* (e.g., education) and to *receive* (e.g., information about where and when accidents might happen or public support when the time comes to buy new gear). Poor perception by the public of your agency greatly enhances the potential for your being taken to court.

A disturbing subset of such actions is the growth of the "We know it all" clique. First of all, no matter how long a person has been in the rescue business, he or she does not know it all.[4] In fact, one item that can be ascertained from such an inflated self-appraisal is that the individual is dangerous to those around him or her. Airs of superiority, as opposed to those of cooperation, do not promote safety on either an individual or group basis, and they interfere with and obstruct learning. Most people have a hard time getting past the personality of a blowhard to mine the potentially important information stored within him or her. Likewise, a person who "knows it all" has a difficult time learning something new. Keep this in mind during the discussion of the importance of being up-to-date in the next section of the text.

If a decision is made to improve public relations, are there any shortcuts outside of the slower but proper processes of sending out news releases, giving speeches, and attending luncheons that may be of value? Yes. The following suggestion is simple, sincere, and synergistic (i.e., a number of aims are met by a single ploy).

> *Think children.* Everyone either has them or has been one and is somehow touched by them.

Any type of interpersonal improvement or relationship generally is centered on what makes all humans alike, not different. Children form communal glue. Set up aquatic safety educational happenings for grade school children, and the following should take place:

- The children learn how not to become statistics by avoiding water hazards. Since when they become slightly older, they would otherwise form a large subgroup of possible drowning victims, you will be attacking the problem at a major source.
- They influence their parents in a number of ways. Having a short session on water safety and sending the children home with simple materials such as coloring books allow them to influence and possibly to teach their parents. (This also spreads public awareness about your department's good works and intentions.)
- They grow up to become informed (influenced) taxpayers and potential recruits for your organization, and they have their own, hopefully safer, children, thereby making your job (you are the department chief by now) that much easier.
- They will ask questions. Children usually are not inhibited by fear of asking "dumb" questions. Most of the answers you will be asked to give will become repetitive. But occasionally you rewardingly will be brought up short by a question about something about which you had never thought. In considering it, you gain more safety insight.

IMPORTANCE OF BEING UP-TO-DATE

After a too lengthy period of dormancy, the field of aquatic safety has seen a number of recent innovations, bringing both good and bad news.

The good news is that we now have a number of modern, safe techniques and informational items both for seeing that people do not get into aquatic trouble and for getting them out of it. The bad news is the more any type of understanding expands, the greater is the difficulty in keeping up with it. This is called the *ram jet theory*, or "The faster it goes, the faster it goes." The word *complacency* has appeared in this text as an indictment of those who have not wanted to keep up. Some individuals working in water safety really have thought, and in some cases still believe, for example, that clothing removal and inflation and drown-proofing (survival swimming) are the absolute ends of the safety spectrum. Although the numbers of these individuals are diminishing, they have left a legacy of similarly oriented individuals. Teaching something new is difficult enough without having to overcome built-in prejudices such as the belief that the mountain top has been reached and there is little that can be added.

One exercise to consider to ensure you do not fall into this trap is to find new ways of approaching water rescue, either in techniques or equipment, and attempt to tell other rescuers about your discoveries (Fig. 13-3).

A principle reason that water safety stagnated into a "business-as-usual, just get your ticket punched, there is *only* one way of doing it" rut is that so few people tried to improve on past procedures. Armed with

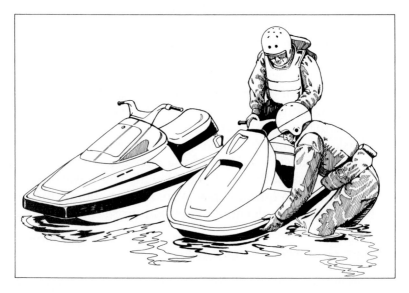

Fig. 13-3 Personal watercraft may represent a new wave in water rescue.

the uncomplicated information in this text, challenge yourself to try to do things better.

Minor hassles might result occasionally if you experiment with innovations, working to stay abreast of the state of the art. But as this whole chapter has attempted to demonstrate, you will acquire a far greater potential for difficulty if you do nothing, letting improvements pass you by.

KNOW WHERE TO FIND IT

The final segment of the text, the appendices, mainly are devoted to providing you with an extended listing of informational resources. Check into them closely, noting what may be available near you. We have explored only rudimentary aspects of the overall field of water safety. A number of specialized courses and informational materials are available in areas such as underwater search, rescue, and recovery; wild or white water canoeing and rafting water safety and rescue; shipboard fire fighting; and powerboat racing and waterskiing safety.

Many of these initial information assets are free. A growing number of learning aids such as books, slide shows, and videotapes are being produced or updated. The resource list provides basic information on major PFD manufacturers in North America. By writing to them, you should be able to obtain their catalogs, price lists, and names of retailers in your area. Manufacturers of other types of water safety and rescue equipment similarly are listed. Among the resources listed in this grouping are innovative, state-of-the-art applications such as Hovercraft and personal watercraft used in search and rescue modes.

The resource list also includes information on various private, state, and federal agencies with materials on water safety that might be of help. Along with this compilation are the addresses of training organizations having courses about water accidents.

A separate section of Appendix I contains information on medical sources, primarily pertaining to protocols dealing with near drowning, hypothermia, and cervical spine injuries. Using all this information in conjunction with the references in each chapter in the text, the reader should be able to develop a fairly extensive background on these items.

TRAINING PLAN REVIEW

Appendix IV lists elementary water rescue training drills and procedures, and the following table refers to sections of the text

Table 13-2 Water Safety and Rescue Drill and Practice Procedures

Title	Chapter	Objective	Equipment
Back floating	5	In-water relaxation and survival	Street clothing, PFDs
Self-extrication	5	Getting self out of water	Street clothing
Heavy clothing flotation	7	Floating in fire fighter's turn-out gear	Turnout gear, hip and chest waders, coveralls, PFDs
HELP	7	Reduced heat loss by one person	PFDs
Huddle	7	Reduced group in-water heat loss	PFDs
Victim extrication (bounce)	7	Removal of victim from water, using one-on-one ploy	—
Elevated entry	7	Entering water from a height	Entry surface above deep water
Tow and throw	8	Moving water self-rescue	Throw bags, PFDs, towing line
Current circle	8	Proper reaction to moving water	PFDs
Breaking seas HELP	8	Reacting to breaking waves in HELP	PFDs and canoe
Swift water ferry	8	Crossing moving water	Flowing stream
Ferry rescues	10	Traverse (span) line placement and use	Flowing stream, lines, boat(s)
Ice rescues	10 and 11	Victim retrieval on ice	Fire hose and inflation gear, dry suits, boats
Low head dam	10 and 11	Victim retrieval in low head dam	Same as for ice rescues
Line search	8 and 10	Shallow water bottom search	PFDs and clear plastic bottle
One-on-one or two-on-one	7	Lifting methods	Line, PFDs
Parbuckle	11	Lifting method	Line, PFDs
Boat rescues	11	Proper use of boats in rescues	Boats, lines, PFDs
Cervical spine immobilization	12	Turning over neck-injury victim	Dry suits, PFDs, backboards, cervical collars

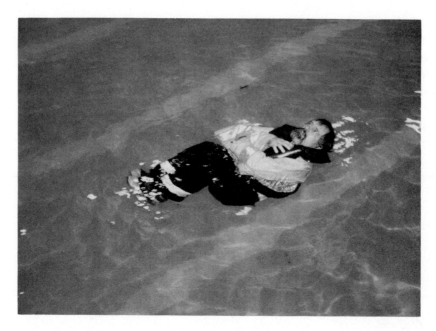

Fig. 13-4 HELP your agency, your community, and yourself to stay afloat by being practiced and prepared.

pertaining to each drill routine and to learning objectives and equipment needed (Table 13-2). Review this table and Appendix IV to make certain you understand and can explain these procedures to others. Note again that safety is a foremost consideration in any of these exercises. Conduct them only under safe, well-supervised conditions, providing specific instructions and flotation devices to all participants as indicated per the information in the relevant areas of the text.

If you understand and accept the principles enumerated in this chapter, acquire resources, and practice (and keep records of) drills, your department's potential for injurious exposure to litigation should be minimal (Fig. 13-4).

CHAPTER SUMMARY

This final chapter of the text has provided information about why water rescues fail, why legal suits follow, and what you might do to ensure your organization's staying out of a court case. In particular, it has examined:

- Failed rescues resulting in litigation.
- Oversights or negative mind-sets that can imperil rescuers.
- The need for on-scene record taking.
- Debriefing pointers.
- Public relations tips.
- Why it is necessary to keep current.
- Information on materials at the end of the text.

PRETEST ANSWERS

1. False
2. d
3. d
4. True

REFERENCES

1. Hollander T: Personal communication, January 20, 1988.
2. Labine R: Personal communication, January 2, 1987.
3. Selling safety education. In Boating safety education, an anthology of the national boating education seminar, Seattle, 1986, National Safe Boating Council.
4. Smith D: Teaching tips, St Charles, Mo, 1988, Smith Aquatics Safety Services, p 38.
5. Teather R: The night before the dive, Dive Rescue International, Ft. Collins, Colo, 1988 (cassette tape).

A P P E N D I X   I

Resources*

AUDIOVISUALS

Films and Videotapes

- *Water: The Timeless Compound* (film, 45 min)
  (Comprehensive, updated look at water safety from the water's perspective.)
  Public Relations Department
  Lutheran Brotherhood Insurance Co.
  625 Fourth Ave.
  Minneapolis, MN 55415

  or

  W.H. Fawcett III
  3305 Highway 101 South
  Wayzetta, MN 55391
- *Man in Cold Water* (film)
  (Immersion hypothermia explained.)
  Media and Technical Services
  University of Victoria
  Victoria, British Columbia
  V8W 2Y2

---

* Retail sales materials listed herein are provided for informational purposes. Their presence is neither a recommendation nor an endorsement by the authors. The reader is encouraged to compare similar items to find the best compromise for the user's particular needs and situation.

- *Cold, Wet and Alive* (videotape, 22 min)
  (Excellent description of common physical processes involved with immersion hypothermia. Describes and illustrates prevention and treatment principles. Primarily intended for canoeists but has wide application.)
  American Canoe Association
  P.O. Box 1190
  Newington, VA 22122-1190
- *The Drowning Machine* (videotape, 20 min)
  (Fire fighters and low head dams; rescue procedures explained.)
  Hornbein Productions
  106 Boalsburg Pike
  P.O. Box 909
  Lemont, PA 16851
- *Drowning Facts and Myths* (videotape)
  (Real-life drowning sequences; classic drowning behaviors explained.)
- *Why People Drown* (videotape)
  (Drowning sequences and behaviors explained plus information on PFDs and pool safety.)
  Both from:
  Water Safety Films, Inc.
  3 Boulder Brae Lane
  Larchmont, NY 10538
- *Judgement on the Water—A Lesson in Small Boat Safety* (videotape, 25 min)
  (Basic outdoor water and boating emergencies explained and defended against.)
- *Survival* (videotape, 28 min)
  (Four real-life outdoor survival situations, mainly focusing on hypothermia, panic, and misunderstanding.)
- *Swept Away* (videotape, 30 min)
  (A guide to water rescue operations.)
  All three from:
  Alan Madison Productions, Inc.
  Red Rock Road, P.O. Box 100
  Chatham, NY 12037

- *Awesome Power* (videotape, 17 min)
  (Actual scenes and interviews with flash flood victims from U.S. Department of Commerce, National Oceanographic and Atmospheric Administration (NOAA).)
  Copies available from:
  Dubs Incorporated
  6360 Delongpre Ave.
  Hollywood, CA 90028
- *Red Cross Water Safety Presentations* (videotape)*
- *Home Pool Safety: It Only Takes A Minute**
  Stock number 329474
  (Home pool safeguards for families with young children.)
- *Emergency Aquatic Skills**
  Stock number 329331
  (Primarily for pool and beach guards but has generally useful rescue information.)
- *Margin For Error**
- *The Uncalculated Risk**
- *Whitewater Primer*
  (The latter three pertain to fast water paddling and rescue techniques.)

Slide Shows

- *Cold Water Near-Drowning: What You Can Do* (basic)
- *Cold Water Near-Drowning: Emergency Care* (advanced)
- *Ice Rescue*
- *Water Proof Your Family*
  All four from:
  Dive Rescue International
  201 N. Link Lane
  Fort Collins, CO 80524-2712
- *Hypothermia and Cold Water Survival*
  Recreational Boating Institute
  University of Tulsa
  600 S. College
  Tulsa, OK 74104

---

*Contact your local Red Cross Chapter. If not available at your local chapter, contact:
American Red Cross National Headquarters
431 18th Street NW
Washington, DC 20006

WRITTEN MATERIALS

Books
Boating

- *Boating Basics—A Small Craft Primer*
  (Most states have their own versions containing safety regulations and basic information on safely outfitting and operating a boat.)
  Outdoor Empire Publishing, Inc.
  511 Eastlake Avenue E
  P.O. Box C-19000
  Seattle, WA 98109
- *Boating Skills and Seamanship*
  (U.S. Coast Guard Auxiliary boating safety and operation text.)
  Commandant (G-NAB)
  U.S. Coast Guard
  2100 Second St., SW
  Washington, DC 20593-0001

Swimming

- Contact your local American Red Cross Chapter; YMCA; YWCA; Boy Scouts of America or Girl Scouts of the United States Councils. Otherwise write:
  American Red Cross National Headquarters
  431 18th Street NW
  Washington, DC 20006

Rescue

- *River Rescue*
  (Excellent text and resource guide on fast and white water rescue.)
  Les Bechdel and Slim Ray
  Appalachian Mountain Club Books
  5 Joy Street
  Boston, MA 02108
- *River Rescue*
  (Training outlines and information for fast water situations, with emphasis on low head dams.)
  Ohio Department of Natural Resources
  Division of Watercraft
  Fountain Square
  Columbus, OH 43224

- *Underwater Diving Accident Manual*
(Divers Alert Network [DAN] — basic scuba accident treatment and
transport handbook.)
DAN
Box 3823
Duke University Medical Center
Durham, NC 22710

Hypothermia

- *Hypothermia — Death by Exposure*
(Comprehensive, easily read text on outdoor and immersion
hypothermia recognition, treatment, and transport. Usually avail-
able in or through most shopping mall bookstores. Also contains the
Alaskan protocol for hypothermia and cold water near drowning.)
Wm. W. Forgey, M.D.
ICS Books, Inc.
1000 E. 80th Place
Merrillville, IN 46410
- *Hypothermia — Causes, Effects, Prevention*
(Explains all aspects of hypothermia simply.)
Robert S. Pozos and David O. Born
New Century Publishers, Inc.
275 Old Brunswick Road
Piscataway, NJ 08854
- *Cold Weather Emergencies*
(Comprehensive but compact reference for emergency medical
technicians. Discusses and explains hypothermic and near-
drowning patient treatment and transport strategies. Best reflects
and incorporates newest American Heart Association CPR guide-
lines.)
Andrew D. Weinberg, M.D., and Murray P. Hamlet, D.V.M.
American Medical Publishing Co., Inc.
P.O. Box 1087
Branford, CT 06405

Alcohol

(Additional handout information is available from sources listed
under "Pamphlets.")

- *Drugs, Society and Human Behavior*
  Oakley Ray
  Mosby–Year Book, Inc.
  11830 Westline Industrial Drive
  St. Louis, MO 63146
- *Alcohol and Diving Performance*
  (Detailed information on many alcohol-induced psychomotor problems.)
  Glen H. Egstrom
  Department of Kinesiology
  University of California, Los Angeles
  Available from:
  National Swimming Pool Foundation
  10803 Gulf Dale, Suite 300
  San Antonio, TX 78216

Pamphlets
Boating safety

- *U.S. Coast Guard Boating Safety Hotline* (800) 368-5647
  (Information on Federal boating safety materials.)
- *Canadian Coast Guard*
  Canada Bldg., Minto Place
  344 Slater St.
  Ottawa, ONT K1A 0N7, Canada
- *Boat U.S.*
  (General information on how to obtain handout materials on boating and location and scheduling of nearest boating safety courses. Ask for *Boater's Six-Pack*. This packet of materials has excellent general water safety, hypothermia, and alcohol information. It also contains a detailed listing of many North American aquatic safety agencies and resources.)
  Boat U.S. Foundation
  880 South Pickett St.
  Alexandria, VA 22309
- *Boater's Guide*
  (Booklet prepared by the National Marine Manufacturers Association and Outboard Boating Club of America. Lists the name, address, and phone number of each state boating law administrator [BLA]. This official can be contacted for information on your state's boating safety materials. Either call the number listed in *Boater's*

Guide or contact the BLA through your state's departments of natural resources or fish, wildlife, parks, and game.)
National Marine Manufacturers Association
2550 M Street, NW, Suite 425
Washington, DC 20037

Outdoor safety (hunting and fishing)

- *Boater's Guide*
(In most states the boating law administrator is also the hunting and fishing safety coordinator. Contact him or her through the process given immediately above. If all else fails, contact Outdoor Empire Publishing, Inc., listed under "Books."

Pool safety

- *National Swimming Pool Safety Committee*
(Clearing house for all types of pool- and spa-related safety information materials.)
c/o U.S. Consumer Product Safety Commission
Washington, DC 20207

Anti-child drowning

- *National Drowning Prevention Network*
P.O. Box 16075
Newport Beach, CA 92659-60754
- *SEAL (Swim Early And Live) Foundation*
c/o Margaret Freemon
Windsor Drive, Route 3
Gallatin, TN 37066

Hypothermia and cold water near drowning

(General nonmedical information is available from state and federal sources as listed above. The following items are for emergency medical providers.)

- *State of Alaska Hypothermia and Cold Water Near Drowning Guidelines*
(A specific, easily understood protocol for field and clinical use. Cost: $2.50)
Emergency Medical Services Section
Division of Public Health
Alaska Department of Health and Social Services
Pouch H-06C
Juneau, AK 99811

- *Emergency Management of Accidental Hypothermia*
(Practical, illustrated monograph presenting protocols for field and clinical use. An accompanying videotape is also available for rental.)
Rodney D. Edwards, Jr., M.D.
c/o Abbott Laboratories
Abbott Audio-Visual Services, D-383
Abbott Park, IL 60064

Maps (detailed, topographical)

- *Areas West of the Mississippi*
Branch of Distribution
U.S. Geological Survey
Box 25286, Federal Center
Denver, CO 80225
- *Areas East of the Mississippi*
Branch of Distribution
U.S. Geological Survey
1200 South Eads St.
Arlington, VA 22202

PERSONAL FLOTATION DEVICES

- Stearns Manufacturing Co.
P.O. Box 1498
St. Cloud, MN 56302
- America's Cup
P.O. Box 244
Madison, GA 30650
- Northwest Environmental Services
911 Western
Seattle, WA 98104

RESCUE AIDS

Immersion (Dry Ship Abandonment) Suits

- *Stearns Manufacturing Co.*
(See above under "Personal Flotation Devices.")
- *Bayley Suit*
900 South Fortuna Blvd.
Fortuna, CA 95540

Rescue (Dry) Suits

- *Stearns Manufacturing Co.*
  (See under "Personal Flotation Devices.")
- *Dive Rescue International*
  201 N. Link Lane
  Fort Collins, CO 80525

Roof Penetrator

- *Bow-Parm, Inc.*
  2443 Hemlock Avenue
  Granite City, IL 62040

Miscellaneous Water Rescue Equipment (Including Rope and Throw Bags)

- *Dive Rescue International*
  (See previous listing under "Slide shows.")
- *The Rescue Source*
  P.O. Box 519
  Elk Grove, CA 95759-0519
- *J.E. Weinel, Inc.*
  P.O. Box 213
  Valencia, PA 16059
- *MARSARS/Great Eastern Marine, Inc.*
  155 Myrtle Street
  Shelton, CT 06484

MEDICAL MANAGEMENT AIDS

Hypothermia Management

- *H.O.W., LTD.*
  (Manufacturers and distributors of a four-part treatment combination, including Micro Temperature Computer [low-reading thermometer and computer]; portable, compact intravenous (IV) warmer; heated drug box; heated and moisturized portable oxygen system.)
  2443 Hemlock Avenue
  Granite City, IL 62040
- *C.F. Electronics, Inc.*
  (Distributors of *portable* oxygen humidifying and warming systems.)
  5 Brayton Ct.
  Commack, NY 11725

- *Trademark Medical*
  (Distributors of IV line insulating jackets.)
  1053 Headquarters Park
  Fenton, MO 63026
- *MTM Health Products Ltd.*
  (Distributors of portable IV warmers.)
  2349 Fairview Street
  Burlington, Ontario
  Canada L7R 2E3

RESCUE CRAFT
Inflatables

- *Zodiac of North America*
  Thompson Creek Road
  Stevensville, MD 21666
- *Avon Boats*
  30 Barnet Blvd.
  New Bedford, MA 02745

Personal Watercraft

- *Personal Watercraft Industry Association*
  923 N. Pennsylvania Ave.
  Winter Park, FL 32789

Air Cushion Vehicles

- *Scat Hovercraft*
  10621 North Kendall Dr., Suite 208
  Miami, FL 33176

ORGANIZATIONS
General Aquatic Safety

- *National Water Safety Congress*
  (National organization working with safety officials on rivers, lakes,
  and other rural environments.)
  Outdoor Empire Publishing, Inc.
  (See under "Boating.")
- *American Canoe Association*
  (Information on moving water rescues.)
  Box 248
  Lorton, VA 22079

- *National Association for Search and Rescue (NASAR)*
  (Oriented to large-scale search and rescue operations.)
  P.O. Box 3709
  Fairfax, VA 22038

Water Safety and Rescue Training

- *Smith Aquatic Safety Services*
  (Basic fire, police, and EMS training in water safety and rescue plus hypothermia and cold water near drowning. Offers traveling seminars specifically designed for sponsoring organizations.)
  61 Broken Oak Court
  St. Charles, MO 63304
- *Nantahala Outdoor Center*
  (White water rescue.)
  US 19W, Box 41
  Bryson City, NC 28713
- *Dive Rescue International*
  (Underwater search, rescue, and recovery.)
  (See under "Rescue [Dry] Suits.")
- *Rescue 3*
  (Advanced white water, surf, and rope rescue.)
  The Rescue Source
  P.O. Box 519
  Elk Grove, CA 95759-0519
- *Ohio River Rescue*
  (See previous listing under "Rescue.")
- *Pennsylvania's Water Rescue Program*
  (Modeled after Ohio River Rescue Program.)
  Pennsylvania Fish Commission
  3532 Walnut Street
  P.O. Box 1673
  Harrisburg, PA 17105-1673
- *Indiana Water Rescue School*
  (Fast water rescue course taught in a unique setting—the middle of a city!)
  Law Enforcement Division
  Department of Natural Resources
  606 State Office Bldg.
  Indianapolis, IN 46204

- *Calgary Fire Department Water Rescue Training*
(Canadian source of comprehensive water safety and rescue information and training.)
Location 50
City of Calgary Fire Department
P.O. Box 2100, Postal Station M
Calgary, Alberta T2P 2M5, Canada

A P P E N D I X   I I

General Glossary*

abutments Supporting structure of a bridge.

aerated Mixture of air and water.

aft Toward the stern or rear of a boat.

ascend To move toward the source of; to go up.

backwash Water moving backward; caused by rapid drop over an obstruction, creating a hole in the surface water directly below and causing water to flow backward to fill in the hole.

belay To secure by a rope; to stop and hold fast.

bight Middle part of a slack rope; a loop.

bilge Lower part of a boat's hull.

bitter end Extreme end of any line.

boil In the hydraulic backwash below a dam, the point where the current splits, flowing upstream and downstream.

bolo On the end of the line, small padded weight that is twirled around the head and thrown to carry the line.

bow Front part of a boat.

broach To turn a boat sideways to wind, waves, or current, frequently resulting in the craft's capsizing or rolling over.

carabiner Ring of high-tensile alloy used to rig or connect lines under tension.

cavitation Slipping or nondevelopment of thrust by a boat's propeller.

chute The clear passage through a rapids in the river.

confluence Flowing together of two or more streams; place where they flow together.

convergence Where waterways come together.

---

* This is an expanded list of common terms used in boat and water rescue. Although a number of these terms do not appear in the text, they are in normal use by those working along waterways.

current differentials   Flow that will have different reactions or results for anything crossing into it; the area where two distinct currents could act at once on a boat (e.g., eddy lines).

descend   To go down, away from the source.

downcurrent   Away from the oncoming flow or push of the river.

downstream   Downriver in relation to the banks; when used synonymously with downcurrent, it can mean away from the oncoming flow, which may not be downriver in relation to the banks (i.e., the flow of an eddy).

downstream V   Clear passage area in a rapids; the upstream points of the V are caused by solid obstructions diverting the water.

eddy   Current of water moving against the main current in a circular motion; found behind solid obstructions where water is forced around (not over) the obstruction.

eddy line   Line between water flowing in an eddy and water continuing downstream.

Eskimo roll   Self-rescue technique used by kayakers and other closed boaters, allowing them to right their boats after capsize occurs.

face   Smooth upright surface of a dam.

ferrying system   Method for moving across a stream.

fluke   Lower arm of an anchor.

ford   Shallow portion of a waterway suitable for allowing crossing.

forward ferry   Boating maneuver in which the bow of the boat is facing upstream and toward the shore where you wish to go. By applying upstream power and using the correct angle to the current, the boat will travel across the main current to the shore without losing headway downstream.

foul   To become jammed, knotted, or immovable.

freeboard   Height of boat gunwales above the waterline.

grade   Degree of rise or descent on a surface.

grapnel   Multipronged anchor.

gravel bars   Large accumulation of gravel caused by slowing of the current in a certain area of the river.

gunnel (or) **gunwale**   Upper edge of the side of a boat.

harness seat   Sometimes called *Swiss seat;* a device into which a climber or rescuer ties himself or herself, which affords both security and comfort. The rope can be tied directly to the seat or hooked in using a carabiner.

HELP   Fetal position assumed in water to reduce heat loss.

huddle   Close gathering of individuals as protection from cold water.

hydraulics (as in hydraulic backwash)   Recirculating current formed when water drops over a large rock, ledge, or lowhead dam.

International River Scale   Classification of difficulty used mainly on Eastern rivers, with Class I the easiest and Class VI the toughest on the scale.

johnboat   Double-ended skiff with a flat bottom.

keeper hydraulic   Perfectly formed recirculating backwash that, because of its uniformity, will hold a buoyant object in its grasp.

leg loops   Portions of a harness seat configuration that allow the entry and support of the legs.

life jackets   See personal flotation devices.

line gun   Device used to shoot a messenger line across an area. Regular gun loads are commonly used as a means of propulsion.

matrix   Graphical approach to problem solving.

neoprene   Soft, pliable plastic-based material used in manufacturing flotation devices.

novice   Beginner.

outwash   Usually refers to water flowing downstream after separating from the backwash in the boil of a hydraulic.

parbuckle   Method for rolling an object or person up the side of a boat or dock.

personal flotation device (PFD)   Traditionally known as life jackets. They come in five distinct U.S. Coast Guard approved types (details of types and uses in Chapter 6).

pike pole   Long slender hooked pole used by boaters to retrieve line and objects from the water. Also known as a boat hook.

pillow   River characteristic formed when water flows over a rock or jutted-upward obstruction.

prusik   Short loop of small-diameter, high-strength line used in rope rigging.

reeve   To pass through.

rescue tube   Buoyant device usually used at the end of a line to extend into dangerous areas to the victim.

reversal   Current differential or eddy; whirlpool action of otherwise straight-flowing current.

ring buoy   Type IV PFD usually made of a hard buoyant material with a line encircling it.

riprap   Bank protection, usually large boulders or rocks, found along the shoreline of some waterways to check erosion; used to fill in the downstream side of some dams to break up the hydraulic backwash.

rudder   Broad, flat, movable piece attached to the stern of a boat; used for steering.

runner   Moving line.

scenario   Outline of any planned, real, or imagined series of events.

sculling   Working a hand, oar, or paddle from side to side to propel a boat or a body forward.

self-rescue position   Position — lying on back facing downstream with the feet in front near the surface to fend off rocks — assumed when in moving water. The victim should use a sculling arm motion to ferry his or her body to safety.

shoaling   Sudden rise in the bottom, shallow waters.

sling   Loop tied from nylon webbing. In vertical rescue slings often are used as anchor attachments.

snub   To apply friction in slowing or stopping a moving (running) line by partially wrapping (bending) it around a stationary object.

souse hole   Hydraulic backwash usually formed behind one large rock or obstruction.

span or **traverse line**   Line going completely across the waterway.

standing wave   Usually found in a chute or downstream *V*; results when water piles on itself in a continuous manner.

static line   Line that, once suspended, is used to support the weight of other active lines in the rescue system.

stern   Back of a boat.

strainer   Obstruction in the river that allows the current to pass through it but does not allow the clear passage of larger objects such as people or boats.

tail water   Slow-moving downstream water directly below an eddy.

tether   Rope or chain fastened in a way that limits one's boundary such as in double-boat tether technique.

thermocline   Dividing line between sun-warmed, upper layers of still water and markedly cooler lower layers.

throw bag   Rescue device comprised of a length of line attached and inside of a storage bag with flotation. End of the line is held in one hand while the bag and remaining line are thrown with the other. The line is stuffed in the bag to feed out freely once the bag is thrown.

tiller   Handle for turning a boat's rudder.

transom   Horizontal panel at the back of a boat.

treble hook   Three-pronged hook used for dragging.

undercut rock   Rock cut allowing water to flow partially under it instead of totally around it.

upcurrent   Against the oncoming flow.

upstream   Up the river relative to the banks; upcurrent.

upstream *V*   Caused when a solid obstruction diverts the water. Apex of the *V* in this situation is upstream.

upwelling   Rising of water from the bottom toward the surface.

viaduct   Long bridge consisting of short spans supported on piers or towers.

wake   Track left in the water by a moving boat.

weirs   Small dam; an obstruction placed in a stream to divert the water through a prepared aperture for measuring the rate of flow.

BIBLIOGRAPHY

Maloney ES: Chapman: Piloting, seamanship and small boat handling, New York, 1989, Hearst Marine Books.

River rescue, Columbus, Ohio, 1980, Ohio Department of Natural Resources.

APPENDIX III

Medical Glossary*

acute Having a brief but severe course; opposite of chronic.

acute (or adult) respiratory distress syndrome (ARDS) Respiratory emergency characterized by breathing insufficiency and failure; also called *shock lung* or *wet lung*.

alveolus Air cell in the lung. Plural, *alveoli*.

anoxia Decreased supply of oxygen to the tissues; literally means "without oxygen."

arrhythmia Variation from the normal rhythm of the heartbeat.

asphyxia (asphyxiation) Lack of oxygen caused by the presence of an unbreathable substance in the lungs.

aspiration Intake of foreign material into the lungs during breathing.

barotrauma Injury sustained as a result of exposure to increased environmental (air, gas, or water) pressure.

bradycardia Slow heart rate of 35 to 60 beats per minute or less.

bronchodilator Drug, hormone, or substance that dilates bronchi to improve ventilation to the lungs.

caloric labyrinthitis Disorientation and vertigo induced by cooling the balancing centers in the inner ear.

cardiac Pertaining to the heart.

cardiovascular Pertaining to the heart and blood vessels.

carotid Principal artery of the neck.

cerebral (cerebrum) Pertaining to the anterior, larger part of the brain.

cerebroskeletal Pertaining to the spinal column.

cervical Pertaining to the neck.

CNS Abbreviation for central nervous system.

coma State of unconsciousness from which the patient cannot be aroused.

---

* This is an expanded list of medical terms commonly encountered in boat and water rescue. Not all terms appear in the text.

comatose   In a condition of coma.

CPR   Abbreviation for cardiopulmonary resuscitation.

cyanotic   Descriptive term for bluish skin color that results from lack of blood oxygen.

dependent lividity   Settling of blood in the lower parts of a corpse.

depressant   Agent that retards any function.

dilate   Enlarge or expand.

diving (dive) reflex (formally mammalian diving reflex)   Slowing of heartbeat and metabolism during which blood is primarily circulated to the brain, heart, and lungs; induced by cold water on the face.

dry drowning   Water death caused by suffocation in which no water enters the lungs.

edema   Swelling; abnormal accumulation of fluid in body tissues.

EEG   Abbreviation for electroencephalogram.

electrocardiogram (ECG or **EKG)**   Graphic tracing of electrical signals in the heart.

embolus   Plug (blood clot, air, fat, or tumor) within a vessel that is carried in the bloodstream until it lodges and becomes an obstruction to circulation.

endotracheal intubation   Insertion of an endotracheal airway through the mouth into the trachea to assure an open airway and to prevent foreign material from entering the tracheobronchial tree.

epiglottis   Cartilage that covers the larynx during the act of swallowing; prevents food from entering the trachea.

evisceration   Disemboweled.

fibrillate   To undergo rapid, irregular, noncoordinated heart contractions.

fibrillation   Chaotic, unsynchronized beating of the heart muscle.

gastric   Pertaining to the stomach or digestive system.

heimlich maneuver   Abdominal thrust mainly designed to aid choking victims. Used to expel objects blocking the breathing passages.

hematocrit   Measure of the packed cell volume of red cells; expressed as a percentage of the total blood volume.

hemodilution   Thinning of blood caused by infusion of water in drowning.

hyperbaric   High pressure; above the normal sea-level atmospheric pressure.

hyperextension   In diving accidents the head is rotated upward and backward.

hyperflexion   In diving accidents the head is rolled forward and downward.

hyperventilation   Abnormally prolonged and deep breathing, resulting in loss of carbon dioxide from the body, causing dizziness and fainting.

hypothermia   Subnormal body temperature.

hypoxia   Reduced amount of oxygen (same as anoxia).

inhalation   Breathing in or drawing in with the breath.

intravenous (IV)   Within a vein.

intubation   Insertion of a plastic or rubber tube past the glottis into the trachea (endotracheal intubation) or into the esophagus (esophageal obturator airway insertion).

isotonic   Maintaining the same tension.

laryngospasm   Spasmodic closure of the larynx.

larynx   Organ of voice production; located at upper end of the trachea.

metabolic rate   Speed at which chemical and physical processes occur in a living organism.

mortality rate   Frequency of death.

myocardial infarction   Heart attack.

myocardium   Muscular substance of the heart.

near drowning   Condition in which a person would have died as a result of being in the water if emergency care had not been given.

neurological   Pertaining to the nervous system.

paralysis   Loss of ability to move voluntarily.

paralytic   Person suffering from paralysis.

paraplegia   Paralysis of half of the body, usually referring to the lower part, including the legs.

peripheral vasoconstriction   Constriction of blood vessels, causing an increase in blood pressure.

peripheral vasodilation   Dilation of blood vessels, causing a decrease in blood pressure.

pharynx   Cavity behind the mouth, larynx, and nasal cavities.

protocol   Specific remedial procedure to follow in dealing with illness or injury.

psychomotor   Having to do with mental-muscular interactions and abilities.

pulmonary edema   Abnormal accumulation of fluid in the intercellular spaces of the lungs.

putrification   Decomposition resulting from death.

quadriplegic   Paralysis of arms and legs.

regurgitation   Backward flow; vomiting.

respiration   Exchange of oxygen and carbon dioxide in the lungs.

sequela   Lesion or affection following and resulting from an attack of disease.

shunting   Diverting.

subcutaneous   Beneath the skin.

suffocation   Lack of oxygen resulting from blockage of breathing passages.

surfactant   Active on the surface.

syndrome   Repeated, easily defined pattern of behavior.

tachycardia   Excessive rapidity of heart's action (>100 beats per minute).

thoracic   Having to do with the chest.

trachea   Tube extending from the larynx to the bronchi; the windpipe.

trauma   Injury; especially damage produced by external force.

vascular   Pertaining to or full of vessels.

vasoconstriction   Narrowing of a blood vessel.

vasodilation   Widening or distention of blood vessels.

ventilation   To resupply with fresh air.

ventricle (ventricular)   Small cavity; normally refers to right and left sides of the heart.

ventricular fibrillation   Spontaneous, independent contraction of muscle fibers in the lower, larger cavities of the heart.

BIBLIOGRAPHY

Urdang L, editor: Mosby's medical and nursing dictionary, St Louis, 1983, The CV Mosby Co.

APPENDIX IV

Skill Drills

These exercises are indicated by the *Skill Drill* notation in Parts two and three of the text. Thoroughly read the chapter containing each exercise before initiating the drills. By doing so, you will understand better how each drill fits into the total chapter progression. Note and use all safety requirements made in both the text and this appendix for each drill.

PRECAUTIONARY NOTE: When carried out properly, the following basic exercises are neither especially difficult nor particularly dangerous. However, since it may be expected that some participants have little or no in-water safety and rescue experience, these points are *paramount:*

- Always conduct these drills under the on-scene guidance of a qualified and experienced aquatic safety instructor.
- Be sure all participants are in adequate physical condition. For example, the drills dealing with extrication of self or others while wearing heavy clothing can be physically challenging to out-of-shape persons, especially those with a potential for cardiovascular difficulties.

Skill Drill 1. Natural Flotation

Goal: In-water relaxation and confidence.

Objectives
A. Self-discovery and reenforcement of innate floating ability.
or
B. Determination that participant *is* a sinker and strongly *needs to wear a PFD.*
C. Initiate learning-to-swim progression in nonswimmers.

Location: Shallow end of swimming pool, with assistant.

Equipment: Light clothing – shirt, pants, shoes, socks.

Procedure
1. Take large breath.
2. Bend at hips.
3. Grab ankles.
4. Hold as long as possible.
5. Determine if participant lifts off bottom of pool.

Skill Drill 2. Nonswimmer Adaptation

Goal: Reassure and prepare nonswimmer for further water experiences.

Objectives
A. Learn to place face in water.
B. Learn to hold breath with face in water.
C. Learn to do simple, facedown float.

Location: Shallow end of swimming pool, with assistant.

Equipment: Light clothing – shirt, pants, shoes, socks.

Procedure
1. Take breath, immerse face and blow bubbles.
2. Take breath, immerse face, and say complete name several times underwater.
3. While holding breath, insert face in water, bend from hips, and place hands on knees.
4. Same as 3 above but grasp ankles. Hold ankles as long as possible. Assistant notes if participant sinks or floats.

Skill Drill 3. Back Float

Goal: Learning to back float.

Objectives
A. Relaxation in the water.
B. (Increased) ability to hold breath and expand lungs.
C. Arching back to aid flotation.

Location: Shallow end of pool, with assistants.

Equipment: Light clothing—shirt, pants, shoes, socks.

Procedure
1. Learner *gently* lies on back in front of assistant.
2. Assistant supports learner by standing alongside learner and placing hands under learner's back and hips.
3. Assistant continually tells learner to relax, arch back, rotate chin away from chest, breathe deeply, expand lungs. Hands and arms remain in water.
4. Learner extends arms in water beyond head and locks thumbs.
5. Assistant slowly removes support, allowing learner to back float.

Skill Drill 4. Breathing

Goal: Proper breathing while back floating.

Objectives
A. Maintaining a back-floating position while breathing.
B. In-water breathing and floating with minimum motion.

Location: Medium depth water (between chest and chin). Assistants needed for less competent swimmers and nonswimmers.

Equipment: Light clothing—shirt, pants, shoes, socks.

Procedure
1. Back float.
2. Gently press arms down while exhaling.
3. Inhale when face elevated above water.
4. Hold breath.
5. Continue back float.

Skill Drill 5. Deep Water Float

Goal: Motionless face-up floating in *deep* water.

Objectives
A. Relaxed face-out-of-water float.
B. Convince shallow water leg sinkers they can float in deep water.

Location: Deep water *by side of pool*, with one PFD-wearing assistant for each learner.

Equipment: Light clothing—shirt, pants, shoes, socks.

Procedure
1. Motionless float with feet straight down, head back (looking straight up), holding onto side of pool with one hand.
2. Inhale, hold breath.
3. *Gently* let go of pool edge.
4. To breathe, repeat Skill Drill 4 above.
5. Alternate method for sinking *swimmers:*
    Take *large* breath.
    Arch back.
    Reach rearward for ankles.
    Hold position with face out of water.

Skill Drill 6. Water Entry

Goal: Proper emergency water entry.

Objectives
A. Defeat torso reflex.
B. Condition learner to land in water with face up.
C. Trap air in footwear as flotation aid.

Location: Waist-deep (3 feet) water with slightly elevated pool deck or dock; assistant in water.

Equipment: Light clothing — shirt, pants, shoes, socks.

Procedure
1. Stand on deck with back to water.
2. Check water behind self for obstructions and people.
3. Take breath; then cover nose and mouth.
4. Fall backward into water. NOTE: Nonswimmers can be talked into doing this from a sitting or squatting position. *Do not arch back. Do not back dive.*
5. Assistant aids learner in gaining surface but does not catch him or her.
6. Back float (do not remove hand from nose and mouth until regaining surface and becoming stable on back).
7. Attempt again with toes of waterproof footwear last to enter water.
8. If confident, repeat in deep water — with PFD-wearing assistants standing by. *Nonswimmers in water deeper than their chests must wear PFDs.*

Skill Drill 7. Small Craft Survival

Goal: Using canoe or johnboat as flotation aid.

Objectives
A. Proper entry into swamped or capsized small craft.
B. Achieving best positioning for survivors in swamped small craft.

Location: Initially in shallow (4 feet) water. All participants wear PFDs.

Equipment: Canoe (16 to 18 feet) or johnboat (10 to 12 feet); extra PFDs.

Procedure
1. Place occupants in craft with extra PFDs.
2. *Warn* occupants to protect heads from rotating gunwale.
3. Capsize craft.
4. Note how people are thrown out but that PFDs stay in or near boat. MORAL: If you cannot swim and are not wearing a PFD, you probably cannot reach for or use it.
5. Turn craft upright.
6. Space group evenly around outside of craft.
7. Starting with largest person, slowly slide in and sit on bottom of boat. (Do not sit on thwarts or seats.)
8. Others stabilize craft and then enter.
9. Do HELP in boat.
10. Note capacity plate. Craft should hold as many people swamped as it does when dry. Both ends of craft should be slightly above water.
11. Try handpaddling boat. (Do not move too fast in pool because momentum of swamped, loaded boat can crack pool's deck tile.)

Skill Drill 8. Self-Extrication

Goal: Simple self-extrication.

Objectives
A. Using minimum exertion to exit water.
B. Using own buoyancy as extrication aid.
C. Not falling through or breaking ice.

Location: Initially in shallow water; then in water over head (alongside pool deck). *Nonswimmers wear PFDs in deep water.*

Equipment: Winter clothing, including coat, hat, boots.

Procedure
1. While holding side of pool or deck, gently bounce up and down.
2. When height above surface allows, gently fold upper torso over edge of deck.
3. Allow water to drain.
4. Slowly slide more of body from water.
5. When legs clear, spread out and roll away from edge.

Skill Drill 9. Turnout Gear Float*

Goal: Relaxed flotation in fire fighter turnout gear.

Objectives
A. Reenforce point of *not* sinking in "heavy clothing."
B. Overcome panic in unexpected immersion.
C. Introduce and practice aids to flotation.
D. Practice self-extrication (bouncing) wearing heavy gear.

Location: Initially shallow end of pool; then move to deep end. Carefully note and review *all* safety guidelines for this drill as listed in Chapter 7. Nonswimmers *must* wear PFDs in deep water.

Equipment: Turnout gear on participants; PFDs on assistants.

Procedure
1. Test helmet buoyancy by pushing underwater. Place helmet aside.
2. Kneel on edge of deck, with body parallel to water.
3. Take breath; cover nose and mouth with one hand.
4. Roll in tuck position into shallow water.
5. Remaining in tuck, roll onto and stabilize self on back. (Do not remove hand from nose and mouth until regaining surface and stable on back.)
6. Keep knees up to chest, grasping collar. Blow into top of coat if feasible.
7. Slowly back paddle to side and *gently* bounce out.
8. Drain boots.
9. Repeat back entry from standing position. Float as before.
10. Repeat standing back entry wearing helmet with loose or no chin strap. Place one hand on top of helmet to stabilize it before entry. Cover nose and mouth with other hand.
11. When stable on back, remove helmet and place brim down on chest. Hold helmet to chest with one hand; paddle with other.
12. Repeat 10 and 11 above in deep water. *Apply all safety notes.*
13. Holding side of pool, place helmet on pool deck.
14. Do Skill Drill 5 wearing turnout gear and flooded boots.

*NOTE: In this drill, instructor repeatedly emphasizes need of *always wearing* a PFD over or under turnout gear. This exercise is a backup should an individual unexpectedly be immersed.

Skill Drill 10. HELP

Goal: Understanding and properly doing HELP.

Objectives
A. Identify primary body heat loss areas.
B. Protect them from excessive in-water heat loss.
C. Practice solo heat conservation strategies using PFD.

Location: Shallow or deep water.

Equipment: Various PFDs. (Trade during drill to test and compare different types.)

Procedure
1. Lie back in water while wearing PFD.
2. Cross ankles; bring knees to chest.
3. Cross arms over chest; grasp throat.
4. Assume tight fetal position with as much of your head out of the water as possible.
5. Counteract sideways rolling by turning head opposite to roll.
6. Counteract forward rolling by extending legs until stable.
7. Hold position for at least 1 minute.
8. Slowly extend arms and legs. Note sudden chilling effect of water, even in heated indoor pool.

Skill Drill 11. Huddle

Goal: Understand and practice group in-water heat retention.

Objectives
A. Slow in-water heat loss of group.
B. Provide improved visual target to rescuers.
C. Aid morale.

Location: Deep water.

Equipment: Initially, all wear PFDs.

Procedure
1. Break into groups of at least two people.
2. Face each other, placing arms around each other's waist.
3. Wrap legs around each other.
4. Hold position for at least 1 minute.
5. Slowly move apart and notice chilling action of water.
6. Some members of group remove PFDs.
7. Reform groups. Note effect on flotation.
8. Place smallest person in center of huddle. Note effect on this person's warmth.
9. Place arms around each other's shoulders. Note sinking effect. Return to arms-around-waists position.
10. Disburse group. Reform with eyes closed, shouting for others as in after-dark situation.

Skill Drill 12. One-on-One Bounce

Goal: To lift immobile person from water.

Objectives
A. Lifting using water buoyancy.
B. Not straining own muscles.
C. Not losing victim.

Location: Deep end of pool.

Equipment: Immobile victims wear PFDs.

Procedure (Note warning regarding cervical spine injury.)
1. Turn victim to face rescuer.
2. Place victim's hands together, with rescuer's hands on either side of them.
3. Gently bounce victim. (Rescuer uses own leg muscles, not back, to bounce victim.)
4. When victim's torso is sufficiently elevated above pool edge, rescuer steps back, bending victim's upper body over edge.
5. Not letting go of victim, rescuer slides hands down victim's body.
6. Grasp victim's clothing and slide victim further onto deck.

Skill Drill 13. Two-on-One Lift

Goal: Two (smaller) persons lift immobile victim.

Objectives (Note warning regarding cervical spine injury.)
A. Allow smaller persons to lift larger, immobile victim from water.
B. Use victim's buoyancy to aid lift.
C. Increase height of lift over one-on-one extrication.

Location: Deep water; may be done on side of pool or with boat.

Equipment: Victim in PFD and wearing clothing sufficient to prevent brush burns from rope; 20 feet of line. (Double smaller lines to prevent rope burn.)

Procedure
1. Turn victim to face rescuers.
2. Pass line under victim's armpits and around his or her back.
3. Holding line at point 12 to 18 inches from water surface, gently bounce victim.
4. When victim's chest is above edge of deck or side of boat, bend his or her upper torso over edge by stepping back.
5. Without letting go of line, slide hands down victim, grasp clothing, and pull victim further from water.

Skill Drill 14. Elevated Entry

Goal: Safe water entry from height.

Objectives
A. Reduce injury potential during elevated entry.
B. Improve orientation during entry.

Location: Off diving board in deep water.

Equipment: Clothing and PFD.

Procedure
1. Place hand over nose and mouth.
2. Lock first arm in place by crossing second arm over it and grasping PFD.
3. Look down to ensure not jumping on objects and people in the water.
4. Look outward to orient body vertically and horizontally.
5. Step off, crossing legs.
6. Enter water vertically, feet first.
7. Do not uncover nose and mouth until regaining surface.

Skill Drill 15. Rescue Jump

Goal: Jumping entry to assist victim.

Objectives
A. Maintain visual contact with victim.
B. Remain on surface during entry from height.

Location: Deep water.

Equipment: PFD with carried reaching aid.

Procedure
1. Watch victim but also determine that no obstructions are in water.
2. Spread arms from sides, palm down.
3. Spread legs, one forward, other to rear.
4. Lean forward so that chest will hit water at least at 45-degree angle.
5. Continue to watch victim. Enter water.
6. On entry, snap arms forward/downward and legs together.

Skill Drill 16. Tow and Throw

Goal: Proper reaction to moving water.

Objectives
A. As victim—assuming proper downcurrent position.
B. As victim—receiving thrown line.
C. As rescuer—throwing line with accuracy.

Location: Total length or width of pool.

Equipment: Tow lines, throw bags or bottles, PFDs.

Procedure
1. Victim, wearing PFD, stands in shallow end of pool and ties tow line around waist.
2. Two or three individuals on far end of line tow victim (at *moderate speed*) across pool.
3. Victim rolls onto back with feet "downstream."
4. Line throwers attempt to heave throw bags or bottles or lines across victim.
5. Victim rolls into line and is pulled to side by rescuers.

Skill Drill 17. Current Circle

Goal: Proper reaction to swift water immersion.

Objectives
A. React to current by getting on back with feet downstream.
B. Orient body by feel alone.

Location: Shallow end of pool.

Equipment: Everyone in a PFD.

Procedure
1. By holding hands, form two large circles in shallow corner of pool.
2. Circles rotate in opposite directions as rapidly as possible, generating outward flowing current between them.
3. On command, participants release hands and lie on backs, attempting to keep their feet pointing downstream with current flow.
4. Repeat with eyes closed to orient self by non-visual cues as might happen during unexpected immersion at night.

Skill Drill 18. Breaking Seas HELP

Goal: To use HELP properly in rough water.

Objectives
A. To experience rotation into waves while doing HELP.
B. To learn to keep hand over face in rough water HELP.

Location: Shallow end of pool.

Equipment: Canoe; all participants in PFDs.

Procedure
1. Group assumes HELP in shallow corner of pool.
2. Canoe is placed diagonally across corner between group and deeper water.
3. Canoe is rocked up and down by alternately pushing down on bow and stern.
4. Waves generated by canoe wash over persons doing HELP.
5. Individuals place one hand over nose and mouth to deflect waves from face.
6. Repeat in deep corner of pool with groups doing huddle.

Skill Drill 19. Swift Water Ferry

Goal: Safely crossing moving water.

Objectives
A. Avoid being knocked down by moving water.
B. Appropriate use of equipment in stream crossing.
C. Group tactics for stream crossing.

Location: Safe but moderately fast-flowing stream, knee to thigh deep. Station several rescue line throwers downstream.

Equipment: PFDs, paddles, oars, poles as required.

Procedure
1. Individuals attempt crossing by leaning on pole and shuffling sideways across current.
2. Try single person ferry by facing upstream; then return facing downstream.
3. Repeat in groups of three or four, leaning in toward center of group, with arms around each other's shoulders. Place larger persons on upstream side of group.

Skill Drill 20. Shallow Water Search

Goal: Finding objects in shallow, obscured water.

Objectives
A. Appreciating difficulty of underwater search.
B. Understanding a basic shallow water search method.

Location: Best in shallow swimming pool; otherwise target may never be located.

Equipment: Clear plastic container of at least 1 quart capacity.

Procedure
1. Fill container with water and place on bottom of pool.
2. Have line of searchers lock elbows and proceed across pool, sweeping bottom with feet.
3. May be repeated in deeper water with surface-diving swimmers on deep end of search line.
4. All persons should be wearing PFDs unless they impede diving attempts.
5. In both cases team leader on shore directs effort, noting areas searched.

Skill Drill 21. Cross-Stream (Line) Ferry

Goal: Safely reach person stranded in stream.

Objectives
A. Passing lines across moving water.
B. Positioning small craft by heaving on or slacking lines.

Location: Moving water, with slow flow until proficient in drill.

Equipment: Messenger line (light), span line (heavy), runner line (moderate to heavy), small craft, carabiner, or pulley.

Procedure
1. Station line handlers on both sides of stream.
2. Pass messenger line across stream, attempting to keep line as high as possible and out of the water.
3. Bend or fix carabiner or pulley to middle of span line.
4. Reeve runner line through carabiner or pulley.
5. Attach small craft to stream end of runner line.
6. Pull span line across using messenger line.
7. Maneuver craft using span and runner lines.

Skill Drill 22. Low Head Dam*

Goal: Safely performing rescues at low head dams.

Objectives
A. Shore-based rescue.
B. Inflated fire hose rescue.
C. Boat-based rescue.

Location: Low head dam.

Equipment: A. Lines, small craft (preferably inflatable), raft, line-throwing gear.   B. Inflated fire hose gear per Skill Drill 24 below.   C. Small craft (two – preferably inflatable), lines, throw bags.

Procedure
A. *Shore-based rescue*
   1. Attempt to talk victim into self-rescue.
   2. Attempt to throw line plus flotation gear to victim.
   3. Constantly watch victim.
   4. Assemble personnel and equipment; prepare lines for running.
   5. Pass line across stream using most expeditious method:
      Pull line across above dam (do not place boat or crew in hazardous situation).
      Pull line across below dam.
      Shoot messenger line across, using line-throwing apparatus.
   6. Place span line against face of dam and pull small raft or flotation gear across face of dam to victim.
   7. Retrieve victim.
   8. For inactive victim, rig float with hooks.
B. *Inflated fire hose*
   1 to 4. Same as *A* above.
   (See Skill Drill 24 *C* for remainder of drill.)
C. *Boat-based rescue*
   1 to 4. Same as *A* above.
   5. Position boats *downstream of boil line* using two-boat tether, with farthest boat downstream acting as anchor for boat closest to boil. (For more information on two-boat tether, see Fig. 11-15.)

*For more information, see Appendix I, Ohio's *River Rescue* (manual) and *The Drowning Machine* (videotape).

Skill Drill 23. Rescue (Dry) Suit

Goal: Use neoprene (dry) rescue suits in water rescue.

Objectives
A. Use in open water rescue.
B. Use in fast water situations.
C. Use in ice rescue.

Location: A. Pool or pond.   B. Slow to moderate current.
   C. Ice.

Equipment: Dry suits for rescuer and backup and extra suit for "victim" in cold water; tethers, throw bags, PFDs.

Procedure
A. *Open water*
   1. Rescuer and line tender don suits and attach tether while watching victim.
   2. Rescuer enters water with PFD and swims toward victim on back as tender points to victim.
   3. When rescuer is within 6 feet of victim, tender makes a circle overhead, telling rescuer to turn around and to aim feet toward victim.
   4. Rescuer extends PFD to victim.
   5. Rescuer talks to victim to calm and reassure him or her.
   6. When victim has stopped struggling, rescuer loops tether around victim and gives "all clear" sign by patting top of head.
   7. Tender pulls rescuer and victim to shore.
B. *Fast water*
   1 to 7. Basically same as open water. However, tender always attempts to keep tether *perpendicular* to current while avoiding snags. Consider using quick-release device on rescuer's tether. Also best to place PFD on victim before retrieval if possible.
C. *Ice rescue*
   1. Same as *A* above.
   2. Rescuer moves out on ice, attempting to distribute weight.

Skill Drill 24. Inflated Fire Hose

Goal: Use inflated fire hose for water rescue.

Objectives
A. Use inflated hose in ice rescue.
B. Use inflated hose in fast water rescue.
C. Use inflated hose in low head dam rescue.

Location: A. Pool or pond. B. Slow or moderate current. C. Low head dam.

Equipment: Several lengths of 2½-inch fire hose; SCBA bottles; male and female caps adapted to take inflator hose coupling; spanner wrench; steering lines; PFD; appropriate pressure-reducing valve-couplings; high-pressure air hose. (See Table 11-1 and Figs. 11-9 to 11-12 for more information on fittings.)

Procedure
A. *Ice rescue*
    1. Lay out 2½-inch fire hose.
    2. Attach steering lines (two), cap, and PFD to waterside end of hose. One steering line runs to right, other to left.
    3. Connect SCBA bottle through valve and couplings to modified hose cap. Tighten all fittings.
    4. Inflate hose.
    5. Push hose toward target or victim, using steering lines to pull waterside end toward right or left. Depending on inflation pressure, may be necessary to twist hose to keep straight or to use double lengths.
B. *Fast water rescue*
    1 to 4. Same as *A* above.
    5. Twist hose into current, allowing it to pivot on shoreside end, with offshore end falling downstream to victim.
C. *Low head dam*
    1 to 4. Same as *A* above.
    5. Push hose as far out into face of dam as possible. Use highest air pressure available to make hose rigid enough to force past debris.

Skill Drill 25. Parbuckle or Net Roll Aboard

Goal: Quickly extricate *noncervical spine injury* victims from the water.

Objectives
A. Easily roll helpless victim into boat.
B. Roll victim up vertical surface.

Location: Initially poolside; then transfer to boat.

Equipment: Length of larger diameter line, net, expanded plastic barrier mesh.

Procedure
A. *Line**
   1. Pass line around or secure midpoint of line to immovable object approximately 6 feet from edge of pool. (In boat, secure midpoint of line to opposite gunwale.)
   2. If no immovable objects available, have two people act as strong backs or posts. Located 6 feet from edge, they face toward victim, placing line behind their backs.
   3. Place victim on back, parallel to pool or boat side.
   4. Run one end of line from secured point or strong back under *middle* of victim's back (starting from pool or boat side outward) and back to bigger rescuer or line hauler.
   5. Run other end of line from secured point or strong back under victim's knees (starting from pool or boat side outward) and back to smaller rescuer or line hauler.
   6. Line haulers or rescuers step inside lines from strong backs. (Strong backs do not move.) Line haulers take slack from outboard ends of line. Grasping outboard lines only, line haulers walk backward, slowly and gently rolling victim out of the water and over pool edge or gunwale.

CAUTION: *Always be sure line initially under middle of victim's back does not move toward his or her neck or throat.* The victim can easily be injured if line wraps around his or her throat. For this reason, line haulers stand *inside lines*.

---

*Use larger diameter line or double line to prevent rope burns or cutting on victim. Also have heavy clothing on practice victims to prevent foregoing.

Skill Drill 26. Boat-Based Rescue

Goal: Safely perform boat-based rescues.

Objectives
A. Accomplish single boat–single victim rescue.
B. Accomplish single boat–multiple victim rescues.

Location: Pond or lake.

Equipment: Boat (preferably inflatable), rescue dummy, boarding net.

Procedure
A. *Single victim*
   1. Crew constantly watches victim.
   2. Boat *slowly* approaches victim with bow *into* wind or current, whichever has greatest effect on boat.
   3. Bow man throws line or throw bag to victim. *(Operator must ensure lines are kept away from screw.)*
   4. Bow man grabs victim as operator stops engine or places engine in neutral or idle, depending on environment and situation *(recommend stopping engine during initial series of drills).*
   5. Crew brings victim aboard, using two-on-one lift, parbuckle, or boarding net. (For practice purposes, suggest doing all three.)
B. *Multiple victims*
   1 to 5. Same as *A* above except crew must maintain contact with other victims. Suggest using dummy for first victim in drills because it may be necessary to leave engine in neutral while first victim is brought aboard.

A P P E N D I X   V

Flood Rescue Planning and Preparation

FLOODING: GENERAL OVERVIEW

Flooding emergencies may be divided into two main categories: static and dynamic. The following lists the primary characteristics of each category plus major planning considerations needed to deal with them.

Static Flooding

Description

- Relatively slow rise in water level.
- Slow current.
- Primary cause: downstream blockage or obstruction of flood waters, resulting in overflow onto surrounding areas.

Hazards and concerns

- Cannot see underwater.
- Everyone, including those being evacuated, *must* wear flotation devices.
- High risk of striking underwater obstructions; boat and heavy equipment operators must be alert.
- Normal routes, roadways, and access areas blocked or impassable; must reroute or preidentify alternate routes *before* flooding.
- Utilities: secure electricity, gas, water, and sewers. Reduce accidental contact dangers, future repair, and outage problems if practical.
- Persons in low-lying areas may need warning or evacuation; need coordinated incident command and agency interaction plan.

Dynamic (Flash) Flooding

Description

- Extremely high flow rate confined to relatively small, restricted area.
- *Very rapid rise in water level; highly destructive water effects on roads, bridges, structures, and vehicles.*

349

- Occurs as result of heavy rainfall in localized, centrally drained area or sudden upstream water release such as dam or levee failure.

Hazards and concerns
- *Tremendous* potential for sweeping away or entrapping in debris persons who may drown.
- Early warning and evacuation paramount.
- Areas possibly subject to flash flooding must be identified and rapid evacuation plans must be in place.
- Fire, police, and rescue team personnel *must* be familiar with fast water equipment and rescue and extrication techniques.

Emergency (Inter) Agency Preparedness
Primary considerations
- Coordination of warning and evacuation.
- *Pre*-incident identification and evaluation of primary hazard areas; key into flood stages and weather forecasts.
- Effective incident command system.
- Communications.
- Backup systems.
- Emergency and nonemergency vehicle rerouting.
- Local resource and personnel identification and marshaling.
- Fast water rescue training.
- Equipment and procedure familiarity and integration.
- Other (extended) agency interaction.
- Use of state and federal resources.
- Regional coordination.

FLOODING: SPECIFIC TACTICAL CONSIDERATIONS

In Flood Relief and Rescue, Think Four As

The four As of flood relief and rescue are awareness, anticipation, access, and awash.

Awareness. Flash flooding is a continuing, if not increasing, hazard in many parts of the country. The primary cause is lack of forested and cultivated lands to absorb rainwaters and the larger areas of paved or blacktopped surfaces increasing the dynamics of rain runoff, mainly in suburban areas. As with many other areas of emergency response, fire fighters and their communications and response capabilities, along with law enforcement personnel, are a community's prime response element. Even with increasing numbers of flood control projects, principally in rural areas, continued population and building expansion indicates the problem will not get any smaller.

Anticipation. Flooding generally has an annual or seasonal pattern that may fluctuate in scope of damage; nonetheless, it is always present to some degree. Do not be caught unaware! Know locations and situations that may become flash flooding problem areas. Scout these areas, and at least consider mental scenarios for dealing with potential incidents; better, commit thoughts to paper in action-plan outlines; and best, periodically run drills, especially if you know from past experience that flooding may seriously threaten your community.

Access. Work out and review plans for entering areas from high ground when normal equipment entry is blocked by high water. Similarly, understand best rerouting procedures when normally used routes are blocked. Obtain topographical charts indicating ground elevations to aid your planning. List water-oriented resources that can supply boats and *experienced* operators as needed. Also list potential divers.

Awash. Train and prepare with the understanding of two main principles. First, you cannot see *under* floodwaters; therefore no one really knows what he or she is crossing. Thus everyone must wear a PFD and must have lots of spare boat propeller shear pins. Second, you cannot accurately predict water dynamics, especially in nonchanneled, rapidly changing areas. *Do not take chances.* Floodwaters can and do rise at unbelievable rates. Moving water 2 feet deep (or enough to cover wheels) can float a small car. *Approximately 500 persons per year die in water-related car accidents mainly caused by flooding.*

Primary Principles

- Be prepared for the potential of flooding.
- Expect and inspect areas of possible high water.
- Be especially aware of entrapment points such as storm drains. Set up plans for safely getting victims out of such hazards.
- Check equipment. Have sufficient PFDs *plus spares for victims.* Check on lines, boats, trailers, and backup communication gear and systems.
- Periodically train personnel in water safety and self- and others rescue procedures. Be sure that people who will back up your personnel are similarly trained.

  Make sure all individuals are aware of specific flooding hazards such as vehicles driving in deep water lose braking ability; barbed wire fencing makes an extremely dangerous entrapment or strainer hazard;

when leaping off moving boat or truck, a person may land in a hole, increasing possibility of being run over or drowned; floating propane or gasoline storage tanks are potentially hazardous and should be secured as soon as possible; and looters may be encountered by rescuers.

- Have topographical maps of area. Lay out alternative access routes, anticipating blockage of main thoroughfares and low-lying bridges.
- Set up "ops normal" check-back communications system in which groups working in isolated areas contact control center on expected, periodic basis.
- Institute system of water-level monitoring and reporting stations. Interact with weather bureau to share and gain information.
- Establish effective public relations networks to keep public aware of dangerous areas and blocked roadways. Be sure public is continually informed of conditions in their specific area and *which rescue and evacuation routes are impassable.* (A number of flooding-related deaths have occurred when individuals have decided to evacuate, only to find their escape route cut off.)
- Position competent communicators to interact with public in both gaining information and disseminating it. Trained and practiced communicators can reduce panic while increasing the quality of information delivered to command centers.

RISK DECISION TABLE

RISK MANAGEMENT CAPSIZING AND FALLS OVERBOARD

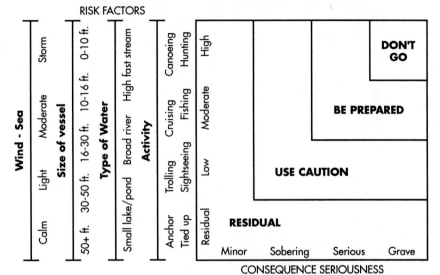

Who is most at risk in which conditions? A sample risk decision table for boating, adaptable to swimming situations. (From Capt. Roger Miller, USCG, Ret.)

BIBLIOGRAPHY

AC Nielson Survey, Swimming pool age and spa merchandiser, October 1982.

About life jackets and EMP, St Cloud, Minn, 1981, Stearns Manufacturing Co.

Accident facts, 1980, Chicago, 1981, National Safety Council.

Accident facts, 1989, Chicago, 1989, National Safety Council.

Accident facts, 1991, Chicago, 1991, National Safety Council.

Alcohol, vision and driving, Falls Church, Va, 1978, American Automobile Association Traffic Engineering Division.

Allman F et al.: Outcome following cardiopulmonary resuscitation and severe pediatric near-drowning, AM J Dis Child 140:6, 1988.

American Heat, St Louis, Jan 1988, American Heat Video Productions (videotape).

American Red Cross basic water safety textbook, Washington, DC, 1988, American Red Cross.

American Red Cross lifeguard training, Washington, DC, 1983, American Red Cross.

Anderson H: Physiological adaptations in diving vertebrates, New Haven, Conn, 1966, John B Pierce Foundation.

Awesome power, Washington, DC, 1987, National Oceanographic and Atmospheric Administration (videotape).

Baker S, O'Neill B, and Karpf R: The injury fact book, Lexington, Mass, 1984, DC Heath.

Barriers for residential swimming pools, spas and hot tubs, Preamble, CPSC Staff Recommendations, Washington, DC, 1990, American Red Cross.

Beach boy spent day drinking, Boston Herald Wire Services, Dec 30, 1983.

Bechdel L and Ray S: River rescue, Boston, 1985, Appalachian Mountain Club Books.

Bernhartsen J: Cold water primer, Washington, DC, J Phys Health Educ Recreat Dance, May 1979 pp. 52-53.

Better think twice . . . A look at alcohol use while boating, Delaware, Ohio, 1985, FlowGraphics Photography (slide/tape).

Boating basics—A small craft primer, Seattle, 1989, Outdoor Empire Publishing Co.

Boating statistics 1987, Washington, DC, 1988, US Coast Guard.

Boating statistics 1991, COMDTPUB P16754.5, Washington, DC, 1992, US Coast Guard.

Bolte R et al.: The use of extracorporeal rewarming in a child submerged for 66 minutes, JAMA 260:3, 1988.

Braude M: Interactions of alcohol and drugs of abuse, Psychopharmacy Bull 22:3, 1986.

Bryan B: Heartbeat found in dead man, St Louis Post-Dispatch, Nov 16, 1990.

BSA Lifeguard counselor guide, Irving, Tex, 1989, Boy Scouts of America, p 2.

Burns M: Alcohol effects on skills performance, Report of Tenth Annual Education Seminar, Tampa, Fla, 1985, National Safe Boating Council.

Burns M: The effects of alcohol on performance, Proceedings from the 1984 conference on alcohol and recreational boating safety, Columbus, Ohio, 1984, Ohio Division of Watercraft.

Children and pool safety checklist, Pub No 357, Washington, DC, Spring 1988, US Consumer Product Safety Commission.

Children and pools: A safety checklist, Pub No 357, Washington, DC, 1990, US Consumer Safety Commission.

Cold water near-drowning: Emergency care, Fort Collins, Colo, 1980, Dive Rescue International (slide/tape).

Collis M: Survival behavior in cold water immersion, Toronto, 1976, The Royal Life Saving Society Canada.

Consumer Products Safety Commission proposes pool barriers to Council of American Building Officials, Newport Beach, Calif, Spring 1989, National Drowning Prevention Network News.

Conway P: Marijuana—Its highs and lows, St Louis Riverfront Times, Jan 8-14, 1986.

Cooper K: Respiratory and thermal responses to cold water immersions. In Proceedings of Cold Water Symposium, Vancouver, May 1976, Canadian Red Cross.

Deep water lifeguard training, Washington, DC, 1988, American Red Cross.

Deluca J: Alcohol and health, Rockville, Md, 1981, National Institute on Alcohol Abuse and Alcoholism, US Public Health Service.

Do you know the facts about drugs?, Hollywood, Fla, 1981, Health Communications.

Driver Magazine, Washington, DC, June 1977, US Air Force.

Egstrom G et al.: Alcohol and diving performance, Los Angeles, 1988, University of California Los Angeles, Department of Kinesiology.

Erwin R: Defense of drunk driver cases, New York, 1981, Mathew Bender.

Experimental evaluations of selected immersion hypothermia protection equipment, Rep No CG-D-79-79, Springfield, Va, 1979, National Technical Information Services.

Fawcett W: Water the timeless compound, Wayzata, Minn, 1980, Fawcett Communications (film).

Federal requirements for recreational boats, Pub No DOT 514, Washington, DC, 1986, Department of Transportation.

Freeman M: Teach your child to swim, Gallatin, Tenn, 1981, SEAL Foundation.

Gabrielson M: Diving injuries, a critical insight and recommendations, Indianapolis, Ind, 1984, Council for National Cooperation in Aquatics.

Guidelines for cardiopulmonary resuscitation and emergency cardiac care, American Heart Association, JAMA 268:16, 1992.

Gulaid J and Sattin R: Drownings in the United States, 1978-1984. CDC Surveillance Summaries 37(SS-1), Atlanta, 1985, Centers for Disease Control.

Haddon W and Baker S: Injury control, Washington, DC, March 1981, Insurance Institute for Highway Safety.

Hafen B and Frandsen K: Drug and alcohol emergencies, Center City, Minn, 1980, Hazelden Foundation.

Harnett RM and Bijiani MG: The involvement of cold water in recreational boating accidents, Rep CG-D-31-79, Springfield, Va, 1979, National Technical Information Service.

Hayward J: Hypothermia update, Washington, DC, 1985, National Safe Boating Council.

Hayward J et al.: Effects of behavior variables on cooling rate of man in cold water, J Appl Physiol 38:6, 1975.

Head and spinal cord injury prevention, Atlanta, July 1988, National Coordinating Council on Spinal Cord Injury.

"He's alive!" cop shouts as 'corpse' sits up, Chicago Tribune, p 2, June 30, 1983.

Hollander T: Personal communication, January 20, 1988.

Hypothermia and cold water survival, Tulsa, Okla, 1980, Recreational Boating Institute (slide/tape).

Ice awareness, Emergency, March, 1984.

Ice rescue, Fort Collins, Colo, 1981, Dive Rescue International (slide/tape).

Johnson R: What research has revealed about drowning and diving accidents, 1984, Indiana, Pa, Indiana University of Pennsylvania.

Labine R: Personal communication, January 2, 1987.

Lanoe F: Drownproofing a new technique for water safety, Englewood Cliffs, NJ, 1963, Prentice-Hall.

Leonard G: The silent pulse, New York, 1981, Bantam Books.

Life jackets, Consumer's Report, Aug 1982.

Lifesaving merit badge pamphlet, Irving, Tex, 1980, Boy Scouts of America.

Lin L: How a medical breakthrough came about — Cold water near-drowning, Ann Arbor, Mich, 1978, Michigan Sea Grant Publications Office.

Madison A: Judgement on the water, Chatham, NY, 1987, Alan Madison Productions (videotape).

Madison A: Swept away, Chatham, NY, 1990, Alan Madison Productions (videotape).

Maiman D: Diving-associated spinal cord injuries during drought conditions — Wisconsin 1988, MMWR 37:30, 1988.

Maloney ES: Chapman: Piloting, seamanship and small boat handling, New York, 1989, Hearst Marine Books.

Martin T: Near-drowning and cold-water immersion, Ann Emerg Med 13:263-273, 1984.

McAniff J: US underwater diving fatality statistics, 1989, Kingston, RI, 1991, National Underwater Accident Data Center.

McKeown W: New ways to fight the chill that kills, Popular Mechanics, Dec 1981.

Miller J et al.: The visual behavior of recreational boat operators, Rep CG-D-31-77, Springfield, Va, 1977, National Technical Information Service.

Moessuer H: Accidents as a symptom of alcohol abuse, J Fam Pract 8:6, 1979.

Mohammed WF: St Francis Hospital, Waterloo, Iowa, unpublished protocol, 1983.

National boating survey, final report, Washington, DC, March 1978, United States Coast Guard.

Nichter M and Everett P: Childhood near-drowning: Is cardiopulmonary resuscitation always indicated? Crit Care Med 17:10, 1989.

North Carolina drownings, 1980-1984, MMWR 35:40, 1986.

NSPI-1 Standard for public swimming pools, Alexandria, Va, 1989, National Spa and Pool Institute.

Operation water watch sample news release No 2, Washington, DC, Summer 1990, US Consumer Product Safety Commission.

Orlowski J: Drowning, near drowning and ice water submersions, Pediatr Clin North Am 34:79, 1987.

Patetta M: North Carolina drownings, 1980-1984, MMWR 35:40, 1986.

Pearn J: Management of near-drowning, Br Med J 291:1447-1452, 1985.

Perspectives in disease prevention and health promotion aquatic deaths and injuries — United States, MMWR 31:31, 1982.

Pia F: Drowning facts and Myths, Larchmont, NY, 1976, Water Safety Films (videotape).

Pia F: The reasons people drown, Larchmont, NY, 1987, Water Safety Films (videotape).

Pia F: Why people drown, Larchmont, NY, 1986, Water Safety Films (videotape).

Pipkin G: Caloric labyrinthitis: A cause of drowning, Am J Sports Med 7:4, 1979.

Podolsky ML: Action plan for near drownings, Physician Sportsmed 9:7, 1981.

Pozos R and Born D: Hypothermia: Causes, effects, prevention, Piscataway, NJ, 1982, New Century Publishers.

Praleck B: Boating for the handicapped, Washington, DC, 1985, National Safe Boating Council.

Present P: Child drowning study, Washington, DC, September 1987, US Consumer Product Safety Commission.

Ray O: Drugs, society and human behavior, St Louis, 1990, Mosby–Year Book.

Recreational boating and alcohol safety information kit, Rockville, Md, March 1985, National Clearinghouse for Alcohol Information.

Recreational boating safety and alcohol, Washington, DC, 1983, National Transportation Safety Board.

Report: A model state recreational injury control program, 1981, Atlanta, Centers for Disease Control.

Report of alcohol use and recreational boating safety conference, Cleveland, June 1984, Ohio Division of Watercraft.

Resuscitation from hypothermia: A literature review, Rep CG-D-26-79, Springfield, Va, 1979, National Technical Information Service.

Resuscitation from hypothermia, Rep CG-D-26-79, Springfield, Va, 1979, National Technical Information Services.

River rescue, Columbus, Ohio, 1980, Ohio Department of Natural Resources.

Safety Tips. In USAA aide, San Antonio, Spring 1982, US Automobile Association.

Saxe T: Drug alcohol interactions, Am Fam Physician 33:4, 1986.

Selling safety education. In Boating safety education, an anthology of the National Boating Education Seminar, Seattle, 1986, National Safe Boating Council.

Shallow water lifeguard training, Washington, DC, 1988, American Red Cross.

Smith D: Accidental hypothermia, Postgrad Med 8:3, 1987.

Smith D: Notes on drowning: The misunderstood preventable tragedy, Physician Sports Med 12:7, 1984.

Smith D: Teaching tips, St Charles, Mo, 1988, Smith Aquatics Safety Services.

Smith D and Smith S: Waterwise, Imperial, Mo, 1984, Smith Aquatic Safety Services.

Spaniol S and Boyd D: Near drowning consensus and controversies in pulmonary and cerebral resuscitation, Heart Lung 18:1, 1989.

Stiehl C: Alcohol and pleasure boat operators, Rep CG-D-1134-75, Springfield, Va, 1975, National Technical Information Service.

Survival swimming: To save a life, Chicago, Ill, 1989, Encyclopedia Britannica Educational Corp (videotape).

Teather R: The night before the dive, Dive Rescue International, Ft Collins, Colo, 1988 (cassette tape).

The drowning machine, State College, Pa, 1981, Film Space (videotape).

Tisherman W: Cardiovascular resuscibility of dogs after up to 90 minutes cold water drowning using cardiopulmonary by-pass, Ann Emerg Med 13:5, 1984.

Underwater diving accident manual, Durham, NC, 1992, Divers Alert Network.

Urdang L, editor: Mosby's medical and nursing dictionary, St Louis, 1983, The CV Mosby Co.

Walbridge C: The best of the river safety task force newsletter, 1976-1982, Lorton, Va, 1983, American Canoe Association.

Webb JQ: Cold to the core, J Emerg Med Serv 14:33, 1989.

Weinberg A and Hamlet M, editors: Cold weather emergencies — Principles of patient management, Branford, Conn, 1990, American Medical Publishing Co.

White water primer, Washington, DC, 1978, American Red Cross (film).

Index

Other Mosby Products
of Interest

BOOK CODE	AUTHOR/TITLE	PUBLICATION DATE
21764	ACLS: Video Series	12/91
21766	ACLS: Airway Management	12/91
21771	ACLS: Arrhythmia Interpretation	12/91
21772	ACLS: Conversion Techniques	12/91
21770	ACLS: ECG Recognition	12/91
21767	ACLS: IV Procedures	12/91
21765	ACLS: Mega Code	12/91
21768	ACLS: Pharmacology, Part 1	12/91
21769	ACLS: Pharmacology, Part II	12/91
23764	Aehlert: ACLS Quick Review Study Guide	9/93
00200	Allison: Advanced Life Support Skills	8/93
07067	American Red Cross CPR for the Professional Rescuer Text	3/93
21231	American Red Cross Emergency Response Text	3/93
21241	American Red Cross First Aid: Instructor's Resource Kit—IBM	3/91
21135	American Red Cross First Aid: Responding to Emergencies	3/91
07405	American Safety Video Publishers: Learning ECGs Video Series	10/93
07172	American Safety Video Publishers: PALS Plus: Pediatric Advanced Life Support	12/92
07296	American Safety Video Publishers: PALS Plus: Pediatric Emergencies	12/92
07257	American Safety Video Publishers: Pass ACLS	12/92
00258	Atwood: Introduction to Cardiac Dysrhythmias	3/90
00383	Auerbach-Geehr: Management of Wilderness and Environmental Emergencies, 2/e	12/88

BOOK CODE	AUTHOR/TITLE	PUBLICATION DATE
00385	Auf der Heide: Disaster Response	6/89
01185	Bosker: The 60-Second EMT	11/87
01808	Bosker: Geriatric Emergency Medicine	7/90
01330	Bronstein: Emergency Care for Hazardous Materials Exposure	5/88
01458	doCarmo: Basic EMT Skills and Equipment	8/88
01473	Emergidose Slideguides: Pocket Adult/ Pediatric Emergency Drugs Guide, 5/e	7/91
01478	Emergidose Slideguides: Binder Adult/ Pediatric Emergency Drugs Guide, 5/e	7/91
01472	Emergidose Slideguides: Pocket Pediatric/Neonatal Emergency Drugs Guide, 2/e	8/91
01471	Emergidose Slideguides: Binder Pediatric/Neonatal Emergency Drugs, 2/e	7/91
01969	Gonsoulin: Prehospital Drug Therapy	9/93
01932	Gosselin-Smith: Mosby's First Responder Workbook, 2/e	10/88
00174	Grauer: ACLS Teaching Kit: An Instructor's Resource	12/89
01979	Grauer: ACLS Volume 1, Volume 2, and Pocket Reference	3/93
07069	Grauer: ACLS Volume 1: Certification Preparation, 3/e	3/93
07070	Grauer: ACLS Volume 2: A Comprehensive Review, 3/e	3/93
01980	Grauer: ACLS: Mega Code Review Study Cards, 2/e	3/93
07685	Grauer: ACLS: Pocket Reference, 1/e	3/93
02002	Grauer: ECG Interpretation Pocket Reference	9/91
02159	Grauer: Practical Guide to ECG Interpretation	9/91
02410	Huszar: Basic Dysrhythmia Interpretation and Management	7/88
02927	Huszar: Early Defibrillation	6/91
03353	Judd: First Responder: Textbook/ Workbook Package, 2/e	10/88

BOOK CODE	AUTHOR/TITLE	PUBLICATION DATE
08077	Kidd: Engine Company: 1st Due Video Series	12/93
08093	Kidd: Rescue Company: 1st Due Video Series	12/93
06195	Krebs: When Violence Erupts	4/90
06138	Lee: Flight Nursing: Principles and Practice	9/90
05853	Mack: EMT Certification Preparation	2/90
03375	Madigan: Prehospital Emergency Drugs Pocket Reference	3/90
05791	Miller: Manual of Prehospital Emergency Medicine	3/92
03351	Moore: Vehicle Rescue and Extrication	9/90
03227	Mosby's Medical and Nursing Dictionary, 3/e	11/89
05854	NAEMSP/Kuehl: EMS Medical Directors' Handbook	8/89
06579	NAEMSP/Swor: Quality Management in Prehospital Care	1/93
04284	Rothenberg: Advanced Medical Life Support	11/87
00443	Seidel: Mosby's Guide to Physical Examination, 3/e	12/90
04894	Simon: Pediatric Life Support	11/88
05321	Ward: Prehospital Treatment Protocols	3/89
03525	Yvorra: Mosby's Emergency Dictionary	10/88